Bodies, Politics, and African Healing

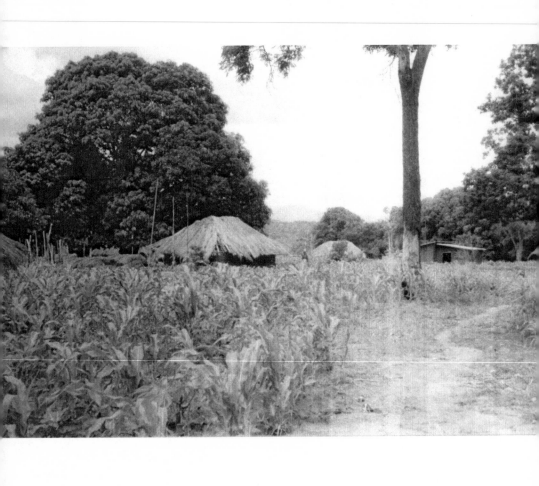

Bodies, Politics, and African Healing

The Matter of Maladies in Tanzania

Stacey A. Langwick

Indiana University Press · Bloomington and Indianapolis

This book is a publication of

Indiana University Press
601 North Morton Street
Bloomington, Indiana 47404-3797 USA

iupress.indiana.edu

Telephone orders	800-842-6796
Fax orders	812-855-7931
Orders by e-mail	iuporder@indiana.edu

*Published with support from the Hull Memorial
Publication Fund of Cornell University.*

⊖ The paper used in this publication meets the minimum requirements of the American
National Standard for Information Sciences—Permanence of Paper for Printed Library
Materials, ANSI Z39.48-1992.

Manufactured in the United States of America

Library of Congress Cataloging-in-Publication Data

Langwick, Stacey Ann.
 Bodies, politics, and African healing : the matter of maladies in Tanzania / Stacey A. Langwick.
    p. ; cm.
 Includes bibliographical references and index.
 ISBN 978-0-253-35527-0 (cloth : alk. paper) — ISBN 978-0-253-22245-9 (pbk. : alk. paper)
 1. Traditional medicine—Tanzania. 2. Medical care—Tanzania. I. Title.
 [DNLM: 1. Medicine, African Traditional—Tanzania. 2. Anthropology, Cultural—Tanzania.
WB 55.A3]
 GN477.L36 2011
 398'.353—dc22
                          2010047853

1 2 3 4 5 16 15 14 13 12 11

For Yanini

Contents

Acknowledgments

The gifts I have received and the debts I have accrued during the course of researching and writing this book are too great to capture in a few pages. Over the past decade, this book has been a medium for deep and intimate relations as well as brief but electric intellectual encounters. These have shaped who I am today not only as a scholar, but as a teacher, a spouse, a mother, and a person. My greatest debt remains to Binti Dadi and Mariamu whose friendship and kinship started in 1998 and who continue to be powerful daily presences in my life. Binti Dadi took a chance on me, shared her life, her medicines, her clients, her heart, and her home with me. This book can only be a partial thank you for this generosity. Her extended family welcomed me and influenced my research and this book. Mariamu, her youngest daughter, grew to be a dear and close friend. As an infant, Mariamu's daughter Yanini was a constant presence during my fieldwork. This family taught me a great deal about living, about kindness and trust, about laughter, and about survival. In addition they made this book possible and so I dedicate this work to Yanini as healing in this matrilineal area moves most often from maternal grandmother to granddaughter.

Many other healers shared their skills and visions with me as well. Although I cannot mention all of their names here, I would like to extend a special note of appreciation to Sheikh Awadhi, Fatu Chenga, F. M. Chinduli, Mzee Haleke, Jambili Hamisi, Mzee Kalimaga, Muhamed Kasim, Mama Libongo, Samato Kiroya Maingo, Habiba Rashidi Mayaula, Mzee Mpende, and B. M. Nampyali. Furthermore, I am profoundly grateful to the many patients as well as their families and friends who shared the stories of their afflictions with me and who welcomed me into the intimate processes of their cures (and sometimes their deaths).

During the course of my research and writing I have been blessed with some great academic teachers. The seed of this book germinated as my doctoral dissertation. It is hard to imagine being able to live up to the generosity that Judith Farquhar has shown me since the first day I walked into her office thinking of applying to Ph.D. programs. Her gifts to me go far beyond the keen analytical eye she brought to my work and the insistence on clarity and rigor that defined my graduate education. Over the years her faith in the power and humility of ethnography, in the import of writing, and the work of words that draw a reader into the pleasures, desires, beauty, and pain of others have inspired me. Margaret Wiener consistently offered her time and provided many careful readings and provocative comments about knowledge and magic. Catherine Lutz, David Newbury, and Barbara Herrnstein Smith each challenged me with useful questions and brought more depth to my arguments here.

Many other colleagues have also served as mentors and teachers over the years. I own Margaret Lock a special thank you. Among other things, Margaret's work taught me what it means to really listen and to capture individual stories of body, of health, of hope, and of healing. The questions she has put to me have opened my analyses to the histories of bodily materiality while she continued to insist on serious and rigorous consideration of scientific knowledge. In 1997, Steven Feierman answered a letter from an unknown graduate student who wanted to better understand the history and literature on African healing and medicine and he generously welcomed me to spend a semester studying with him. I continue to learn from Steve in every conversation I have with him. Each page of this book bears witness to the usefulness of Bruno Latour's provocative writings far beyond laboratory science. His early faith in my work and the possibilities of research in Africa shaped the direction of this book. Julie Livingston not only read an earlier version of this book, her careful review spurring important revisions, but she then also re-read pieces of this argument and spent hours on the phone and in various conferences helping me to make sense of the stories here. Even more than this, however, Julie and her work constantly remind me that research on embodiment is important insofar as it makes possible a powerfully empathetic scholarship, one that refigures the forms of difference that undergird modern global, class, gender, and race hierarchies and one that opens up the possibly for new sorts of solidarity.

This book was written both at the University of Florida and Cornell University. I was gifted with smart, sensitive colleagues at both institutions. Gwynn Kessler thought with me through issues of gender, politics, and writing as well as teaching and all the most important questions of life, family, and career. I hope many motorcycle rides are still in our future. The Center for African Studies at the University of Florida turned me into an Africanist. The enthusiasm and sense of intellectual community at the center under Leonardo Villalón's charismatic leadership was inspirational. The extended and rich conversations with Apollo Amoko, Brenda Chalfin, Hansjoerg Dilger, Abdoulaye Kane, Todd Leedy, Fiona McLaughlin, Sue O'Brien, Renata Serra, Alioune Sow, and Luise White created an exciting place to work and think. Luise White also read this entire manuscript and gave me thoughtful and important feedback. Peter Malanchuk is the kind of librarian that all African Studies scholars dream of working with. His generosity extended to my time at Cornell. My graduate students at the University of Florida were exceptional interlocutors as well. I would specifically like to thank Traci Yoder for the hours she spent reading microfilm and Jennifer (Jai) Hale-Gallardo for her help copyediting and formatting the final version of this manuscript.

At Cornell I have been blessed with a supportive and intellectually stimulating department. I owe a special debt of gratitude to my Mellon writing group of 2008–2009 focused on the theme of De-centering Africa, which included Judith Byfield, Johanna Crane, Jeremy Foster, Sandra Greene, Dan Magaziner, and Dagmawi Woubshet. Their comments on an earlier version of the introduction of this book were immensely helpful as were Dominic Boyer's. Rachel Prentice read this manuscript, some parts more than once, and each time brought the sensitive way she thinks about the phenomenology of bodily care and knowledge to the text. Thank you all.

So many others have helped me think through pieces of this work in scholarly communities in the U.S. and abroad. Lisa Richey saw my interests unfold from the early days of my master's degree in public health. From Chapel Hill to Tanzania to our many meetings and bottles of wine in between, she has grappled with me over the most interesting and difficult issues of medicine and gender in Africa. I thank her in particular for invariably making me laugh in the situations when laughter was needed most. Tim Choy's friendship, intellectual solidarity, and always encouraging yet radical questioning not only deeply influenced this book but also were some of the greatest joys of writing it. Over the past decade he has read and re-read this book as well as many other articles and conference papers that I have written. I thank him for the many cups of coffee and for the possibility of meandering as a methodology. Linda Helgesson has been a comrade in all senses from our African dance lessons to sharing the southeast as our field site, to the refuge, laughter, and parties of the always-welcoming home that she and James have created together in Dar es Salaam. Susan Shaw's subtle analyses of power and fierce critiques of inequality call me to better and more engaged scholarship. I am deeply grateful for the insights she has shared during our many hikes in Vermont that influenced my career and research far beyond this book.

Revisions of this book occurred during my associateship at the Max Planck Institute. Our meetings have been particularly productive for my thinking on medicine in Africa. For this I thank Richard Rottenburg and the Law, Organization, Science, and Technology group he has brought together including P. Wenzel Geissler, René Gerrets, Sheila Jasanoff, Julie Laplante, Margaret Lock, Babette Mueller-Rockstroh, Vinh-Kim Nguyen, Trevor Pinch, Ruth Prince, Susan Reynolds Whtye, and Julia Zenker. In addition, critical to this book has been the advice from, and conversations with, Ned Bertz, James Brennan, Susan Cook, Maia Green, Todd Hasak-Lowy, Nancy Rose Hunt, Sarah Jewett, Ann Kakaliouras, Jeremy Leibowitz, Tracy Luedke, Kristine Peterson, Anne Marie Stoner-Eby, Kaushik Sunder Rajan, Harry West, and Katherine Wildman (may she rest in peace). Annemarie Mol also took the time for a walk with me in Maastricht that opened up the conclusion of this book and helped me find its purpose.

Many Tanzanian colleagues at the University of Dar es Salaam advanced my thinking. I cannot mention all by name here but would like to extend my warmest gratitude to Ruth Meena, Rose Mwaipopo, and Rose Shayo. At the Institute of Traditional Medicine at the Muhimbili University College for Health Sciences I would like to recognize the conversations with Edmund Kayombo over the years. His commitment to healers has fortified me and his belief in the generative possibilities of their engagements with science has challenged and inspired me.

Many friends in Newala helped me understand life and health in the area. Their humor and care brought warmth to each day. A few deserve special mention. Sophia Mpende and her family welcomed me to festivities like a sister. The Magahemas fed me physically and spiritually, offering me friendship, refuge, and good stories. Julie Atkins and Sollo sustained me over the many years in innumerable ways through their lively conversation, thoughtful commentary, welcoming homes, and fabulous seafood dinners.

This research was supported by the University of North Carolina (through FLAS grants, an International Studies Center pre-dissertation grant and a CLAS dissertation grant), the National Science Foundation, a Fulbright Foundation Fellowship, the University of Florida (including through a UF Humanities Grant), and Cornell University. Middlebury College gave me the space to write as a visiting scholar. The Tanzanian Commission for Science and Technology (COSTECH) granted and renewed my research clearance for this work. Dr. Rugumamu in the Institute of Development Studies at the University of Dar es Salaam acted as my sponsor. The staff at the Tanzanian National Archives was uniquely helpful. The District Commissioner of Newala not only welcomed me warmly to Newala but also opened his files to me. At many levels, the Ministry of Health in Tanzania facilitated the process of this research. Peter Riwa in Dar es Salaam organized all the necessary letters of introduction. Dr. Budeba, the Regional Medical Officer in Mtwara and Mr. Mbava, the District Medical Officer for Mtwara (urban) helped orient me to the southeastern part of the country and directed me toward Newala. I benefited greatly from the openness and assistance of the staff at the Newala District hospital. Dr. Msengi, Mr. Kilemba, Mr. Chibwana, Mama Chibwana, and Mr. Mdeka deserve special thanks. Each of them at different moments offered me their time, offices, and expertise. My understanding of the practical aspects of incorporating Traditional Birth Attendants into the health care system was greatly improved by conversations with Zainabu Abdallah Alawe, Saidia Dibaki, Fatu Hali, Halima Masudi Kayidi, Lukia Lada, Angela Mnichelewa, Somoye Yusuph Mpunga, Bibi Salum, Georgina Sefu, Anna Selemani, and Amina Athumani Tepende. Many nurses and nurses' aides throughout the Newala Hospital and the surrounding dispensaries made me feel welcome, expressed enthusiasm for this research, and took an active role in shaping it. The staff of the Office of Traditional Medicine in the Ministry of

Health always offered provocative conversation. I am particularly grateful for the insights of Sabina Mnaliwa.

Two chapters contain material previously published elsewhere. Portions of chapter three appeared in *Medical Anthropology*, and an earlier version of chapter seven appeared in *Science, Technology, and Human Values*. Dee Mortensen was a supportive and skillful editor. The book is much better for having been in her care and that of the staff at Indiana University Press.

I appreciate Sheryl McCurdy's and Linda Helgesson's help in obtaining permission to use the George Lilanga print on the front. I thank the Lilanga family for their permission to use this print. I thank the community in Lincoln, Vermont, that held me during so much of my writing and especially Mesa Dobek who worked on the citations.

My family has seen me through this book and much more. My mother's appreciation of a good mystery, my father's love of travel and of powerful argument, my sisters' affection, and my cousin Laura's enthusiasm all mark these pages. Judy and Mark Bercuvitz have taken me in as a daughter and they and their clan have supported me unconditionally. My dear sweet Grandma Jean passed away before she could see this book, but her delight in the world, her skill in telling a good story, and her faith in me made it possible. Tsadia Jessie Langwick Bercuvitz imbued the last phases of this project with tenderness and she gave deeper meaning to the relationships that are captured here especially as she cemented my kinship with Binti Dadi. At a very early age she also showed great generosity, not least of all when she went for hike after hike with her father so that I had a quiet house in which to work.

Above all, I thank Jeff Bercuvitz who was part of this project from its earliest formation. Thank you, love, for co-creating our life in Tanzania, for listening to the passions that drove this research, and for helping me craft the arguments that might best translate them into ink on paper. Thank you also for the hours upon hours that you carved out for me to work by taking on more than your fair share of the details of our lives only to then receive requests for more editing! While I can only hope to do justice to your gift for compelling narrative in these pages, you have influenced me and this project in infinite ways not least of all by making life immeasurably better with your humor, music, and excitement for living fully.

A Note on Translation

The names of plants and trees used by healers are all in Kimakonde. All other foreign words are Kiswahili unless otherwise noted. A glossary has been included in the back of the book for the reader's reference. All translations are the author's.

Bodies, Politics, and African Healing

Prologue

AIDS, Rats, and Soldiers' Belts

Frozen by her doubts, Binti Mayaula did nothing as she watched a man die of AIDS. She had had a dream in which she had been told to collect the root *dying'weo* and make it into a tea to cure just such a patient. When she awoke, however, Binti Mayaula was uncertain. She knew this root, having used it in the past to make a medicinal paste to apply externally to sores. The sores had dried up and that patient had healed. But now she was called upon to administer the medicine orally. Anxious that the concoction would be toxic, she hesitated. The man with AIDS, who had come to her for help, passed away. She worried: Had her reluctance to follow the directions she received from her familiars cost him his life? Was she implicated in his death? Months later she dreamed about *dying'weo* again. This time her familiars and spirit guides revealed that her cousin, Binti Dadi,[1] would come to know this cure for AIDS. The next day, she met her cousin while they helped their uncle harvest his cassava. As they worked side by side, Binti Mayaula recounted her second dream, which indicated that Binti Dadi would come to know this new medicine when her anthropologist returned.[2]

In 1998, I made a home in the town of Newala in southeastern Tanzania in order to conduct research on healing. During my first year of fieldwork, I worked increasingly closely with Binti Dadi, a well-known healer in the area, spending many hours each day with her collecting plants, talking with patients, and helping her prepare and administer medicine. In late 1999, I left Newala for a few months. It was my intended return in 2000 to which Binti Mayaula referred. Shortly before I arrived in March, the *mashetani* said to rule (*kutawala*) Binti Dadi came to her in a dream to tell her to collect *dying'weo*. The process glossed as "dreams" (*ndoto*) by these healers references a deep engagement with ancestral shades and other familiars.[3] Dreams serve as a medium of communication between visible and invisible realms, between present and past, between the human and nonhuman. In this dream, Binti Dadi's grandmother instructed her to pound the *dying'weo* roots and to prepare it as a porridge (*uji*). As she told me about this vision, she confessed that like her cousin, she also was reluctant to administer the concoction orally for fear that it might be poison.

About a month later Binti Dadi fed a bit of mashed *dying'weo* to a rat. The rat did not die—an indication, she suggested, that it may not be poisonous to humans. Her *mashetani* then brought Mzee[4] Mohammed Salimu to Binti Dadi for help. The *mzee* suspected that his son had contracted AIDS. Sores covered his son's body. A particularly high concentration of these sores gathered on his head. The young man complained that his whole body hurt and that it was extremely itchy. He suspected that he had similar sores inside his body running from his throat to his genitals. He had gone to the hospital, but he left without any clear diagnosis. When the *mzee* came to Binti Dadi seeking advice for his son's treatment, she told him about *dying'weo* and suggested that he collect it himself. The *mzee* gathered the root, boiled it, and applied it to the sores on his son's skin. The sores dried up. Then the *mzee* pounded the medicine and cooked it like porridge. He gave it to his son to drink in order to dry up the sores on the inside of his body. The *mzee's* son did not die after drinking this medicine, and Binti Dadi was further convinced that *dying'weo* was not toxic. Before my next trip to Dar es Salaam, Binti Dadi asked me to take some of this medicine to have it tested (*kupima*) at the government-run Institute of Traditional Medicine in the Muhimbili University Center for Health Services, the primary teaching and research hospital in Tanzania. She also insisted that I carry a portion to the United States to be analyzed.

Binti Dadi and those who seek help from her—like many throughout Africa—are confronting new configurations of affliction. Thanks to public health campaigns, national radio shows, and international development projects, knowledge of—as well as fear of—AIDS is widespread. It shapes the complaints of people who seek Binti Dadi's help; even a healer who specializes in children's illnesses and women's reproductive problems such as Binti Dadi is compelled to address the biomedically defined syndrome of AIDS directly. Notably, the medicine that she tentatively tried did not emerge through connections to a hospital or a chemist's shop. Something subtler was captured in this search for a "traditional medicine." The new medicine began to take shape through a complex set of relations with relatives during a cassava harvest, with ancestral shades through a dream, and with rats and an anthropologist in her courtyard. Each set of interactions moved a complicated set of translations forward. The partial emergence of this new medicine reveals the inseparability of science and nonscience in contemporary healing in Tanzania.

This book is about therapeutic practices in southeastern Tanzania and the ways that people come to know, intervene in, and transform the world. These issues emerge most clearly through juxtaposition. On the other side of town, a different medicine was materializing through the work of Mzee Kalimaga. Officials in the district commissioner's office first directed me to Kalimaga. They told me that when they wanted to know something about the past in Newala, he was the person they consulted. Kalimaga, who had worked with the colonial government and had been active in the movement for independence, was a well-known figure in the town of Newala. He had moved in prominent circles at a dramatic time in the nation's history. An affable, gregarious man with twinkling eyes and a warm, ready smile, he had come to be known as a storyteller—one who knows history as well as being a piece of history himself. Yet when I first arrived at his home, as well as on subsequent visits, Kalimaga was interested in talking about medicine. In retirement, he was refashioning himself as a healer.

His story of his interest in medicine always included his late wife's sister's marriage to Dr. Leader Stirling. His brother-in-law had been a mission doctor in the area, had built the first hospital in Newala in the late 1930s, and, after independence had risen to become minister of health (1975–1980). Mzee Kalimaga, who describes himself as a Christian, an educated and modern person, and a lay historian, consciously strives to re-shape healing practice, to advocate for its grassroots modernization through the incorporation of scientific knowledge into the work of local practitioners. For him this has meant separating herbal medicine from its links with ancestral shades, devilish spirits, and possession. His passion comes from loving trees. "Some love to tend chickens or cows," he told me. "I love trees."

A few years ago, while Kalimaga was in the forest, a particular tree caught his attention. He was taken by its size and beauty.

> I looked at it, and wondered why. *Maana yake ni nini?* What is the meaning
> of this big, *safi*[5] tree? There was white coming from it. I sat beneath the tree. I
> looked at where this kind of tree was growing and saw that it was there . . . and
> there . . . and there. I thought, "Why is this tree like this?" Suddenly, I realized,
> "Oh, it is medicine." I took the leaves. I did not know what they were medicine
> for, however.[6]

When Kalimaga "thinks" about a tree, when he searches for the "meaning" of the tree, he contemplates its name(s). He turns over the name of the tree in his mind. As an mYao[7] who married an mMakonde woman and conducted his professional life in both Kiswahili and English, he often has a number of names at his disposal to ponder. For Kalimaga, names serve as clues to the plant's past relations, as instantiations of ancestors' experiences. The meaning of this particular tree soon found its way to his doorstep.

> Then one day the agricultural officer arrived explaining that his wife was sick
> and asking me if I could I cure the illness. I said, "No." The agricultural officer
> asked, "What can we do then?" I told him to ask his wife to come by at ten in
> the morning the next day. A woman came wrapped in a *kanga*, including her
> head. She was bent over and shuffling. . . . I told her to go through to the back of
> the house. When she sat down and took away the *kanga*, there were pus-filled
> pimples all over her back and sides and stomach and arms. I looked at them and
> I thought. Then I knew that I had to use this medicine. But what to do? I realized

that I must grate the leaves by hand and put them in water for her to drink. After I started grating, I tasted a little. It was bitter. It was truly *dawa* [medicine], so I continued grating. And also what? Ahhh, to wash them [the pimples]. I took the feather of a chicken [dipped it in the solution] and brushed. She was to continue taking this medicine for five days, three times a day, and then come back to see me. But on Sunday [three days later] she appeared at my house. I said, "Why are you here? It is only Sunday." She was wearing a dress and looking very smart. She said that she was able to eat and to sleep. Her husband told her that she must come and show me. She came to the back of my house and showed me the pimples. They had dried up. There was no more pus; they were just scabs. When I asked her if they itched, she said "No." I told her to come back at 4 PM. I sent someone to buy castor oil. I roasted some of the medicine in castor oil. She came back at 4 PM and I rubbed the *dawa za kuchoma* [roasted medicine] onto her scabs. They healed up completely.

By mid-May 2003, Kalimaga claimed to have treated over 200 people with a similar condition: ninety before February 2003 and about 120 between February and mid-May of that year. In a school notebook he kept a careful list of those to whom he tended. He saw this work as preparation for his own drug trials. Kalimaga refers to the affliction as *ukanda wa jeshi* (soldier's belt) because it starts around the waist and then spreads up over the shoulders and across the back, like the holsters soldiers wear. He maintains that people started coming to him after they failed to find relief from hospital treatments. He is confident that biomedical practitioners cannot cure this condition.[8]

What interests Kalimaga are the cognitive processes through which he imagines scientific thinkers work. "I just think," he says, "and then I know." He thanks God for his intelligence, which allows him to decipher the meaning of trees. He claims that his revelations are the product of his mental work. They reside in his mind. Kalimaga does not see his revelations as a process of "channeling" or "speaking with" God, spirits (Christian or otherwise), or ancestors. He accuses those who talk about spirits as just being out to get people's money. In contrast, he represents himself as honest through his "scientific" work. Kalimaga stresses that he conducts research (*utafiti*). By initially testing this medicine on four people, he established "proof" of his medicine's efficacy.

Many contrasts could be drawn between Binti Dadi—a Muslim, mMakonde, illiterate woman—and Mzee Kalimaga—a Christian, mYao, educated man. For the moment, however, I would like to highlight the ways that *knowing* differs in these stories of emergent medicine. For Kalimaga, knowing is an act of an autonomous mind. He meditates on a name, a clue left behind by those of the past. His extensive knowledge of local history helps him with the task of deciphering, but the important point here is that he is deciphering. For Binti Dadi, knowing is an extension of relations between her and her kin, those dead and alive. Knowing is not a product of her "mental" (*akili*) work; it is a result of her embodying, dreaming, and engaging her ancestral shades and a range of other salient humans and nonhumans. She is experimenting with ways to include scientific institutes and an anthropologist into this set of relations. These alternative ways of knowing plants and medicine shape what they are. For Kalimaga, plants are entities out there in the world, some of which have medicinal properties that might be exploited for the benefit of the afflicted. For Binti Dadi, plants are one form of matter that when called upon by ancestors and devilish spirits through a healer in the name of an afflicted person might be transformed into medicine—that is, into substances that might be able to influence relations critical to embodiment.

As Kalimaga seeks to (re)discover the medicinal properties he sees as inherent in some plants, names act as communal memory banks, ways of passing a discovery on through time. His "thinking" depends upon (re)inscriptions of temporal distance. He searches the remains of the past to discover new uses for the future. He criticizes practices that fail to explicitly assert a linear relation between the past and the future as dishonest. He establishes a particular modern spatialization of time—living in a world with history—as a moral difference between his medicine and those of others who work with devils, ancestral shades, and other nonhuman actors.

Intrigued by Kalimaga's practice, I began puzzling over names myself. As I was passing the hours between collecting and preparing medicine, treating and watching patients at Binti Dadi's, I often worked on learning Kimakonde. I was delighted when I learned that the word *numbi* in Kimakonde means *ukoo*, or maternal clan, in Kiswahili. I immediately connected this *numbi* with *numbinumbi*, one of the important plants healers use to address difficulties with conception that have been brought on by *uchawi* (witchcraft). Feeling that I was hot on the trail of something, I discreetly asked about words that make up *nembelembe*, another key ingredient in these treatments. *Nembe*, I discovered, means *nataka*, or "I want." *Nilembe* is translated as *nitake* (the subjunctive tense of first-person wanting), while *nilembela* is *nimetafuta*, meaning "I have looked for" or "searched for." I presented my friends with the product of my deciphering: hidden in the name of *nembelembe* is the clue that it serves as a medicine for those looking or searching for something that is wanted. When combined with *numbinumbi*, this suggests a search for the *ukoo*. In this historically matriarchal area, that search is the desire for a child who will continue the lineage. The combination of *numbinumbi* and *nembelembe* is a medicinal concoction that will help a woman conceive, help her add to the *ukoo*, the maternal clan. The memory of its efficacy, I concluded, is embedded in the names of these trees. When I revealed my sleuthing to Binti Dadi and her daughter, Mariamu, they burst out laughing. My thought experiment clearly tickled them. They adamantly insisted, however, that there was no such meaning hidden in the names of plants used for medicine. *Numbinumbi,* they declared, was just the name of a plant. It had nothing to do with *numbi* as in *ukoo*. For them, the technique I had learned from Kalimaga might be an interesting game with which to while away the hours of a hot afternoon, but it was not a technique for treating serious complaints. For Binti Dadi, such word games circumvented the real matter of medicine: that it is an active extension of relations. Plants, for her, are transformed through interaction, and medicine emerges through social connections, not mental efforts.

Interestingly, few in Newala saw Kalimaga as a healer, or *mganga*. That did not mean they refused his medicine. Kalimaga remained a valued historian and a wise and respected elder, so it was easy to believe that he knew a few valuable herbal treatments. What are we to make of such people, who know medicine, distribute medicine, indeed are interested in treating people but who are denied the status of *mganga*? I take up the issue of what a healer is and how she or he is called into being by particular discourses in chapter 3. For the moment, I would just like to note that the distinction some made between Kalimaga and others, such as Binti Dadi, lies in an ontological difference between the medicines they use.

Critical to understanding Binti Dadi's medicine is that its very being is distributed through a series of events. It is not an object that mediates relations as much as it is a dynamic extension of relations. In contrast, Kalimaga articulates his medicine as a pragmatic answer to an inquiry into what a plant "means." Both remedies stand in contrast to the forms of therapeutic intervention that are derived from biomedical research, which examines plant materials for their efficacy against known pathogens. Yet by (mis)recognizing themselves and their medicine in the discourse of medical science—Binti Dadi through her use of a test rat and Kalimaga through his amateur clinical trail—both healers sought to recast their medicine in light of biomedical concerns. They strove to make it possible for their treatments to travel differently and potentially farther. For Binti Dadi, this travel necessitated addressing an explicitly biomedical disease entity. Kalimaga sought to craft a modern, secular medicine derived from "indigenous" knowledge. These are not simple tales of biomedical hegemony, the encroachment of modern thought, or the corruption of traditional values. Both these stories ask us to think about the micropolitics of knowledge, and both suggest that objects—in this case medicine—consolidate particular assemblages of actors, moments in time, and structures of relation. The origins of this book lie in such stories about worlds born of encounter and knowledges that desire to intervene.

1

Orientations

This book is a study of healing practices in southeastern Tanzania and the worlds they render meaningful and concrete. The World Health Organization (2002) estimates that 80 percent of Africans have sought out traditional medicine and states that many depend on herbal remedies as a critical aspect of their primary health care.[1] Some African health professionals, including the district nursing officer in Newala, where I conducted the majority of the fieldwork for this book, suggest that the use of traditional medicine is on the rise due to the inadequacy of health care services under the growing economic pressures of neoliberal reform. The incorporation of traditional medicine and healers into health development goals raises the question of how to describe the efficacy of such therapies. This includes how to account for happenings that are salient to many therapeutic experiences but are discounted by biomedicine. Often the entities that healers claim to be treating—mischievous spirits, troublesome devils, disgruntled ancestors, the embodiments of human jealousies and greed—are not recognized by medical science, and the transformations that healers effect cannot be confirmed through biomedical procedures. Yet when Binti Dadi tests the toxicity of a new potential medicine on a rat and when Kalimaga keeps careful records of those who use his medicine in the name of "clinical trials," these healers refuse to observe the familiar boundaries between science and nonscience.[2] Rather they reflect the ways that colonization, missionization, postcolonial state building, international development, and transnational capitalism have shaped the practices known as healing in Newala today.

In this book, I argue that the epistemological problem of postcolonial healing can be fully addressed only through a radical rethinking of the ontological ground of therapy. As healers in Tanzania strive to intervene in affliction, misfortune, and a range of undesirable states, they are crafting not only a new lexicon at the intersection of traditional and modern medicine but also new objects and entities toward which their care is directed—from enchanted parasites to biomedical devils. In so doing, healers in a rural district near the Tanzania-Mozambique border—an area known among staff of the regional hospital as a place "full of powerful witchcraft and traditional medicine"—offer innovative contributions to questions that lie at the heart of social theory and anthropology today: Who can assert which things legitimately constitute the world or, more specifically, the matter of the body and bodily threats? Which experts have the ability to generate new objects of care? Which entities have the right to exist in the postcolony? What sorts of politics are possible when we recognize the forms of power that legitimate some kinds of existence and not others?

My approach to these questions is shaped by the rich historical and anthropological studies that have offered nuanced understandings of therapeutic logics in Africa and the cosmological, symbolic, and social worlds that shape them. I am particularly inspired by careful studies that historicize phenomenological experiences of healing in Africa.[3] I am also interested in the ways that experience and the specific forms of the experiencing subject emerge as effects of political, technological, ethical, and cultural relations over time. The objective of this book is, however, a little different. I strive to add to these studies by turning an eye to the ways the experiential is intimately entangled with the production of the objects and entities created in therapeutic practice—that is, to the matter(s) of African maladies.

Careful attention to healing practices in Tanzania complicates disciplinary trends that locate the study of bodily materiality in the natural sciences and the study of cultural meanings in the social sciences and humanities. Taking seriously healers' articulations of corporality, substance, palpability, and sentience means lifting the "critical immunity" often granted to biomedical materiality.[4] Medical practitioners and social scientists often translate devils into parasites, see jealousies as a way of talking about social inequalities, and read angry ancestors as disturbances in the psyche. In so doing, their accounts fail to recognize the materiality of (so-called) traditional therapies and the objects of healers' therapeutic care. This investigation into the therapies of healers in southeastern Tanzania has been shaped by recent work in science studies that explores the co-emergence of matters and meanings.[5] The chapters that follow illustrate how the matter of the body and of bodily threats that are salient to contemporary therapies come into being through practice.

By exploring the semiological and praxiological nature of matter, science studies scholars have countered traditional philosophical representations of transcendent entities unmoored from their histories of becoming.[6] Genealogies of "new" scientific and medical knowledge—which illustrate the temporal specificity of the objects and entities said to make up the world (and their significance)— have upset notions of ontology as a property of things.[7] These histories of natural objects argue that ontolog*ies* are distributed through practices of knowing and intervening.[8] This book is inspired by this focus on the practices through which the world is rendered explicit as it strives to articulate an analysis that is "true to objects that are at once real and historical" (Daston 2000). In Tanzania, any examination of ontological commitments in therapeutic practice requires attention to the material worlds both of and beyond science. Throughout this book, I linger over the times and places where the ambiguities and frictions of postcolonial healing practices hold open the possibility of rendering the world in different ways. It is in these in-between spaces that the stakes over which assertions count as knowledge, which substances count as objects, which people count as experts, and which threats deserve attention are most apparent.

Bodies, Politics, and African Healing strives to account for the kinds of being allowed to exist in the space and time of the postcolonial. It is, in short, an exploration of ontological politics.[9] Ontological politics glosses the processes of making and unmaking—assembling and disassembling—the objects about which history is written and over which struggles are articulated. When taken up in reference to postcolonial healing, the analytical frame of ontological politics draws attention to the ways that particular remedies, bodies, and threats are brought to life, elaborated, propagated, destroyed, and allowed to fade away. These processes sit at the heart of the structures of governance, the strategies of popular resistance, and the techniques of subject formation that support transnational power.

Nowhere are the stakes over being and existence higher than in the arena of medicine and healing. Here the ways that the world is made explicit are immediately and intimately tied to questions of well-being, debility, and survival. And nowhere do the contemporary politics around medicine and healing appear starker than in Africa, where diseases thought to be manageable (if not curable) elsewhere kill millions each year. The "truth" of traditional maladies and the "fact" of traditional medicine is a risky negotiation about which practices, knowledges, institutions, experts, bodies, and threats will dwell in the world. It is not only about who and what has the ability to transform states of being; it is also about whose presence is licit, what is considered real, and which states of being matter.

The Social Basis of Healing Matters

While diverse therapies to address affliction and misfortune existed across Africa long before European explorers and missionaries traversed the continent, these therapies came to be seen as homogenous only in their opposition to biomedicine. First colonial prohibitions and later postcolonial developments elicited traditional medicine as a coherent category of knowledge and practice.[10] Each passing wave of economic optimism has invigorated this modern category of traditional medicine. In the 1960s and 1970s, traditional medicine offered a solution to global inequities in wealth that had been deepened by Cold War divisions. Evoked as the basis of an indigenous pharmaceutical industry, traditional medicine promised to release African states from the devastating burden of supplying their expanding network of health services with foreign medicine that could be purchased only with hard currency. More recently, compelled by different desperations—in particular, those shaped by neoliberal restructuring and the insistence of international financial organizations that the poorest of countries produce their way out of poverty—traditional medicine has emerged as a new way into the global economy. Tanzanian officials are joining other African countries in a chorus that welcomes the commercialization of traditional medicine as a prospective path into the global market of herbal medicine, which the World Health Organization (2002) estimates to stand at USD 60 billion and growing.

Both early postindependence efforts to commodify medicinal plants and minerals as pharmaceuticals for a socialist health care system and later postsocialist efforts to (re)commodify medicinal plants and minerals as herbals have anchored knowledge of traditional medicine in laboratory investigation. The materialist claims of laboratory science hold that the substance of plants, animals, and minerals exist independent of local forms of social organization, ethics, and politics.[11] This book, however, situates the substance of postcolonial therapeutic practices in a broader historical and political narrative. The contemporary healers I met in southeastern Tanzania are acutely aware of their relation to a modern notion of traditional medicine that is defined by medical science and health bureaucracies. They grapple with the fact that laboratory investigations into the medicinal value of plant, animal, and mineral substances draw distinctions between the natural and the social, make ahistorical assumptions about the boundaries between the material and immaterial, and invest in the separation of matter and spirit. Even as they become further entangled with modern science, healers remain unsympathetic to and are unconvinced by such clear divisions between the material and the metaphysical. Rather, through their work, they expand, transform, refigure, and offer diverse and sophisticated alternatives to national and international articulations of traditional medicine. They do this most profoundly through practices that render the therapeutic properties of plant, animal, and mineral substances scientifically explicit and articulate afflictions as spaces of intervention. For instance, as I discuss in later chapters, some forms of *uchawi*, or witchcraft, inhibit biomedical diagnostic technologies or block the efficacy of pharmaceuticals. By removing the blockage, healers' treatments allow hospital-based technologies and medicine to work, as in the case of treatments for malaria (see chapter 7). In these actions, which simultaneously acknowledge the biological body and challenge biomedicine's access to it, healers ground postcolonial healing in a politics of matter. Their treatments offer analytical leverage on biomedicine's claim to fundamental knowledge of the physical body. Healers' entanglements with medicine and medical science capture the tensions of postcoloniality as they reveal the stability of biological explanations (and the entities they entail) in an area that has seen over one hundred years of biomedicine and as they simultaneously generate innovative new ways of articulating the body and those things that threaten it. Postcolonial healing offers a dynamic space in which to investigate the continuities and discontinuities of imperialism and the life of other kinds of power.

The limits of language, especially in translation, have created challenges for those who write about postcolonial healing and attempt to capture the subtleties of complex subjects and objects whose genealogies lay claim to both scientific and nonscientific forms of medicine and whose matter is deeply physical and social, tied up in body and in kin. To keep my account open to multiple ways of knowing the world, I refer to the complaints and concerns of people in southern Tanzania who find themselves in undesirable, painful, and often debilitating states of being as "maladies" (as opposed to diseases, illnesses, or sickness). The English word "malady" resonates more strongly with the meanings and the connotations of the Kiswahili word *ugonjwa* than "disease" or "illness." Coming from the Latin *male habitus,* meaning "out of condition," derived from *male* (badly) and *habitus* (held, the past participle of *habere,* to hold), "malady" posits undesirable states as poorly executed acts.[12] Being badly held suggests an unfortunate interaction with another, a relationship gone bad, an undesirable positioning. In Tanzania, a malady is a state of not being held well by the seen or the unseen world, by spirits or kin or neighbors, or in relation to other things in the world. According to *Webster's Unabridged Dictionary,* "malady" means not just "any sickness or disease; an illness," but also "moral defect or corruption." Even in its more recent configuration, then, this word does not force us to make the problematic separation between natural disease-causing entities and the social expression of illness. The concept of malady holds biomedical and nonbiomedical discomforts, disabilities, and other undesirable states of being in the same frame. The description of a malady traces the practices—of bad holding, violent encounters, unpleasant relationships—that constitute it, be they between viruses and immune systems or the "shadow" of a deceased older sibling and his newborn brother.

"Malady" references the ways that ontologies embed moral concerns as well as political power into the stuff of the world. By giving form to those things that threaten life and livelihood, healers frame narratives of accountability and legitimate regimes of obligation. For example, while living in Newala in the late 1990s, my neighbors' adult daughter returned home to her parents swollen and weak. Several years earlier, her husband had gone north to Tanga for work. After some time, he stopped returning to Newala and stopped sending money to support her and their children. Eventually, the news that he had married another woman made its way south. When my neighbors took their daughter to a healer, they learned she was debilitated by *uchawi* and that this husband must return to Newala to participate in (and pay for) an *ngoma*, a ritual healing ceremony that often lasts several days. He refused, and his wife died. The diagnosis of *uchawi*, the conversations it generated within the family, and the accusations against the distant husband not only pointed to the objects and workings of witchcraft but also wove together a narrative of accountability that included gender relations in southeastern Tanzania, the ethics of engaging in multiple marriages, and the politics of economic survival that necessitates that men travel far from home. The speculation that the wife might have had cancer did not dampen these other trajectories of blame or negate the forms of neglect that framed her death.

Tanzanians discuss, debate, and reconfigure the kinds of things that can be said to exist in the world as they address the maladies, debilities, and misfortunes they and their kin face. In the complexities of everyday life, that which constitutes the body and that which threatens its thriving are never certain. A friend exemplified this one day when he stopped by my home unexpectedly as he was traveling through the town where I lived. He was a Christian from the northern part of Tanzania who worked for a well-established international nongovernmental organization in the provincial capital and whose impressive résumé included fluency in Kichagga, Kiswahili, English, Cambodian, and Russian and work for the United Nations. He found my presence in a small town in southeastern Tanzania and my interest in healing provocative and amusing. Although we had had many conversations about my research in the past, he came that day with a specific articulation of his thoughts. Shortly after settling into a chair he announced that he "chose not to believe" in the power of traditional healers. He claimed that this lived belief did not rule out the possibility of witchcraft, devils, and invisible realms. In fact, for those who chose to engage such entities, he was fairly confident that relationships with them were possible. Rather, his refusal to believe was an explicitly Christian stance that he hoped would place him outside such relations in the predominantly Muslim southeast where he lived.[13] Devaluing, indeed refusing to take part in, particular forms of individual and collective existence reveals the moral nature of worldly terrains.

While ontological refusals such as my friend's are important to healers, doctors, and nurses (see chapter 8), most of my attention here is focused on the ways that ontologies are created through therapeutic practice. Healers and other therapeutic practitioners must establish a working set of commitments to the things that matter for treatment. Their therapies include practices that bring into being (and temporarily stabilize) specific versions of the body and bodily threats in order to facilitate intervention. Ethnographic investigations into these processes of becoming offer a method for revealing the play of power within ontologies. For instance, as I discuss in Part 1, efforts to justify the medicinal value

of particular plant, animal, or mineral substances through laboratory identifications of "active ingredients" must be understood in relation to colonial policies
on native medicine and socialist-era relations with China. The import of assertions of clinical practitioners that a traditional malady known as *degedege* "is"
malaria, which I outline in chapter 7, reveals itself only in light of broader public
health goals to reduce a disease responsible for a third of all hospital admissions
and the difficulties of maintaining microscopes and stocking staining solution
in the local hospital. Assertions and conflicts about the forms of existence that
matter reveal how ontologies have been explicitly politicized within colonial,
postcolonial, and global economies of ideas, objects, and technologies. In the
pages that follow, I use historical and ethnographic evidence of struggles over
the bodies and threats that can be said to exist in southern Tanzania to account
for the dynamics of postcoloniality.

The Ethnographer and the Truth

The ontological complexity of postcolonial encounters about medicine and healing were first brought to my attention in 1998 soon after I arrived in Mtwara,
the capital of Tanzania's southeastern most province to begin my fieldwork on
healing. A young artist named Mohammed Balozi appeared at the guesthouse
where I was staying with a gift to welcome me to the area. Extrapolating from
his experience as a research assistant for a Dutch woman who had studied traditional healing there several years earlier, he anticipated my work in a drawing.
In the image he presented to me, a thin woman with a pointy nose labeled with
my name stands with her arms crossed in front of a man who sits on a wooden
stool, having donned the headdress and cloth of one who specializes in medicinal
therapies. He is labeled as an *mganga*, a healer. Bottles of medicine lie at his feet.
In this cartoon depiction of fieldwork, "I" ask in English, "Truthfully?" or more
precisely "Is [it] true?" The iconic healer simply holds up a bottle and declares
in Kiswahili, "This medicine is for the stomach." His offering seems to be both
the statement that provoked the question of the woman in the drawing and the
answer to her question.

This gift haunted me through the research and writing of this book. The exchange between "Stacey" and "the *mganga*" highlights the awkward search for
channels along which communication about healing might be possible. "Stacey's"
concern with truth claims embodies what this Tanzanian artist has witnessed or
imagined as the voice of the formally educated, of science, of the World Health
Organization and the World Bank, of the Tanzanian elite, of prospectors for pharmaceutical companies, of a Dutch anthropologist, and of myriad global and local
others who are increasingly interested in the possibilities of plant-based medicine
produced in so-called Third World countries. The healer refuses to answer her

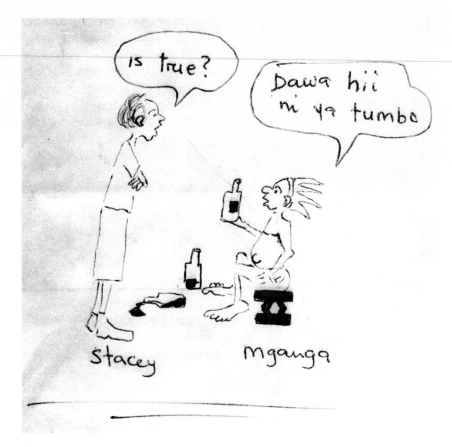

Figure 1.1. Drawing by Mohamed Balozi, 1998.

question directly. He avoids taking a position for or against Truth. Instead, he offers a bottle of medicine for stomach pains to his skeptical visitor.

Unlike my pen-and-ink namesake, I do not seek to assess the truth or falsity of healers' claims or the efficacy of their medicine. I am deeply interested, however, in the dynamics of the encounter and in the kinds of communication that are possible. I am drawn to the space held open by "Stacey's" failure to name the subject of her pursuit—the unspoken or unspeakable "it" that is absent from her question. This simple opening highlights the struggle to translate healing and the insufficiency of the category of traditional medicine that has been created through legal prohibitions, scientific investigations, and bureaucratic management. It also suggests that conflicts over the legitimate objects of postcolonial healing are deeply entwined with debates about the material and the "real."

In order for the medicine in the bottle and the stomach it cures to answer the inquisitor's question about truth, the substance of the threat that links them must be agreed upon. The uncertainty that hovers over this still image is an effect of this lack of agreement. In the outstretched hand of "the *mganga*," Balozi captures the contemporary moment in which science has not (yet) fully disciplined the relationship between the matters and meanings of traditional therapies. This book takes its lead from Balozi's *mganga*, who suggests that the most significant encounter that defines traditional medicine in Tanzania today is that which brings the truth of its matter under inquiry. I argue that this encounter is about a struggle over "what is," over ontological possibilities.

Efforts to develop traditional medicine in contemporary Tanzania privilege science as the medium through which traditional medicine might be recognized by national and international institutions. That is, medical science promises to materialize, to render speakable, the missing "it" from my namesake's question. As others have persuasively argued, however, scientific solutions to problems of knowledge are deeply entwined with moral solutions to problems of political order (e.g., Shapin and Schaffer 1985) and social life (e.g., Franklin 1997). Balozi's drawing then must also be read in light of the fact that Tanzanians regularly engage healing through debates over the objects and entities that make up the world. Such arguments among Tanzanians meld science, religion, family dynamics, and political economy.

Healing in the Space of the Postcolonial

I seek to bring the lessons of science studies into closer conversation with the new forms of history required by postcolonial critique (Chakrabarty 2000; Hall 1996; Prakash 1999). By exposing the ambiguities that lie at the heart of colonial representations (Bhabha 1994) and drawing out the subaltern voices that were hidden, marginalized, and at times erased in colonial records (Spivak 1987, 1990), postcolonial scholars have revealed the tenacity of colonial categories (nation, indigeneity, science, etc.) in articulations of the substance of history.[14] This book contributes to the growing interest in what some now call postcolonial science studies, which suggest that radically new relations of power and privilege require one to be able to imagine not only new categories of historical knowledge but also new objects of scientific controversy.[15] I share the goal of scholars who strive to move through descriptions that disrupt modernist attempts to separate nature and society, bodies and ideologies, and to continue on by developing modes of analysis and forms of action that do not assume that beginning or ending with these dualisms is inevitable.

Efforts to "enframe"[16] traditional medicine have sought to articulate socially relevant differences through the separation of practices as scientific or nonscientific and their corresponding relegation to the modern or the traditional. Connections or crossings between science and nonscience are not unusual, however. In fact, the ways that medicine shapes modern subjects and modern lives is the very ground of possibility for postcolonial healing (Comaroff 1985; Comaroff and Comaroff 1997).

Biomedicine's intimate relation with both colonial expansion and postcolonial development as well as the clinic's role in shaping modern subjects makes it difficult for Tanzanians *not* to be interpolated into technoscience today.[17] Difficult even for *waganga* (healers) in rural Tanzania. They may position themselves as similar to hospital medicine, as dealing with afflictions that clinical practitioners do not know about, or as working against biomedical ignorance and arrogance. Regardless of their stance(s), however, they are compelled to deal with biomedicine and the bureaucratic health systems that support it. Healers address the concerns of patients who are suffering the side effects of pharmaceuticals as well as patients who have found no relief from the medicine the clinic distributes. They confront complaints about specifically biomedical diseases such as AIDS, cancer, tuberculosis, and malaria. Healers are well aware that if patients or their kin do not see and appreciate the effects of their treatment they are likely to abandon it for hospital medicine. They are as knowledgeable about the remedies that are available at the local chemist as they are of the remedies that are available through other healers, including Islamic prophets, Christian exorcists, and Maasai herbalists who visit the local markets. Their success often has as much to do with their skill in influencing the ways that patients and their kin negotiate these options as it does in providing specific treatments. Furthermore, healers are sensitive to the work of bureaucrats who seek to organize them into a national association under the auspices of the Ministry of Health and to international development schemes that attempt to train them as outreach workers and birth attendants.

Science, like the modernity it promises, is "at large."[18] It is everywhere and inescapable, even if deeply controversial. Those who would advance arguments about postcolonial healing must pay attention to the borderlands—that is, to the spaces that not only regulate traffic between modern and traditional medicine but also hold out the possibility of life in between. The emergence of complex subjects and objects that have been forged in the fire of modernist dualisms gestures toward new forms of assemblage and new moments of articulation that mark the potentialities of postcolonialism and not merely its fragmentations. The healers and patients I describe in the chapters that follow pose questions for anthropology from these in-between spaces, from the interstices of powerful systems of materialization. They mediate between two or more powerful ways of enacting bodies, medicine, and threats to life and well-being (Hess 1994).

The term postcolonial, then, describes not only the temporal frame of this study but also the starting assumption that modern and traditional knowledge are co-produced, as are the experts and forms of expertise related to these types of knowledge. Drawing on postcolonial scholars, I start from the position that science and its others (magic, witchcraft, religion) not only coexist but also exist *inside one another*.[19] For example, ancestors and devilish spirits strive to address biomedical disease entities, healers argue for the inclusion of ancestors in the memoranda of understanding outlining the scope of scientific research and public health projects,[20] and nurses diagnose traditional maladies after evaluating the effects of pharmaceuticals.[21] This book pursues the ways that arguments about the interdependence of modern and traditional knowledge challenge accounts of the encounter between diverse therapeutic practices, objects, experts, and medicine in Tanzania. In so doing, it joins work that historicizes how therapies are compared (Adams 2001; Langford 2002), considers how treatments are coordinated (Scheid 2002), analyzes how scientific knowledge about traditional medicine emerges (Adams 2002; Hayden 2003), and chronicles how bodies, threats to bodies, and the medicine used to treat bodies change over time (Farquhar 2002; Livingston 2005; Lock 1993a, 1993b, 2002).

Efforts to capture the dynamism of the categories of traditional and modern medicine as they are being negotiated, elaborated, maintained, or allowed to fade away call for ethnography. This project grounds itself in ethnographic research about the relations between medical science, clinical practice, and the range of "traditional" therapies available in Tanzania. I am particularly interested in the way that practitioners both transform and coordinate traditional and modern medicine as they articulate objects of therapy.[22] This interest has guided my attention to the times when and spaces in which biomedical science and practice interrupt traditional medicine. These interruptions and interferences challenge healers (as well as biomedical practitioners) to formulate new objects of practice or to stake out spaces of strategic difference. This focus draws me into an analysis of the micropolitics of postcolonial healing through an examination of the "generative capacities" of healers (Verran 2001).[23]

The pages that follow highlight the techniques that make things visible, audible, tangible, and knowable in Tanzania. Healers are not faithful to the ontological differences between them and their clinical counterparts that public health campaigns articulate. Often the things that healers claim are palpable or material, biomedical practitioners consider immaterial. The crux of the book probes this disjuncture. At first sight, there is no ground for mutual intelligibility or translation. Yet the project of making a national traditional medicine, as Tanzania is doing, is invested in building the associations and connections that might constitute bodies and afflictions that are compatible with both modern and traditional medicine and are intelligible to both modern and traditional healers. For instance, the ultimate goal of the Institute of Traditional Medicine in the Muhimbili University Center for Health Services is to put biomedically effective "traditional medicine" in the hands of doctors and nurses. If we abandon the assumption that traditional healing is frozen in time in the African past and tune our analytical senses to the shifting claims and practices of contemporary healers, other translations also become evident.[24] A focus on healing practices reveals a variety of ways that bodies and afflictions are—at times—made compatible with both modern and traditional medicine. The fact that the translations healers have made about the maladies they see often differ from those that state scientists and bureaucrats who investigate traditional medicine have made reflects both technological and epistemological differences and the tenuous relationship healers have with the government's project to develop traditional medicine. Healers are seeking alternative spaces from which to negotiate the place of their medicine and expertise. As they position themselves in relation to biomedical tests, medicine, and knowledge, healers are cultivating new techniques of discerning the matter of the body and its threats. They are shifting the axes along which traditional and modern medicine might be said to admit comparison. And in so doing, they are refiguring the forms of difference that are essential to the postcolonial state.

Historicizing the ontological divide between traditional and modern medicine makes talk of "integration" slightly awkward and halting, for there are no sides that are un-integrated to begin with. Rather, it draws attention to specifically situated forms of "knowledge assemblage" (Turnbull 2000). Traditional medicine is articulated in Tanzania through grounded acts of comparison, coordination, translation, and transformation.[25] Accounting for the ways that (in)commensurabilities are being formulated through these acts reframes differences that have been seen as intractable (Pigg 2001). This approach also allows for the complicated, subtle, and often unpredictable ways that people position themselves and describe the world in order to survive, to move forward, to do something in the face of threats to mortality, painful disorders, and profound discomforts. This is true not only for the efforts of healers and patients and their kin but also for those of nurses, doctors, and bureaucrats. Such ethnographic attention opens up ways of describing how particular experts, practices, knowledges, medicine, technologies, and afflictions emerge "in a piece" (Verran 2001) through the processes of assembling therapeutic ecologies.

This approach takes us away from debates about pluralism and the implicit "cross-cultural" comparisons these debates evoke. Rather than making implicit or explicit comparisons between traditional and modern medicine, this book takes acts of comparing and contrasting by healers, nurses, scientists, politicians, and bureaucrats as its point of departure. I examine how these acts of comparing and contrasting structure interventions into traditional medicine. For example, public health posters printed by the Ministry of Health assert that the *ukanda wa jeshi* treated by Kalimaga (see the prologue) should be translated as herpes

zoster. Some nurses advise against seeking treatment from healers for this affliction, calling the effort a waste of money. Kalimaga asserts that the clinic neither
knows what this malady is nor knows how to treat it. He advises against seeking
treatment from the hospital for this malady, insinuating that the trip would be
a waste of time. For the nurses, a healer's treatment of patients with *ukanda wa
jeshi* and the clinic's treatment of patients with herpes zoster are comparable; for
Kalimaga, they are not. These declarations of similarity and difference are both
about access to bodies and influence over bodily practice. My primary concern is
not the ways that types of medicine, therapies, experts, or affliction *are* the same
or different but rather *when* they are made to admit comparison, *how* they are
translated, and *who* declared the differences (un)bridgeable. Ontological politics
captures the frictions that emerge when different people compare therapies in
different ways (chapter 6), when maladies are deemed mistranslated (chapter
7), or when experts disagree about how bridgeable differences are. My focus on
such politics includes a concern about the gaps created by refusals to compare,
refusals to see, and refusals to translate (chapter 8). Where, when, how, and by
whom bodies and threats are rendered insignificant is as important as where,
when, how and by whom they are rendered central to therapeutic knowledge
and practice.

The postcolonial context points to a concern with politics and the complicated
struggle for new forms of politics that might break away from negotiations over
more traditional objects of colonial history (such as indigeneity, especially as it
emerges in relation to formulations of nation and tribe). It suggests a deep interest in what sorts of new objects might be possible and what sorts of politics they
might compel. My articulation of postcolonial ontological politics joins a host of
other analytical tools that have opened up novel ways of pursuing these questions
by drawing attention to moments of partial connection (Strathern 1991/2004),
translation (Latour 1987, 1988; Callon 1986/1999), fractionality (Law 1999), and
interpolation (Haraway 1997). These approaches tell alternative stories about
the workings of power. They suggest that processes of discerning affliction and
techniques of formulating the world are both the product of modernist projects
of colonialism and nationalism, and the basis for generating new relations. They
propose methods for tracing the continuities of power without being blinded
by accounts of hegemony. For instance, how might we understand Binti Dadi's
use of a rat to test the new medicine she was contemplating and Kalimaga's
self-described "clinical trials"? How can ethnographic accounts articulate a
concern about openness and the possibility of alterity without being trapped by
conservative calls for the conservation of indigenous knowledge or cornered by
anxieties of pollution of the traditional by the modern? I draw on the work of
science studies and postcolonial studies to open a space in which to contemplate
the politics of difference enacted through postcolonial healing. Ultimately, this

book strives to convey a picture of the therapeutic landscape that highlights the
ontic and epistemic elements that would need to be negotiated for alternative
forms of politics to occur in Tanzania.

When Objects Come to Matter

"*Mashetani* have always been with us," Binti Dadi explained. "They used to
live in the trees. But now all the big trees have been cut down and they have
nowhere to live. So they come and live on us." *Mashetani*, as they are known in
Kiswahili, both provoke affliction and promise cures. These mischief-makers
play with children, exciting dangerous, sometimes fatal, afflictions, and they
penetrate pregnant women in order to stimulate miscarriage. These encounters
drive hot, weak, convulsing, and worried people from all over the Makonde
Plateau to Binti Dadi for care. Over time, Binti Dadi has garnered a great deal
of experience with *mashetani*. Healing requires "talking with" (*kuongea*) the
mashetani and encouraging them to reveal effective medicine. *Mashetani* have a
complicated history on the Makonde Plateau.[26] They share some kinship with the
beings that populate the elaborate hierarchies of the spirit world on the Swahili
coast, but they more often act like the roguish gangs of nonhumans captured in
George Lilanga's paintings (example on cover).[27] The plural, *mashetani*, connotes
Islamic evil spirits and demons and the singular, *shetani*, is translated as the
Christian Satan. Today, *mashetani* also include many other unseen actors—those
who have crossed into or live in invisible realms, be they ancestral shades or
nonhuman creatures who call on their human counterparts. While *mashetani*
do not provoke all maladies on the plateau or even all the maladies treated by
Binti Dadi, the existence of these meddlesome devils[28] illustrates one of the
more intractable dilemmas in anthropology and in the current development
of traditional medicine in East Africa. How should we talk about and engage
such actors that are so salient to healing and yet so unintelligible to medical
science? How can we articulate the substance of devils and the matter of their
meddle?

One of the obstacles to such research has been finding a language in which
to frame questions.[29] Above, I suggested that "malady" is a better translation for
the Kiswahili *ugonjwa* in that it captures what Bruno Latour has referred to as a
form of "nature-culture" and explicitly mixes subjects and objects, matter and
words. Throughout this book, I use terms that reject a priori divisions between
nature and culture, the physical and conceptual, the material and the immaterial, knowledge and belief. My concern with the ontologies at play in healing is
a concern with how such differences are delineated and the effects these delin-
eations have on bodies and survival in Tanzania. To this end, I draw on terms

from science studies literature that invite attention to the ways that particular forms of otherness—those that inhere in biomedical knowledge and practice and those that might be assumed by the reader—come into relation with life on the plateau. Because these terms can ring awkwardly the first time that one encounters them, I introduce a few of the most important here: nonhumans, actor/actant, and entities.

In the chapters that follow, I use the word nonhuman to talk about a range of actors—including creatures that approach through dreams and visions, *mashetani* that play with children, and the bacteria, parasites, and fungi that are made visible under microscopes—in an effort to highlight moments where the human and its others are being articulated in practice. The work of scholars such as Michel Callon, Donna Haraway, Bruno Latour, and John Law illustrates that differences between humans and nonhumans are historical; they can be traced through grounded acts of discerning, comparing, separating, and ordering; and they have political economies, technical realities, and social lives. The breadth of the term nonhumans leaves open the possibility of different articulations of otherness. For example, people in southern Tanzania refer colloquially to spirits and disembodied entities as *wanyama* (literally, animals). For these speakers, *wanyama* stand in relation to the human—the healer and the patient—as a generic other. Referring to *mashetani* as *wanyama* makes a distinction between *mashetani* and the human bodies they climb on, startle, and play with. Yet the direct translation of *mashetani* as animals in English connotes a history of difference between humanity and animality that is not the same as is found in Kiswahili. The unfamiliarity of the word nonhuman, then, provides a more faithful analytic.

Actant is a term science studies scholars have borrowed from semiotics to cover the agency of both humans and nonhumans. This initial collapsing of the kinds of agency that might be enacted by humans and nonhumans constitutes a refusal to ground analysis in a priori assumptions about their difference, instead allowing characteristics that distinguish humans and nonhumans to emerge through practice, interaction, and effect. While the word "actor" may connote human agency, "actant" refers to anything or anybody that shapes, influences, or modifies another entity through interacting with it. In chapter 6, I introduce the clinical cards that track the monthly visits of all children under the age of five who attend the maternal and child health clinic as "actants" because they have a profound effect on the way children move through the clinic and the way the clinic defines "normal" children's bodies. Entities, in contrast to actants, come to be known as they register the world; that is, their defining characteristics emerge as they respond to stimuli. Entities can be accounted for through descriptions of the ways they change as a result of their interaction with actants.

The difficulty of approaching the reality of *mashetani,* however, is not just an artifact of language. Traditional analytical distinctions between the objective and the subjective, the physical and the experiential, and the natural and the cultural have been reinforced by methodological differences in the study of those things that are deemed knowledge and those that are deemed belief. Distinctions between knowledge and belief convey claims to "realness" in the eyes of the speaker. They are also always distinctions between "us" (a group making a claim to the truth of the world) and "them" (those with different claims on the world). Yet if medical science cannot be unproblematically identified as a different order of knowledge, then biomedicine cannot provide a grounding point for ethnographic explanation.

Byron Good (1994) recommends that medical anthropologists interested in comparative work avoid problematic distinctions between knowledge and belief by focusing on the "formative processes" through which discomforts, misfortunes, and afflictions come to be defined as the target of therapeutic efforts. Not only biomedicine but all forms of healing, he asserts, formulate objects for discussion and intervention. "Healing activities shape the objects of therapy—whether some aspect of the medicalized body, hungry spirits, or bad fate—and seek to transform those objects through therapeutic activities" (69). These processes of shaping and transforming the object of therapeutic attention are the basis for ethnographic inquiry. In his own work, Good explores biomedical practices at Harvard. He advocates breaking down distinctions between knowledge and belief, between nature and culture, by tracing how biomedical diagnostic and treatment procedures shape the bodies of patients. Objectification, in his work, captures the processes that make the body perceivable, speakable, actionable. The anthropologist's task is to examine processes of objectification; that is, to examine the emergence, circulation, and growth of therapeutic objects in practice.

I draw on Good's notion of objectification, but ask: what might it look like to follow his early gesture toward the symmetry of ethnographic studies of different therapies? Good's suggestion that diverse therapeutic practices admit comparison as they construct objects for discussion and intervention opens up the possibility of new articulations of relations between traditional and modern medicine. I expand Good's examples of objectification to include those processes in therapeutic practice on the Makonde Plateau that mobilize treatment in relation to a complaint. Healers, for example, use medicine to define the boundaries of bodies, making them less permeable to *mashetani.* Medicinal baths, rubs, and ropes tied around waists and arms establish the body of the patient as discrete. Bodies that are bounded medicinally in this way become defendable and treatable.

Sustained attention to therapeutic practices inside and outside the clinic quickly illustrates that there are many bodies and many versions of the body at play in any given therapeutic interaction. One way to capture the entanglements of materiality and sociality is to trace the relations through which bodies as objects of therapy achieve durability, fixity, and coherence (see Butler 1993 and Law 1999), at least long enough to sustain a particular treatment. Annemarie Mol's (2002) empirical philosophy expands on Good's call for attention to the "formative processes" of medical practice. In *The Body Multiple,* she describes the many versions of the body that are "enacted" in the treatment of a particular vascular leg disease (atherosclerosis) in one Dutch hospital. Her account weaves together the many specialists, technologies, needs, and desires that bring bodies into being as objects of medical practice. In this way, she considers the sociomaterial reality of various medical bodies. Because medicine is a decidedly interventionist discipline, she privileges the ordering and coordinating of the bodily enactments of vascular surgeons, radiologists, pathologists, patients, and others as they work to intervene in the pain or disability that frames the original complaint. She describes the institutional structures, epistemological hierarchies, and expert skills that momentarily stabilize multiple enactments of the body in the hospital, thereby producing an effect of singularity that makes treatment possible. Bodies, for Mol, are carefully choreographed events. Opening Good's notion of "objectification" and his description of bodies as medical objects to Mol's notion of "enactment" and bodies as events (moments of ontological coordination) provides a richer and more dynamic point of comparison with postcolonial healing practices on the plateau.

Yet any attempt to account for the body in Tanzania must consider regional histories of "the body" as a focus of diagnosis and treatment and an object of healing.[30] While the matter of the body is inescapable when talking about healing in the early twenty-first century in Africa, it is not uncontroversial. Struggles over the ontological status of the body and its threats and its medicine have been (and remain) at the heart of efforts to (re)shape the therapeutic landscape. Over the past hundred years, missionization, Islamicization, colonization, the development of a national health care service, and (more recently) the demands of structural adjustment policies have reconfigured the practices through which bodies and afflictions might be enacted in Tanzania (Feierman 1985).[31] Furthermore, part of this controversy has been about the centrality of the body itself. In any accounting of the objects of therapeutic practices in Tanzania, it quickly becomes difficult to remain rigorously focused on "the body." In the diverse fields of healing in Tanzania (and many other places in Africa), treatments do not necessarily work on or treat discrete bodies bounded by skin or necessarily bodies at all. Rather, treatments may focus on ancestors, kin, residential units, jealousies, devils, or other mischievous agents (Ademuwagun et al. 1978; Giles 1987, 1999; Devisch 1993; du Toit and Abdallah 1985; Feierman and Janzen 1992; Janzen 1982; Turner 1967, 1968, 1975). This book considers a range of objects that materialize in therapeutic practices on the Makonde Plateau in southeastern Tanzania, including parasites, devils, jealousies, and numerous versions of the body. I describe, for instance, how healers discern the hunger, desires, and needs of the *mashetani* by satisfying or appeasing them with medicine. As healers evaluate *mashetani*'s responses to their medicinal offerings, they make claims about what *mashetani* are. Through the skilled use of protective medicine, *mashetani* take shape. Their character and substance emerge as a series of events, partly orchestrated by healers.

Some of the practices that bring ancestors, kin, jealousies, and devils into being as objects of therapy are the practices that were violently oppressed or secreted underground during colonialism. As the viability of these objects of therapeutic practice was threatened, a space opened for the elaboration and expansion of the biomedical body. Today, healers remain conscious of anti-witchcraft laws. When Binti Dadi sees that someone is afflicted with *uchawi*, she attempts to remove the witchcraft but no longer names the instigator. While she claims to know who sent the *uchawi*, she argues that the government forbids her from accusing that person directly. As a result, her treatments do more to articulate the body of the patient and the polluting substance than to reconfigure the relations that led to the jealousy and violence. Furthermore, translations of the body physical have spread from biomedicine to other treatment modalities through the training of traditional birth attendants and other processes that produce "traditional medicine" as a supposed alternative to the hospital. Contemporary attention to the body in postcolonial healing practices must be situated in histories of colonial and postcolonial law and biomedicine.

Mashetani and bodies that are sensitive to their mischief are just some of the entities that are central to postcolonial healing. They serve well however to introduce how accounts of healing in Tanzania can contribute to contemporary debates that rethink ontology by insisting that arguments in these debates remain alert to the asymmetries of lived relations. Articulating the dynamics and tensions in postcolonial healing requires us to critically reassess the regulatory norms that support or diminish the meaningfulness of certain kinds of bodies and worldly matter (Butler 1993; Haraway 1997; Lock 1998). In a region declared "underdeveloped" and considered part of the "Third World," the normative conditions that establish epistemic and ontic possibilities are often not of the making of the people who live there. The hegemony of certain "First World" norms becomes apparent in any direct attention to the production of objects of therapy in Tanzania. For this reason, *Bodies, Politics, and African Healing* does not stay tightly focused on objects of scientific investigation or medical technologies. Rather, it takes in the ground on which medical science has carved its channels, linking bodies, medicines, and imperialisms (Tsing 2005).

The wide-angled lens I have chosen for this book does more than capture the interdependence, the dynamism, and the shifting material realities of the therapeutic landscape in Tanzania. Bringing African therapeutics and lifeways to bear on discussions of ontology raises new questions for science studies scholars. Good's focus on medical education and Mol's description of the multiple versions of a patient's body that circulate in a hospital might be taken to imply that their notions of objectification and enactment (respectively) link epistemologies and ontologies.[32] The necessity for this linkage, indeed the politics of this linkage, are made more apparent in a turn to Africa. Students of healing in Africa have long noticed that decisions about treatment are made by a loose group of kin, what Janzen (1978) originally termed a "therapy management group." The treatments these groups choose do not reflect any one person's "self-interest," nor are they easily explained as "rational" from the perspective of a particular actor. As I sat in healers' courtyards on the plateau, patients, their kin, their neighbors, and other people who were either waiting to see the healer or were visiting a member of the healer's family contributed to discussions with and about the afflicted. The itineraries of those seeking therapies for stubbornly resilient illnesses and the epistemic objects that the multiple treatments bring into being are the result of complex negotiations—and the social hierarchies, irrationalities, and power plays of which they are a piece. The specific practices I describe in this book and the specific healers I portray are part of these collectively negotiated healing itineraries.

The emergence of objects of therapeutic attention as a product of collective action rather than cosmological coherence or secular rationality was further illustrated when Binti Dadi would at times hand the mother of a sick child a plate of different roots, a stone, and a cup of water so she could grind her child's medicine. In this way, mothers participated in the making of their children's remedy. On any given day, a mother may grind more or less of one root, not because she has some conceptualization of "dosage"—indeed, on the plate many roots look very similar and she likely does not know what she is grinding. Rather, she may be talking and may grind one root for a long time or a particular sample of root may be small and tricky to grind without hurting her fingers so she may stop sooner; she may like the feel of one in her hand or she may suspect that one with yellow bark or red skin is particularly potent so she will add more or less of it to her child's concoction. As for Binti Dadi, sometimes she asks the mother to grind the medicine so that the mother's own "power" is in the medicine or sometimes she does so because she is too busy to do it herself. Such scenes resist any reduction of the ways that treatments proceed and the objects of their attention emerge to merely a question of the politics of knowledge. Rather, the ways that epistemologies (knowledges) are (or are not) intertwined with ontologies (matters) becomes an ethnographic question. And the politics become more complicated.

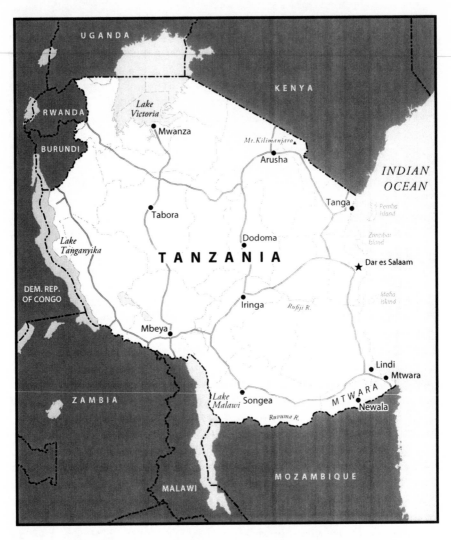

Map 1.1. Tanzania. Newala is located in the southeastern province of Mtwara.
Detail excerpted from *Map of Tanzania. Central Intelligence Agency,
United States, 2003.*

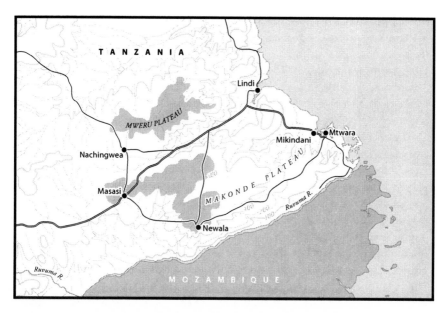

Map 1.2. Detail excerpted from *Dar es Salaam, Africa* (Sheet 28). Washington, D.C.: U.S. Army Topographic Command (LU), 1969. Altitude in meters. *Courtesy of the University Libraries, The University of Texas at Austin.*

Location as Relation

Just as objects of therapy materialize through their relations, including those enacted in clinical investigations, healers' treatments, political machinations, and anthropological analyses, so locations also materialize through relations. I approach ontological politics as they emerge in struggles over the translations of bodies and their threats that are central to therapeutic practices conducted in the district of Newala in southern Tanzania. Although I have provided maps, Newala is not understandable as a place to live or a field site in such two-dimensional renderings. Newala consists of its relations, layered as they are over time, through historical transitions, agricultural practice, shifting tensions with colonial and postcolonial governments, migrations, and wars.

The town of Newala, which is the capital of the district by the same name, sits on the southwestern corner of the Makonde Plateau. As one comes from the east, from the older trade centers of the Swahili coast or from Mtwara, the current capital of the southeastern most region in Tanzania, the Makonde Plateau rises gradually. When one reaches the town of Newala, the western and southwestern escarpments drop off sharply for a steep descent of approximately 1,000 feet. The dry plateau stands between the Ruvuma and Lukuledi rivers and their accompanying valleys. From the grounds of the Newala District Hospital, one can see over the south-facing escarpment, across the twenty-five kilometers of flat, green, and often-swampy farmland to the Ruvuma River. On the other side of the river, the mountains of northern Mozambique rise, suddenly defining the horizon. If one walks along the edge of the escarpment for a kilometer or so, the hills of Masasi about seventy kilometers northwest of Newala come into view.

These views made Newala a strategic location during the wars, slave raids, and ivory hunting of the eighteenth and nineteenth centuries. The unique location attracted a variety of inhabitants despite the challenges of life on the waterless plateau. The people living on the plateau today embody this complicated history of migrations. In addition, more contemporary movements for economic, personal, and political reasons continue to shape the demographics of the population. Although the majority of people living on the plateau identify as Makonde, the town of Newala is home to a range of diverse ethnic and language groups.[33] In the town and its nearest villages, people often speak three or more Bantu languages. The most commonly heard are Kimakonde, Kiyao, and Kimakua as well as Kiswahili, which is one of the two official national languages (the other is English).

Despite the rich diversity of lifeways and histories on the Makonde Plateau and the changes they have stimulated over time, this region has been considered one of the most "underdeveloped" areas of the country throughout the twentieth century and into the twenty-first century. The origin of this region's marginality is often traced to early German colonialists' frustrations with rule in southern Tanganyika and their preferences for land in northern Tanganyika.[34] After World War I, the British took over the administration of colonial Tanganyika (1918–1961). Their regional predilections followed those of the Germans. The British administration concentrated their minimal efforts to develop the infrastructural and economic capacities of Tanganyika outside the southeast. Some have linked the colonial frustrations in the southeast—in particular, the decentralized resistance to imperial rule and the difficulty of implementing taxation policies—to descriptions of the area as one populated by stateless matriarchal societies (e.g., Iliffe 1979). The stigma of statelessness seems to have followed southeasterners into the present.[35] Their reputation of having been resistant to colonization refigures in their more contemporary reputation as being "resistant to development."[36]

As Binti Dadi's comment above about the new habitations of the *mashetani* "on us" rather than "in the trees" suggests, the physical landscape of the plateau has changed dramatically. Although Newala is a rural district, it is densely populated. The vast majority of these people are subsistence or small-scale farmers.[37] While it appears from the Newala District Books[38] that there may have once been old-growth forest on this plateau, by the time British colonists arrived, only small pockets of forest remained and most of the Makonde Plateau was covered with a dense thicket of secondary growth. In fact, Makonde is said to mean "people of the thicket" (Liebenow 1971). Now, however, much of that thicket, too, is gone. Over the past century, farming practices have changed to accommodate the growing number of people living on the plateau. Whereas today farmland is scarcely ever left unused, in the past the rotation of crops was critical to maintaining the fertility of the soil. One district officer in the 1940s penned an essay on "bush fallowing" in the district books in which he noted that people typically planted for three years and then left land to lie fallow for six to nine years.[39] By 2000, although there were patches of bush, these were more infrequent and the natural vegetation was not particularly dense. It was unusual to see land left fallow. Perhaps if a woman who gave birth around planting time had the support of her family, she would leave her land uncultivated for a season. Instead of boosting productivity by allowing land to lie fallow at regular intervals, farmers now rely on the increasingly heavy use of fertilizer. Even so, crop yields are shrinking. Because so much of the land on top of the plateau has been continuously planted, healers often go to the edges of the plateau where the steep banks have been left uncultivated to collect the wild plants needed for medicine. Sometimes they even transplant medicine in or near their courtyards or fields. One healer purposely left an area of her farmland uncultivated so she could collect common medicinal plants there.

In addition to the corn, dry rice, cassava, millet, pumpkins, and beans that farmers commonly grow on the plateau, many people in Newala also tend cashew trees. The sandy loam on the dry plateau has proven excellent ground for this cash and export crop. This important crop is the primary way the plateau has inserted itself into the national economy. Yet, the impact of cashews on the local wealth is circumscribed. Although individual farmers grow and sell raw cashews, the majority of the transport companies are based in Dar es Salaam and the majority of the buyers are from India. At one time, the government built and attempted to manage cashew processing plants. One still sits vacant in Newala. It operated from 1976 to 1978. I rented one of the workers' residences from the Cashew Nut Board of Tanzania during my fieldwork. Today only a few small cooperatives in the area process cashew. Frustrated with the limitations on their agricultural futures, young men on the plateau complain about the lack of jobs. Many make trips back and forth across the Mozambique border working as small-scale traders. Others go to Dar es Salaam to look for work. Young Makonde boys in Dar es Salaam, referred to as *machinga,* can often be seen selling clothing on the street in a consignment-like arrangement with local stores. Most men and women, however, continue the backbreaking work involved in coaxing food for their families from the tired soils of the plateau and selling raw cashews each season.

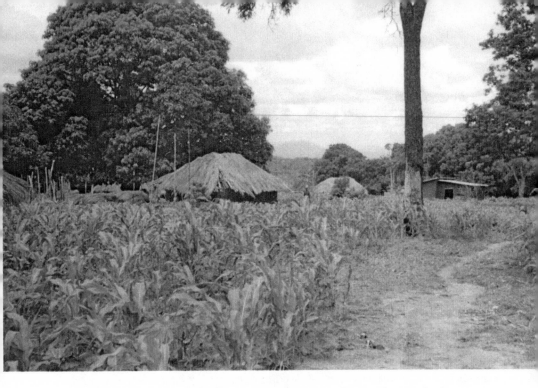

Figure 1.2. Domesticated landscape of the Makonde Plateau. The view looks over the northwestern escarpment toward the Masasi hills. *Photo by Jeff Bercuvitz, 1999.*

The challenging agricultural conditions as well as the lack of roads, the poor schools, and the deficiency of other infrastructural resources all feature prominently in the bitter complaints of government employees who find themselves assigned to a post in Newala. In contrast, for those who live in urban areas far from Newala, the stereotype of the Makonde as primitive, rural, and undeveloped seems to be explicitly linked to the lack of water that has historically characterized the plateau. Until relatively recently, men and women had to carry water from below the escarpment up the 1,000-foot slope and then often as many as twelve miles across the plateau to their homes. A water scheme was initiated in the 1950s, but it took several decades to get it working and to keep it maintained with any regularity. By the late 1990s, piped water was available (for a price) most of the time. These historical everyday struggles not only conjure "backwardness" in the national imagination but also "strength" (*wana nguvu sana*). The Makonde residing in this area have a reputation for being able to endure hardship. This toughness—sometimes described as stoicism and sometimes as scrappiness—is a point of pride on the plateau.

These conditions not only shape the afflictions found on the plateau and the services available to treat them, they also link Newala with traditional healing in a broader national imaginary. Tanzanian government officials, for instance, often tie their accusations that those on the plateau are "resistant to development" directly to Newala's equally strong reputation as an area of powerful healers and powerful medicine. In the southeast, the Makonde are popularly known as "the ones who know medicine." The senior health care practitioners in the regional hospital in Mtwara encouraged me to conduct my research on traditional medicine in the district of Newala. This reputation as a place of both feared and effective healers is not just crafted from the "outside"; Makonde healers too put forward such claims when arguing for the strength of their medicine.

Newala also has an interesting history with biomedicine that has influenced the national structure of health care. The first hospital in Newala was built in 1939. The man responsible for building this hospital, Dr. Leader Stirling, later rose to the position of minister of health in independent Tanzania.[40] Before he left the area for more prestigious positions, his hospital trained the first nurses in the colony. Moreover, the first school for village midwives was started in Newala in the 1950s (Stirling 1947, 1977). After independence in 1961, this training grew to influence the national-level training of low-level dispensary staff to promote public health for women and children.

Today the health care institutions on the Makonde Plateau tend to be less cutting edge. In 2003, the district nursing officer argued that the government hospital at Newala was working with only 42 percent of the staff it needed. As underfunded as it is understaffed, the hospital often runs out of medicine halfway through each month. Perched on the edge of a dry plateau, it has also run out of water at times. Even when medicine and water are available in the hospital, the poor roads in southern Tanzania make it difficult for many to get to any hospital, particularly in the rainy season. Due to structural adjustment programs and their fee-for-service initiatives, seeing a doctor is beyond the means of some. The shortage of nurses means that the Newala District Hospital cannot afford to have the staff feed and bathe patients; therefore, family members must leave their fields and livelihoods to care for someone who is admitted into the hospital.

The financial struggles of the Tanzanian health service make the conditions of the work in the Newala District Hospital unenviable. In an attempt to distribute medical expertise throughout the country, the Ministry of Health assigns Tanzanian doctors to service in Newala. During the years that I have been traveling to and living in Newala, these well-educated practitioners, many of whom have studied abroad, have rarely had any interest in living on the plateau or in the kind of toughness needed to craft a life there. I heard many stories of doctors who avoided or tried to avoid this placement. Indeed, in 1998 the head of the Newala District Hospital fled the country rather than remain stationed in this small southeastern town. He told his colleagues that he was going to Mtwara for supplies and would return in twenty-four hours. Many in the hospital believe that he went to Botswana to establish a private practice. What is certain is that he did not return, despite the fact that this abandonment of his post likely means that he can never practice medicine in his home country again. These issues are not the focus of this book, but they are clearly not trivial matters. They are the very real context in which healing happens in Newala. In the face of these conditions, people (the afflicted, their family members, nurses, doctors, and healers) do the best they can to negotiate meaningful lives and, if necessary, deaths that are as comfortable as possible.

To account for the matters of therapeutic concern on the Makonde Plateau, this book draws on fieldwork carried out between 1998 and 2008. Most of this time was spent in the district of Newala interviewing, observing, and working with healers and hospital staff. In my efforts to account for the historical and contemporary pressures that have shaped healing on the plateau, however, I was also drawn into regional capitals, national headquarters, and a variety of archives in Tanzania and the United States. Due to the sensitivity of information about medicine and therapies, I did not use a research assistant. I conducted multiple intensive interviews with over thirty healers and traditional birth attendants in the district of Newala; the majority of nurses, nurses' aides, administrators, and doctors in the Newala District Hospital and those in key positions related to maternal and child regional health care in the Mtwara Regional Hospital; and well over a hundred patients. While my initial interviews with healers were often conducted formally, my subsequent conversations occurred while collecting medicine, preparing therapies, treating patients, or waiting—waiting for people to come, for afflictions to unfold, for patients to respond.

Central to my arguments in this book are these extensive observations of healing practices. I learned to identify and collect herbal medicine. My knowledge was "tested" by healers, and I was sometimes asked to prepare and/or administer therapies. I worked particularly closely with Binti Dadi and her daughter Mariamu. I spent many hours each day with them for ten months in 1998–1999, two months in 2000, and two months in 2003. I continue to visit them during my trips to Tanzania and, as I describe in the epilogue, Binti Dadi treated me in 2008. Therefore, it is them, their treatments, and the collective of therapeutic objects and entities they draw together that receive the most detailed attention in the pages that follow. The life stories and practices of the broader range of healers that I interviewed and observed are used to illustrate commonalities in healing practices as well as unique aspects of these healers' work. The mother-and-daughter team, however, are situated the most thoroughly in my analysis of colonial and post-independence histories and development initiatives. Over the past decade, my relationship with Binti Dadi and Mariamu has come to resemble a loose form of apprenticeship. They have taught me to attend to and care for the entities that are central to their therapies. We also have come to attend to and care for each other quite deeply. My account therefore reveals that the process of formulating objects of therapeutic attention—what I call objectification—is an act full of intimacies. Ontological politics is about the struggle to bring attention (touch, prayer, love, and healing) to matters of mutual concern.

Outline of the Book

The history of traditional medicine as a modern category of knowledge and practice runs through colonial, socialist, and postsocialist regimes, reshaped with each turn as a new solution to problems of both society and knowledge. It refracts imperial violence and postcolonial dispossession. It is the ground on which any investigation of the ontological politics of healing in Tanzania must begin. Part 1 traces the emergence of the category of traditional medicine in Tanzania. Over the past hundred years, legal prohibitions have shaped its contours and scientific investigations have defined its content. I locate the conditions of possibility for the modern life of traditional medicine in two historical moments. The first is colonial rule and the redefinition of harming and healing—of witchcraft and medicine—in the service of imperial power (chapter 2). The second is the post-colonial globalization of traditional medicine, with its socialist roots and its neoliberal possibilities (chapter 3).

These legal, scientific, and bureaucratic efforts to define traditional medicine transformed the figure of the healer and his or her relationship with structures of governance. Contemporary practitioners on the plateau strive to influence the institutional relations that are bringing them into existence as modern traditional healers and traditional birth attendants. Part 2 considers those experts commonly referred to as traditional both by the state and by the practitioners themselves. I investigate how healers (chapter 4) and traditional birth attendants (chapter 5) develop their expertise. Caught in the opposition of the witch and the doctor, the traditional healer and birth attendant capture changing notions of those practices known as healing and expose the limitations of the official category of traditional medicine. At issue in these chapters is what has come to constitute legitimate therapeutic knowledge.

Part 3, the ethnographic core of the book, investigates the ways that healing renders the world speakable and actionable. Chapters 6, 7, and 8 look closely at therapeutic practice and focus most directly on Binti Dadi and her daughter Mariamu. I account for the emergence of postcolonial healing at the intersection of different orders of knowledge—what some have called culture and medicine. I train attention on the comparisons that healers draw between traditional and modern medicine, the new objects of therapeutic attention that materialize through these comparisons, and the spaces of (un)intelligibility that they create.

Chapter 6, "Alternative Materialities," turns directly toward the elaboration of different objects of therapy. In this chapter, I exploit the benefits of a methodologically symmetrical approach to therapeutic practices. David Bloor (1976) drove the development of a field referred to as the sociology of scientific knowledge (SSK) with a call to methodological symmetry. This call and the responses to it have come to shape a range of debates within science studies and have framed this new field's first serious engagement with anthropology. The symmetry principle suggests that all assertions of truth or fact, whether they are judged to be rational or irrational, accurate or inaccurate, possible or impossible, should be approached by the sociologist in the same way. SSK scholars were disturbed by a pattern they saw in studies of the development of knowledge, particularly scientific knowledge, in which accounts of the emergence of beliefs that in retrospect were deemed true proceeded through a series of internal and rationalist explanations and accounts of the emergence of belief that in retrospect were deemed false proceeded through external or social explanations. They challenged such unequal handling of accounts of the development of knowledge and proposed that a commitment to methodological or analytical symmetry would ensure more equal accounts. In chapter 6, I juxtapose the articulation of objects that are central to biomedical preventive care with the articulation of objects that are central to nonbiomedical protective care through a case study of the therapies used to secure the health of one child during the first two years of her life. For Tanzanians—patients, kin, healers, and nurses alike—differences in the objects of therapeutic attention during preventative treatments and protective treatments mark differences in modern and traditional medicine. This chapter demonstrates how the movement of patients between healers and among healing modalities elicits multiple objects of therapy and generates a field of coexisting practices.

As the stories of Binti Dadi and Kalimaga in the prologue illustrated, however, methodological symmetry in the study of traditional and modern medicine has its limitations. While this analytical approach challenges divisions between culture and nature, society and science, belief and knowledge, it does so by illustrating how claims to one or the other are established (Barnes and Bloor 1982). The focus of symmetrical studies is necessary during the times when and in spaces where the world is separated and purified into (modernist) units of analysis. Healers, however, are not necessarily dedicated to this work of purification.[41] Therapeutic objects that are constituted through healers' attention and treatment, therefore, do not always evade each other as easily as they appear to in chapter 6, and sometimes they conflict with each other. The stakes over "object conflicts" (Hess 2004) often include not only the legitimacy of particular objects of therapeutic care—from biomedical bodies to the medicinal bodily boundaries enacted by healers, from parasites to devils, and viruses to jealousies—but also the forms of expertise and kinds of relations that sustain particular objects of therapeutic care.

The final two chapters, then, explore the spaces where it becomes difficult to maintain methodological symmetry.[42] They describe the ways that one set of practices and claims interrupts or disrupts another.[43] Chapter 7 examines the struggle between traditional healers and clinical practitioners over the bodies of convulsing children. In this chapter, I consider when and how different actors compare and translate the "traditional" affliction *degedege* and the modern disease malaria. I am particularly interested in how therapies, knowledges, medicine, and bodies interfere with one another; how doctors and healers refigure patterns of inclusion and exclusion; and how therapies start to create complex hybrid objects of practice. Chapter 8 examines concerns that cannot be biomedically translated. These include certain vaginal growths, unclean breast milk, bodies that are "drying out," adulterous spouses, and children with large heads. I describe the asymmetries that support not only incommensurability but also incomparability. I draw attention to the times when and the spaces where symmetry slips between our analytical fingers. The stakes are not only the status of belief and knowledge and claims to truth or falsity but also the right of healers to focus their treatments on certain kinds of bodies, types of threats, and forms of misfortune and discomfort. When the right of healers to formulate their objects of therapeutic attention is challenged, then the right of some bodies and some bodily threats to exist is also challenged. These chapters illustrate the demand that postcolonial healing creates for new strategies of analysis that account for the particular bodies and threats at stake in the pluralisms bred by scientific, legal, institutional, and therapeutic practices and in the sorts of differences that articulations of pluralism strategically elide.

This book argues that opening notions of materiality to the practices through which healers, patients, nurses, and bureaucrats formulate objects of therapeutic attention—that is, to the generative processes of objectification—describes the ground on which power is working. It forefronts questions about which bodies and which bodily threats are allowed to exist as a focus of therapeutic practice, as well as where they are allowed to exist and what relationships enable them to exist. A rigorous ethnographic examination of the processes of becoming that are critical to therapeutic practice unsettles normative descriptions of medical pluralism. It challenges us to consider how medicine comes to admit comparison, how modes of comparison define particular historical moments, and, perhaps most important, what this means for the sorts of politics that are possible now.

Part 1

A Short Genealogy of Traditional Medicine

It is apparent that primitive medicaments to certain common diseases have been deteriorating in the past five decades just because more sophisticated ones have been introduced by more developed countries. This does not by any means prevent the Scientists from investigating the old or indigenous ways of curing diseases and hence developing new ways of curing.

—J. N. R. Kasembe, research officer from the Tanzanian Ministry of Agriculture and Cooperative Development, *Report on the Symposium of African Medicinal Plants* (1968)

All people who took witchcraft seriously anywhere in the country were usually lazy, jealous, and deceitful liars who have to be shunned by other members of society.

—Ndugu Jumbe, second vice-president, "Witchcraft a Waste of Time," *Daily News* (Dar es Salaam), 24 January 1975

2

Witchcraft, Oracles, and Native Medicine

In 1999, the district commissioner of Newala—feeling a little guilty, I believe, that the "district archives" to which I had requested access were a heap of termite-eaten, mouse-inhabited papers in a warehouse that was partially open to the elements—invited me to read the current files in his office on traditional medicine. Healers' appeals to work in the district dominated these files. The Tanzanian government mandates that all healers in the country register with the Ministry of Health and requires that healers declare on the record, in any and every district they intend to work, that their therapies do not involve "witchcraft." As healers sought permission from the district office to sell medicine in Newala, they declared that their trade was different from divination and from the practice of mass distribution of medicine to identify witches or protect whole communities from witchcraft. A common letter giving healers permission to sell their medicines reads:

> The District Commissioner has consented that this comrade mentioned by name above has been given permission to sell traditional medicine here in the town of Newala, and not to divine or to give all people medicine to drink . . . [Period for which permission has been granted is stated] . . . S/he will sell medicine to those who want it, not make it obligatory.[1]

In these official letters, the practices legally prosecutable under the 1928 Witchcraft Ordinance, which is still in effect in Tanzania today, are made explicit.[2] The prohibitions against divination and the practice of distributing medicine to whole communities are artifacts of colonial efforts to separate witchcraft (uchawi) from healing (uganga) in ways that mapped over European understandings of medicine and magic and in ways that supported colonial governance.[3]

The British, all too aware of the political nature of African medicine, introduced a witchcraft ordinance into each of their colonial territories. The task of translating imperial policy on the ground fell to provincial and district officers. In colonial Tanganyika, revisions of the witchcraft ordinance and companion policies concerning native medicine divided African therapeutics into practices to be disciplined by law and those to be disciplined by science. These legal statutes cast witchcraft as fraud and witches (as well as the healers that combated them) as charlatans, while leaving open the possibility that herbalism was a protoscience and that herbalists were custodians of knowledge obtained over the centuries by trial and error. These attempts to separate African therapeutics into witchcraft and herbalism generated the forms of skepticism and kinds of evidence that continue to shape debates about traditional medicine in Africa today.

Colonial violence against healers and the legal statutes that altered the status of witchcraft (*uchawi*) in the colonies delegitimated entities and persons central to the material life and social organization of much of Sub-Saharan Africa. At the same time, biological and medical sciences introduced new forms of expertise in the colonies and new ways of articulating bodies and the matters of affliction. By privileging certain forms of evidence, colonial courts and laboratories authorized some threats and afflictions and declared others illicit. In short, colonialism transformed who and what had the right to exist in Africa. It made existence itself a political question. Courts and laboratories became central sites for generating colonial ontologies. This chapter's account of the birth of traditional medicine as a coherent category of knowledge and practice calls particular attention to debates and policies that established law and science as the languages through which existence of particular bodies and bodily threats could be justified in the colonies.

Legal solutions to the problem of witchcraft and scientific answers to the questions of African medicine were also solutions to problems of imperial governance. At times, debates over what sorts of legal and scientific solutions would be most politically efficacious were explicit. In colonial Tanganyika, such moments emerged during the translation of witchcraft ordinances and native medicine policies passed down from the metropole. Debates about which forms of being healers and healing practices should be allowed to address became the ground for larger political debates over how the British government could control its African subjects. Colonial administrators intervened into the substance of affliction and the reality of threats with policies and laws that aimed to disrupt notions of cure based on obligations to kin, to community, or to indigenous sovereigns. They displaced forms of justice founded on practices to eliminate evil with forms of justice founded on evaluations of individual rights and bodily integrity. While British administrators often seemed baffled by what *uchawi* and *uganga* were, their confusion and even their misrepresentations are less salient than the effects (both intended and unintended) of their interpretations and interventions. As provincial and district administrators strove to implement imperial policies on witchcraft, they formulated a politics of matter that supported and made colonial governance possible.

The Political and Social Basis of Medicine

Scholars of African healing have long recognized that the ethnographic and historical category of medicine is unruly at best. There was no singular understanding of what constituted medicine or legitimated a healer in precolonial East Africa (Feierman 1985). Healing and harming—and the various types of medicine and forms of expertise that facilitated both—could not be separated from political and social power. Yet the relationship between sovereign powers and those with the abilities to heal and harm varied across the territory and over time. In some areas chiefs themselves held esoteric healing knowledge, in others healers worked with a king's court, and in still others healers engaged in less established and therefore less predictable relations with political leaders, sometimes supporting, sometimes challenging, and sometimes redirecting their power (Feierman 1974; Janzen 1982, 1992; Tantala 1989; Vansina 1972). Throughout the region, however, those known as healers shaped investments in various forms of (re)production. Through their influence over where communities should settle, when rains would come, when planting or harvesting should begin, and how kinship relations should be managed, healers mobilized medicine to intervene in a range of affairs that affected the coherence of groups, the organization of social networks, and the vagaries of illness. Some have referred to these interventions as forms of "public health" (e.g., Waite 1992).[4]

Gus Liebenow's study of the political practices of the Makonde (1971) hints at the complicated and multifaceted role that medicine played in political life on the plateau in the middle of the twentieth century. While his description is filtered through a modernist division of science and spirit, medicine and magic, he alludes to a range of activities (e.g., initiation and witch finding) and relations (e.g., with ancestors and other disembodied powers) that grounded political power among the Makonde. The "mystical powers" and "ritual paraphernalia" of initiation specialists shaped the founding moments of Makonde male political socialization (49–52; see also Harries 1944). The *mkulungwa* (leader of a "vaguely territorial" grouping (42), sometimes translated as chief; pl. *wakulungwa*) harnessed "spiritual powers" that involved communicating with ancestors, protecting the community against disaster, and eliminating evil (54–55). Finally, traveling witch-finders challenged *wakulungwa*, who dared not refuse them for fear that such would be taken as evidence that the *mkulungwa* was a witch him or herself (61–62). In practice, these activities and relations overlapped with practices that have come to be known as healing. Initiation specialists, *wakulungwa,* and witch-finders negotiated with disembodied entities in invisible realms and/or had knowledge of *dawa* (medicine, in the broadest sense of the word). Liebenow's account suggests that medicine among the

Makonde mediated efforts to both consolidate political and social power and disrupt that consolidation.

This reading of Liebenow links the role of medicine with the relatively flat social structure and horizontal political leadership that was the focus of his study. The decentralized or "polycentric" character of Makonde political authority that he outlined reflected the strength of matrilineal kin groups (*litawa*), the effect of overlapping identification with political or territorial groups (*chirambo*), the density of the thicket on the plateau that always held out the possibility of groups breaking apart and smaller units withdrawing, and the system of cultivation the Makonde employed (Liebenow 1971, 41–45). As mentioned in the previous chapter, the Makonde let their fields lay fallow after three years of planting in an effort to accommodate the fragile soils on the plateau. This technique necessitated relatively frequent movement and resulted in the widely scattered distribution of homesteads. A Makonde proverb that healers and others repeated to me ("When you can see your neighbor's fire, it is time to move") reinforces this notion that precolonial residences were dispersed across the plateau and suggests the difficulty any chief or headman would have had in maintaining tight control over the population. These conditions fostered diffuse forms of leadership and multiple ways of settling disputes on the plateau. Medicine, at times, contributed to the cohesion of groups and the organization of collective action within this relatively flat or horizontal social structure. It had the ability to galvanize people and things, dispense justice, and transform alliances.

Medicinal Water and the Crisis of Colonial Rule

Before the British acquired the territory of Tanganyika in the settlement following the Allied victory in World War I, the area was part of German East Africa (1986–1919). The Germans quickly discovered that control over East Africa required control over medicine.[5] The Maji Maji Rebellion of 1905–1907 was a particularly influential lesson. In 1905, a form of medicinal water, said to dissolve bullets and thereby make men invincible in the face of European weaponry, circulated through the southeastern part of colonial Tanganyika. Experts referred to as *hongo* carried this "water" (*maji*) from one region to another, sprinkling it on groups of warriors. Seemingly unallied groups of African men began to rise up against German rule.[6] Over the next two years, as the *maji* moved farther inland, the rebellion spread west, from the southeast to the southern highlands. The solidarity that the distribution of the medicinal water coordinated lent the uprising its name—the Maji Maji Rebellion.

The German forces eventually crushed the Maji Maji Rebellion and proceeded to institute stricter administrative controls throughout the southeast (Liebenow 1971). After the uprising, for instance, the German administration stationed a permanent officer in Newala for the first time. This German resident (accompanied by thirty African guards) managed the area alone until 1913, when a colonial police officer was also posted to the Newala station. Although these numbers seem relatively small, they represent a considerable change in the attention of the German colonial administration toward outlying areas. Even more significantly, fear of another Maji Maji instigated German initiatives to circumscribe the deeply political nature of medicine in Tanganyika. The fact of the rebellion shaped the kind of control that colonial officials felt they needed in this territory. In particular, so-called native or indigenous practices involving witchcraft and healing became subject to more systematic colonial intervention.

Well over a decade later, when the British took control of the territory, the movement of medicine still made colonial administrators anxious. The British in Tanganyika rationalized their fears of healers and traditional medicine through their reflections on the experience of the Germans during the Maji Maji Rebellion. Medicine seemed to lurk outside British authority, threatening to organize another rebellion against imperial power.

Maji Maji serves as a particularly instructive instance of the political and social power of medicine, both because it directly shaped British concerns with medicine in colonial Tanganyika and because it remains iconic in Makonde illustrations of the power of their medicine. As I worked on the plateau at the turn of the twenty-first century, healers still evoked Maji Maji, claiming that they knew the secrets of this medicine and the process of its production.

Accounting for the power and efficacy of the medicinal *maji* in 1905 necessitates situating it in a broader network of circulating medicine, including medicine used for poison oracles. The medicinal *maji* mobilized the rich set of networks, expectations, and obligations established through the widespread use of oracles. Broad regional acceptance of poison oracles resulted in a shared conception of medicine and healers among the Makonde and throughout southern Tanganyika. Those who distributed the *maji* expanded on the forms of expertise and styles of treatment that were central to the oracles in order to organize a disparate array of groups across large territories.

The *mwavi* poison ordeal most likely entered the territory from central Africa and spread throughout the southern two-thirds of Tanganyika in the nineteenth century.[7] Over time, as colonialism, the slave trade, shifting allegiances among indigenous groups, and the ivory trade (among other things) created new social divisions, witchcraft as well as treatments to eliminate it and protect people from it changed. Iliffe (1979) suggests that the use of *mwavi* to evaluate the innocence or guilt of those accused of *uchawi* may be the "chief innovation" in efforts to control witchcraft at this time (82). The oral histories Wembah-Rashid (1974, 1975, 1976) collected in the early 1970s confirm that people in southern Tanzania remembered the *mwavi* poison ordeal as one way to determine responsibility in the face of serious allegations such as those concerning witchcraft, theft, and adultery. He explains that a specialist would grind up the bark of a *mwavi* tree (*Erythrophloem guiniense*) and mix it with water (Wembah-Rashid 1974). A person accused of being a thief, adulterer, or *mchawi* (a witch or sorcerer; pl. *wachawi*) would be required to drink the solution. First, the accused would be forced to announce the consequences of the solution: if he was guilty as accused, then he would be affected by the drink, and if he was not guilty, he would not be affected. While standing in the midst of the community he was thought to have offended with his misdeed, the accused would then drink the *mwavi* solution. If he became intoxicated and incoherent after drinking it, then he was considered guilty. If the accused remained calm and unaffected, then the "healer" (*mganga*) declared that the accused was not an adulterer, a thief, or a *mchawi*. In some cases and in some places, a chicken was used to represent the person accused. The accused would be declared guilty if the chicken died as a result of ingesting the *mwavi* and would be declared not guilty if the chicken lived. The ordeal was never a singular institution, however. Even as *mwavi* gained popularity in southern Tanganyika, other ordeals continued to be used, including giving the accused a medicinal porridge to drink, demanding that she pick a ring from the bottom of a pot of boiling water, or forcing her to handle a red-hot iron (Wembah-Rashid 1974, 15). The meanings of these ordeals were not in all cases simply evidentiary. Chanock (1998), drawing on a 1969 essay by Vansina on the Bushong, noted that the aim of the ordeal was "to 'eliminate evil and death', i.e. to struggle against witchcraft itself, and the ordeal is in essence a ritual in this struggle between good and evil in the community, and not simply a sort of judicial procedure" (86). Medicinal *maji* drew on such understandings of medicine as a medium through which serious wrongdoings could be identified and managed.[8]

Furthermore, widespread familiarity with these oracles, including the *mwavi* ordeal, set the context for the circulation of the medicinal water that coordinated the Maji Maji Rebellion. Although the Germans cracked down severely on the use of poison oracles early in their administration, the *hongo* were able to rely on both the social-material networks and the widespread understanding of the symbolism of poison oracles to obligate masses of diverse people to consume their *maji*. By linking their bullet-melting treatment to witchcraft, the *hongo* compelled people to accept his medicine and the resulting rebellion. One district officer reported how the *hongo* instructed those who received his medicine:

> No white magic or witchcraft was to be performed, no charms or medicines of any kind must be kept in their houses but all [must be] destroyed by fire.[9]

Persons who refused medicine to prevent witchcraft or left town when a healer arrived to identify witches in the area were sometimes accused of taking these actions because they were guilty of using witchcraft. By forbidding the use of witchcraft (at least in some places) as part of the practice of distributing his *maji*, the *hongo* suggested that anyone who refused to accept his treatment might invite suspicion of witchcraft on himself or herself. As one person in the Southern Highlands explained:

> When the *mwavi* expert arrived at some headman's, he was obliged to send people thought to be witches to go to take the medicine. Very often the medicine was very effective. The witches died and those who were not witches survived. For this reason, when Hongo's medicine came and was distributed, it was difficult for people to refuse it.[10]

The medicinal water of the Maji Maji Rebellion, capable of protecting warriors against bullets, became compulsory because of its relationship with medicine that rooted out *wachawi* (those who conducted *uchawi* or those who used medicine to harm or to bring suffering and death; sing. *mchawi*).

After the Maji Maji Rebellion, controlling *uchawi*, or more broadly controlling evil by poison ordeal became a riskier endeavor due to the increased German presence in southern Tanganyika and the greater attention German officials paid to the workings of medicine. The German administration's harsh punishment of those accused of being witches and those who administered poison ordeals to detect witches compelled people in the region to search for other ways of dealing with these social problems. Iliffe (1979) sees the emergence of witchcraft eradication movements as a response to the German administration's violence against those accused of being *wachawi* and those who administered poison ordeals. Eradication movements simultaneously offered a way to manage the problem of people using medicine with the explicit desire to harm others and avoided reprisals from colonialist administrators.[11]

Rather than identifying those doing harm, eradication movements protected all of the potential victims. Leaders in various eradication movements claimed that their medicine worked by making whole populations invulnerable to *uchawi*. The medicine of the witchcraft eradicator not only protected individuals against attacks of witchcraft but also served as a disciplining technology. Eradication experts claimed that anyone who took protective medicine without first giving up his or her practice of *uchawi* would die. Ranger observed that witchcraft eradication movements resembled some aspects of the circulation of the medicine that had been key to the Maji Maji Rebellion.[12] Notably, both Maji Maji and the eradication movements involved experts who moved from village to village in a region, demanding that people bring all implements and medicine of witchcraft to a central location to be destroyed. Thus, while *hongo* offered villagers medicine to make them invincible to colonial bullets, eradication experts offered villagers medicine to make them invincible to *uchawi*.

The first recorded witchcraft eradication movement in Tanganyika took place in the northeast, the rural area under the strictest German control, during the period 1906 to 1910 (overlapping with the end of the Maji Maji Rebellion in the south). After Maji Maji, numerous witchcraft eradication movements also sprang up in southern Tanganyika. In the southeast, the most influential movement was called Ngoja, after the famous eradicator Ngoja bin Kimeta. This specialist and his disciples used medicine to transform *wachawi* and protect others against attacks. Ngoja's campaign drew explicitly on beliefs surrounding the Bokero water cult, which had initiated the Maji Maji Rebellion, as well as on Islamic forms and rituals (Iliffe 1979, 367). Witchcraft eradicators and their medicine became increasingly important targets of colonial intervention because officials feared that the eradicators could organize another rebellion like the Maji Maji uprising. Colonial administrators interpreted the fact that the eradication movements drew on idioms that resonated with Maji Maji as evidence of the reality of this threat.

First German and later British officers believed that other *waganga* (or healers) who mobilized village after village in a region were more threatening to the administration—and therefore more important to control—than "witches" who mobilized forces against an individual person, family group, or community. Colonial administrators saw such medicine as political because it threatened the success of colonial governance. Yet the Germans failed, as did the British after them, to realize that the social life of medicine among the people in the southern part of their territory rested on its explicit role in controlling those who threatened the life of individuals and the well-being of communities; that is, medicine's role in eliminating evil. This misunderstanding generated the productive confusion that led to the making of witchcraft.

The Magic of Making Witchcraft

At the end of World War I, agreements made between the Belgians, Portuguese, South Africans, Americans, and British at the Paris Peace Conference of 1919 brought the administration of Tanganyika under official control of the British Empire. Immediately after the British acquired the territory from the Germans, large movements to eradicate witchcraft attracted their attention. The British distributed the first circulars concerning "witchcraft" in the colony that same year. By 1922, British policy had evolved into An Ordinance to Provide for the Punishment of Persons Practicing or Making Use of So Called Witchcraft.

British officers in Tanganyika defined "witchcraft" as a legal category of offense in response to the witchcraft eradication campaigns. They designed the 1922 ordinance to prevent another Maji Maji rebellion by separating medicine that could coordinate resistance against British colonial rule from medicine that was

considered benign or even useful. The British did not see all witchcraft eradication campaigns as threatening. While recognizing that the mass administration
of medicine to eradicate witchcraft could be a means of organizing against the
government, some colonial officials believed that this process could also be a
means of managing Africans' fear of witchcraft. At times, the British viewed
witchcraft eradication campaigns as a way of limiting the agitation that *uchawi*
created among credulous natives. They hoped that allowing, even fostering, the
expansion of select eradication efforts would prevent problematic levels of fraud
and violence (Larson 1976).[13] In strategically elaborating the 1922 ordinance over
time, British officers sought to create a legal tool that was both subtle enough
and strong enough to help them suppress healing practices that were threatening
to the colonial administration while supporting those that were helpful to the
colonial administration.

The "witchcraft" that the British prohibited was not immediately or easily
identifiable in colonial Tanganyika. In his work on the historical roots of contemporary witchcraft in Tanzania, Mesaki (1993) argues that the differences
between "European witchcraft" and "African witchcraft" made it difficult for the
British to prosecute witches. He situates these differences in the history of the
relationship of witchcraft in Europe to the church. Witchcraft was constituted
as an object of bureaucratic control within the legal machinery that drew the
church into the affairs of European states of the seventeenth century (85). He is
correct that in Tanganyika, three centuries later, this specific condition did not
exist. Rather, the British colonialists confronted the social, material, political,
and ethical machinery of *uchawi,* the Kiswahili term that Mesaki translates as
"African witchcraft." He argues that the most notable differences between "European witchcraft" and "African witchcraft" were that the latter neither implicated
devils or demons nor required prayer or worship. Rather, "African witchcraft"
involved mobilizing specialized knowledge in an effort to cause harm to others and did not include the concepts of "spirits" or "religion."[14] Chanock (1998)
adds an important addendum, noting that the imperial policies on witchcraft
in Anglophone Africa drew on British statutes that had stopped the conviction
of witches for cavorting with Christian demons and instead sought to punish
people for pretending to be witches (94). The witchcraft ordinances imposed
by colonial law sought to construct a secular category of witchcraft. However,
uchawi was neither Christian nor secular, in the sense that this later word has
in the context of European history.

Below I build on arguments that "European witchcraft" was a colonial category;
it was embedded in British history and translated into Tanganyika through colonial administrative practices, bringing with it a complex mixture of religious
and secular ideas from Europe. However, I question ahistorical assertions of
equivalence between *uchawi* and witchcraft. Translations of *uchawi* as witchcraft

(even if or perhaps especially when such "witchcraft" was qualified as specifically African) were central to the process of constituting a legally meaningful category of "witchcraft" in colonial Tanganyika. It is this work to translate *uchawi* and its counterpart *uganga* that requires consideration. These translations established "witchcraft" as a new category and transformed the existing complex of healing and harming. The side effects of colonial efforts to discern and codify witchcraft—the distortions, losses, new connections, and new meanings that were enacted by translations of *uchawi* as witchcraft—had a profound effect on which practices were to continue to be considered healing and which materials were to continue to be considered medicine.

The magic of British efforts to construct a category called "witchcraft" was that it simultaneously remade healing. In their efforts to interpret and enforce the 1928 Witchcraft Ordinance, British officials strove to define the relationship between colonial notions of witchcraft and medicine and Kiswahili concepts of harming and healing. In their struggle to draw the analogy that *uganga* was to modern medicine as *uchawi* was to European witchcraft, colonial officials fragmented the contours of local categories of practice.[15]

Initially, district-level officers bore the brunt of the work of mediating the encounter between European witchcraft and the matrix of practices known as *uchawi* and *uganga* in Tanganyika. As they took up their posts, these new colonial officials found that the 1922 Witchcraft Ordinance did not provide them with an effective administrative tool to control disruptions attributed to witchcraft. Some called for a stronger law (Liebenow 1971, 61). In response to such concerns, Donald Cameron personally took up the task of drafting a revision of the 1922 ordinance when he became governor of the Tanganyika Territory in 1924. Four years later, the Legislative Council passed a new ordinance that expanded the definition of "witchcraft." Acts of "sorcery, enchantment, bewitching, or the *purported* exercise of any occult power, or the *purported* possession of any occult knowledge" (italics mine) remained an offense. In addition however, under this legislation, witchcraft included not only acts "with the intent to cause injury or misfortune" but also so-called occult knowledge and practices that were not intended to cause injury or misfortune.[16] This revision forced the issue of healing onto center stage, where it has remained for more than seventy-five years.

The definition of witchcraft in this later version of the law pivoted on the use of hidden knowledge or references to special powers. Reliance on the term "occult" facilitated the conflation of practices of *uchawi* and (some) practices of *uganga*. People committed offenses when they called on objects and entities that were unrecognizable and unknowable for colonialists. The law had nothing to do with assessments of the effects of such practices. It created a space for the category of "witchcraft" by focusing on activities that could be examined by colonial officials. Efforts to sort through the confusion that resulted from the British administration's conflation of practices that were intended to harm with practices that were intended to protect people from harm (referred to by many Africans as healing) resulted in an important renegotiation of categories of activity.

The administration's reliance on terms such as "occult" and "superstition" made it possible for colonial officials to include a broad range of African practices under the single rubric of "witchcraft." This legislation thus conflated practices of *uchawi* with some practices of *uganga* that called on entities and agents that colonial administrators did not recognize as legitimate. The definition of healing and the authority of healers were at stake in the colonial officials' articulations of witchcraft.

British officers in the field immediately found it difficult to implement the new ordinance and its distinctly colonial category of witchcraft. After only a few years of attempting to enforce this legislation, the colonial government began considering how to amend the ordinance again. In 1934, the British secretariat sent a letter to selected officers requesting that they "submit their opinion as to how the present law meets its objective and how it should, if necessary, be amended."[17] The responses from these officers provide some insight into how colonial officers understood the uniquely European term "witchcraft."

Each of the respondents grappled with the distinction between the two local categories of *uchawi* and *uganga*. The candid and frustrated response of one colonial official succinctly captures the awkwardness of defining (much less imposing) this new category of witchcraft in Tanganyika.

> But to give a definition of witchcraft which would fit in with native thought is impossible as two separate and very distinct aspects of native belief are involved—"uganga" (the art of the known native doctor and general spiritual benefactor to the community) and "uchawi" (the cult of the unknown and feared ghostly enemy of the community). These two terms are sometimes translated as white and black witchcraft or benign and malignant witchcraft. These latter terms give the idea of a connection between these functions which does not exist. The two are mutually antagonistic and "uganga" might be translated as physical, spiritual and mental healing while "uchawi" is a cult of bringing evil on people by willful and occult means.[18]

Translations of *uganga* and *uchawi* as a good and a bad version of the same thing—benevolent witchcraft and malevolent witchcraft—created a false similarity. This conflation constructed witchcraft as an unwieldy, administratively clumsy category of practice in the field. The official argued that greater precision was necessary. A more practical witchcraft ordinance needed to better articulate the distinctions between *uganga* and *uchawi*.

Other officials agreed that the difficulty in interpreting and enforcing the Witchcraft Ordinance lay in the fact that the colonial category of witchcraft did not map neatly or easily onto any previously existing category or categories in the territory. In an attempt to better translate the relationship between *uganga* and *uchawi*, Kitching, a provincial commissioner, mobilized another dualism.

> "Uchawi" is the black art, whatever the intentions of the person exercising it. "Uganga" is a science, practiced no doubt by many charlatans and not always with benign intentions but nonetheless a science.[19]

He distinguished these Kiswahili categories of practice through an analogy to English categories of practice: *uchawi* is to art as *uganga* is to science. Kitching suggested that this comparison would enable the colonial government to interpret the Witchcraft Ordinance more strategically. Unlike his colleague quoted above, Kitching did not aim for absolute distinctions between the categories of *uganga* and *uchawi*. Rather, he offered an analogy that would figure the boundary between *uganga* and *uchawi* as a partial and shifting line. He suggested that such flexibility would enable the colonial government to separate practices that they found beneficial or harmless from those that they found problematic by identifying the former as "scientific" and the latter as "black art." An ordinance that did this would, he claimed, still

> never have any value as a piece of social legislation or assist in any way towards the eradication of the beliefs and fears which haunt and obsess the minds of natives and oppress their lives as nothing else does. . . . [However,] a "Witchcraft" Ordinance intended to be brought into use only when the maintenance of peace order and good government are at stake is a different matter and is, I think, an administrative necessity.

Kitching argued that a witchcraft ordinance would be useful to administrators insofar as it could be directed at and used to control practitioners of *uganga*. For Kitching, the Witchcraft Ordinance did not need to be amended as much as its purpose needed to be reconceived. He saw this legislation as an administrative measure to prevent disorder when "from time to time a Mganga emerges who is believed to have discovered a panacea for 'Uchawi' and conditions of great social excitement and even unrest may then arise in native areas." At such times, "Intervention becomes necessary and if it is to be efficacious, must be downright and prompt."[20] In Kitching's view, because European witchcraft failed to map neatly over *uchawi*, the colonial government needed to use the Witchcraft Ordinance to constrain the activities of healers whose efforts to organize villages, communities, or regions made colonial officers uneasy.

Kitching's strategy offered a novel interpretation of the spaces that awkward and slightly vague translations could open up for imperial power. He recommended exploiting new distinctions between practices of *uganga* and practices of *uchawi* in order to criminalize some of the practices central to African concepts of healing. Indeed, colonial interpretations of this law expressed little concern with the harm done to individuals who were attacked by *uchawi*, instead expressing more concern with the threat to the colonial state by those who organized events inciting African subjects. The primacy of British officials' concern with the peace and security of the state led to a focus in the law on the dangers of secrecy and the occult.

The Occult and the Real

The term "occult" not only connotes what is hidden from view, it also connotes forces "not apprehensible by the mind."[21] Therefore, when colonial law came to define witchcraft through the occult, *uchawi* came to refer to more than "special knowledge" that was used in networks unknown to the colonists. Because the British did not believe in *uchawi*, they articulated it not only as clandestine practice but also as unknowable and therefore unreal. Witchcraft was the practice of making false claims to be able to manipulate evil forces of jealousy, greed, and hatred through herbs and other treatments. The British deemed anyone claiming the power of a witch to be a fraud and a charlatan.[22] Under British colonial law, the secretive practices of those claiming to be witches did not conceal work with actual "hidden forces."[23] Rather they played on superstitions. The work of the law, then, was not to reveal or uncover the substances and mechanisms through which *uchawi* worked. The law deemed the very existence of *uchawi* impossible. Witchcraft emerged in British law as the manipulation of individuals and groups through purported and false claims to access to "occult powers."

The prosecutable offense in the 1928 version of the Witchcraft Ordinance was shaped by what counted as evidence in the eyes of the court. "Witchcraft" in Tanganyika, as opposed to *uchawi*, came into being through specific colonial ways of seeing. Evidence that could be seen in a court of law became the legal evidence that traced an individual's association with witchcraft. Colonial courts did not accept ways of being and knowing that were not transparent under the British gaze. For example, the results of divination could not be submitted in colonial courts as evidence that supported conviction or pleas of innocence.[24] Similarly, the results of witch-finding efforts were inadmissible in court as legal evidence. The limitations on the types of legal evidence that were admissible in court made it difficult for colonial officials in Tanganyika to prosecute "witches" because witches acted in ways that were not intelligible to the scientific or judicial procedures of the officials administering the colony. However, *waganga* worked in the presence of a community of people when they were curing a person of the effects of witchcraft, rehabilitating a witch, or protecting a community against the effects of witchcraft.[25] As a result, authorities could collect the kinds of evidence called for in a court of law against healers: eyewitness accounts of the movement of individual healers, healers' use of visible artifacts, healers' collection of money or property, and the occasional visual evidence of bodily harm that healers had purportedly inflicted.

Unlike healers who knew how to locate sources of and protect against *uchawi*, colonial officials fought representations of witchcraft. In denying that *uchawi* existed in the physical natural world and defining witchcraft as fraud,[26] they relegated the battle to the domain of ideology and belief.[27] In 1944, the district commissioner of Newala argued that "there can hardly be a Government Officer or enlightened Native Authority who would not take every opportunity which presented itself . . . to impress on the natives the futility and perversity of a belief in witchcraft."[28] By making "belief" the central issue in combating witchcraft, the government declared insubstantial the threats Africans referred to as *uchawi*.[29] The Witchcraft Ordinance cast the substance of threats as a political question and challenged the rights of people to protect themselves from forms of being not recognized in British colonial courts of law.

The 1928 version of the Witchcraft Ordinance made the possession of "instruments of witchcraft" and the activities of certain specialists illegal. Tools, amulets, horns, and clothing could be seen and seized. These "instruments" became legal evidence that the person who owned them claimed to be a witch and perhaps was guilty of assaults such as poisoning, beating, and creating psychological stress. Ironically, criminalizing the instruments of witchcraft made the law more similar to the witch-finding and witch eradication techniques that were practiced in various East African communities. The difference, of course, was that for the *mganga* seeking to eradicate *uchawi*, the instruments collected provided evidence of *uchawi* (i.e., use of medicine to inflict harm or death), whereas for the government they provided evidence of the fraudulent claims to access to occult knowledge or to use occult powers.

The Witchcraft Ordinance and the forms of evidence that it legitimized served as a mechanism through which the government could control forms of therapeutic knowledge that it deemed threatening.[30] In the process, it catalyzed a shift in the types of ontological claims that grounded officially sanctioned notions of medicine and efficacy in East Africa. As *uchawi* became a rational impossibility under colonial law, *uganga* (healing) was divided into the categories of "witchcraft" and "native medicine." The former delineated practices to be controlled through bureaucratic prohibitions, and the latter delineated practices to be managed through scientific discipline. In addition, the legal distinctions between witchcraft and native medicine relegated the effects of practices that were undesirable to the colonial government to the realm of belief and made the effects of practices that might be profitable to the government the domain of empirical evidence and knowledge.

Native Medicine and Colonial Science

Although the British did not articulate the category of "native medicine" as carefully or extensively as they did the term "witchcraft," they did study the plant-based medicine used in the territory. The scope of this research illustrates which qualities colonialists demanded of substances they were willing to consider medicine and which transformations they felt constituted healing. Intrinsic to the changing conceptions of medicine and healing this research motivated was a change in how the British conceived of healers and which roles they saw as legitimate for healers.

The oldest and most prominent center for the investigation of medicinal plants in the territory was the East African Agricultural Research Station in Amani, northeastern Tanganyika. This facility dates back to 1902, when the German government established an environmental research station at Amani. British forces took over this station in 1916, and the first English director assumed control in January 1920. Shortly thereafter, the British Department of Agriculture assumed responsibility for the administration of the Amani research station. Little research was conducted, however, until 1927. At that time, under the leadership of a new director, the Amani research station acquired a range of staff, including an entomologist, a plant pathologist, a soil scientist, a biochemist, a plant physiologist, a plant geneticist, and a systematic botanist. The botanist who began work at Amani in April 1928, P. J. Greenway, developed a strong interest in medicinal plants. Although he focused most intently on improving agricultural production in the territory, Greenway's knowledge of locally available plants and their uses evolved over the decades that he worked at the station. He eventually published several editions of a Kiswahili-English dictionary of plant species as well as lists of plants in numerous local vernacular languages.

As Greenway developed some knowledge of local languages and was able to talk with residents about plants, his awareness of their indigenous uses grew. In 1932–1933 he identified plants that local fisherman used to poison fish and hypothesized that they might be useful as insecticides. In 1933–1934 he identified plants he suspected were poisonous to humans and were used in cases of criminal poisoning. In the 1934–1935 annual report of the research station at Amani, he noted that some of the medicinal plants natives used might be useful in European pharmacology. In 1935–1936 he worked with the Medical Department of Tanganyika to collect and investigate "native medicinal and poisonous plants of the territory." By 1937, he had published two papers related to native medicine. The first concerned fish poison and the second was an article in *The East African Medical Journal* entitled "Artificially Induced Lactation in Humans" (February 1937).[31]

Although scientific research on medicinal plants remained marginal to the central concerns of colonial administrators, native medicine did begin to receive a little political attention in the mid-1930s. In 1933, the chief secretary of the colonial government wrote to the director of medical and sanitary services of the colonial government's medical department that herbal practices to cure things that the colonial government recognized as physical ailments were to be considered outside the prosecutable categories of witchcraft. He wrote that:

> Generally speaking, it is not considered that there is any political or social significance attached to the activities of these native herbalists who, it is thought, are quite distinct from practitioners of witchcraft, though they may take some advantage of the superstitious nature of their patients in a harmless way.[32]

The category of native medicine emerged as a space that was shielded from certain kinds of prosecution and colonial violence. It allowed for the existence of therapeutic practices that were not threatening to the state. The category of native medicine held open the possibility that some practices of *uganga* exceeded categorization as witchcraft.

Policy discussions about native medicine focused on the pharmaceutical potential of plant, animal, and mineral substances. Therapies suitable for scientific investigations worked on individual bodies, not on communities or rain clouds. They were typically curative. They neither sought retribution nor implicated others. British officials judged their efficacy in terms of biological and chemical agents.

This narrowed, materialist view of medicine marginalized the position of the healer. While healers served as informants to individual scientists and colonial officers, the government explicitly refused to acknowledge them, much less organize them. The chief secretary of the colonial government argued against the suggestion that such practitioners be registered because "registration would, in fact, accord them Government recognition and greatly strengthen their position."[33] The government agreed only to turn a blind eye to practices that it deemed of no "social or political significance" (or, as illustrated by the colonial administration's tentative support for some witchcraft eradication movements, those deemed potentially beneficial to it). Government officials assumed that modernization would slowly discredit treatments that did not conform to notions of scientific efficacy.[34]

Through the separation of medicine into practices that were a political threat to the colonial administration and those that were not, healers explored the possibility of (re)negotiating their legitimacy. For example, in 1933, one healer who was having trouble with some members of his local Native Authority wrote to the provincial commissioner asking for a letter that would "give him the authority" to continue his therapeutic practice. The awkward position of the provincial commissioner was eased only slightly by the advice of his higher-ups, who suggested to him "that the applicant should be informed that no license is required for the practice of native medicines, nor does Government interfere with such practices unless the native practitioner breaks the law. Should he break the law, he will be liable to prosecution."[35] At this initial point, the colonial administration was unprepared to respond to the creative and productive efforts of healers to use the category of "native medicine" to shape new positions.

By the late 1930s, Lord Hailey's *An African Survey* (1938) had catalyzed a broader policy discussion of "native medicine." In it he suggested:

> Not all those who practice native medicine in Africa can be dismissed as witch doctors; many are much respected, and it is indeed possible that a study of the herbs used by some of them might add to the list of remedies, such as quinine, which the pharmacopiea owes to primitive medicinal practices. (1198)

This excerpt was circulated during the Conference of Directors of Medical Services held in Nairobi in July 1939. The proceedings from the conference stated:

> The Conference found itself in full agreement with Lord Hailey's views . . . and desired that it be recorded that so far as the study of native medicines was concerned the East African Medical Departments had been working along the lines indicated by Lord Hailey for a long time past, and that the subject was still on the East African Research Program.[36]

In addition to the continued work at the Amani research station and herbarium, analytical chemists on staff in the colonial government's medical department began examining plants and medicine sent to them by officers and researchers in the field. They attempted to identify known chemical compounds in these (mostly) botanical substances. Colonial officers on and off the continent considered native medicine useful insofar as it provided insight into new modern medicine—or, in Greenway's words, insofar as it was of "interest to European pharmacology." Yet colonialists often reacted to this interest with skepticism. As the acting director of medical services in Zanzibar stated: "It is possible that a study of native medicines may produce some material of value. [But] in my own experience I have never encountered any which were of any practical value and many were definitely harmful."[37]

At the same time that the Witchcraft Ordinance worked to re-categorize acts of *uchawi* and certain acts of "occult" healing, "native medicine" came to be distinguished as a separate category of knowledge and practice. Policy debates as well as botanical and chemical investigations brought this category into existence. Whereas witchcraft was conceived of as a problem of social control, native medicine was conceived of as a problem of natural resources. Whereas solutions to the problem of witchcraft were sought through law, solutions to the problem of native medicine were sought through science. Native medicine emerged as witchcraft's Other.

The Legacy of Colonial Ontologies

The British recognized the political nature of medicine early on. Yet while they worried about the power of some medicine to organize local resistance to colonialization, they demonstrated little concern for or understanding of the ontologies at work in African therapies. For this reason, colonial efforts to map "witchcraft" and "native medicine" over existing representations of harming and healing generated confusion among government officials. Legal definitions intervened in and exceeded local categories of practice. In the end, the awkwardness of colonial translations and the murkiness that they cultivated created the space for establishing a legal category of "witchcraft" that targeted healers. Kitching's interpretation of the Witchcraft Ordinance as a useful intervention in practices that sought to eliminate witchcraft took hold. Practices that Africans once evoked in the name of justice, safety, and healing became punishable under law.

The designation of some practices as "witchcraft" and their distinction from "native medicine" articulates a historical shift in the substance of dangers. Because the British government did not believe in witches or witchcraft by the early twentieth century, the evidence accepted in colonial courts and laboratories did not allow for the revelation of actual *uchawi* in African territories. It could be used only to prosecute those making false claims to the reality and use of *uchawi*. The Witchcraft Ordinance and policies on native medicines cast talk of entities that could not be seen by a British judge or a scientist as claims to "occult powers." The framing of witchcraft as pretense, deception, and fraud denied the existence of those things invisible to law and science and challenged the right of people to protect themselves from those things that escaped the colonial gaze. The colonial administration preserved its interest by invoking the authority of the types of visibility that could be apprehended in the courtroom and the laboratory.

Policy debates about the definition of witchcraft and its distinction from *uganga* not only shaped which practices came to be considered healing but also transformed the figure of the healer. The healer became suspect as knowledge of witchcraft, including that which facilitated its eradication, became prosecutable as fraud. Yet at the same time, the healer became redundant as medicine became the focus of scientific investigations. Plant, mineral, and animal substances could travel more easily and productively between the African territories and Britain than African healers could. Colonial scientists collected medicinal plants in regional herbariums and grew them in metropolitan botanical gardens. The institutionalization of the colonial-era division of witchcraft and native medicine is critical to understanding the postcolonial development of traditional medicine with its focus on medicinal substances and its marginalization of healers from modern forms of bureaucratic governance.

In 1974, Wembah-Rashid, a Tanzanian intellectual who worked with the National Museum of Tanzania to record indigenous practices and ideas (especially in the southeastern regions of the new nation-state), attempted to clarify "witchcraft" from an African perspective. He defined witchcraft as that which does bodily harm to another person or destroys another's property.[38] In a 1974 paper on "traditional religions," Wembah-Rashid categorized three different types of witchcraft: witchcraft that used organic substances, witchcraft that manipulated body parts, and witchcraft that materialized hatred or jealousy. Conducting his research soon after independence and in the context of the strong socialist rhetoric of the first administration, Wembah-Rashid argued against colonial categories of practice and thought. He reasserted more subtle articulations of *uchawi* (medicine used to harm, to bring death) and clarified its distinction from *uganga* (medicine used to heal, to support life) in the face of the confusion inaugurated by colonial legislation against witchcraft. Wembah-Rashid did not consider, however, that delineating some practices of *uganga* as witchcraft under British colonial law was more than simply a poor understanding of an African phenomenon propelled by imperialism; it was a technique of governance. Colonialism conjured "witchcraft" in an effort to refigure African therapeutics into realms of practice that could be disciplined by law and science. Colonial notions of witchcraft situated questions of existence in courts and laboratories. It rejected the reality of entities that the eye of the state could not perceive, thus denying certain forms of being the right to exist.

3

Making Tanzanian Traditional Medicine

In 1968, a research officer in the Tanzanian Ministry of Agriculture and Cooperative Development attended the first Symposium on African Medicinal Plants, which was held in Senegal. Upon his return, he claimed for scientists the role of transforming "the old or indigenous ways of curing diseases" into "new" forms of modern treatment (see first epigraph to Part 1). His argument for transforming "primitive medicaments" through scientific investigation reflected the broader recommendations crafted during this gathering of the Organization of African Unity (OAU) member states (Kasembe 1968). The symposium marked a shift in emphasis from the colonial prohibition against some healing practices to the funding, research, and legalization of traditional medicine in postcolonial Africa.

The ontological implications of the colonial separation of belief and knowledge, spirit and substance, and harming and healing have structured the postcolonial search for the scientific truth of traditional medicine. The newly independent Tanzanian government focused its attention on the commodification of plant, animal, and mineral products that might enable Africa to better position itself in a variety of global relationships. The idea that science might convert plant, animal, and mineral products into desperately needed pharmaceuticals found purchase in the highest levels of the first post-independence administration, led by Julius Nyerere. Stocking the new network of clinics and dispensaries that comprised the fledgling national health care service with pharmaceutical drugs ate up a significant proportion of the nation's hard currency reserves. Tanzanian leaders hoped that scientific research into medicinal plants would offer a solution to the economic challenges cash-strapped African countries faced. By recasting plant material as a resource for an indigenous pharmaceutical industry, traditional medicine held out the promise of greater economic independence.

Over time, the ideological and epistemological projects that gave life to this postcolonial (and pan-Africanist) category of traditional medicine have shifted. In the past twenty-five years, economic liberalization and the pressures of global capitalism have transformed earlier dreams of a self-reliant Tanzania that could exploit its natural and cultural resources in the service of a socialist state's commitment to health care for all. Today, talk about traditional medicine is animated by a spirit of entrepreneurship, a desire to break into the global market for herbal medicine, and the demands of the elite. Even as the politics of modern traditional medicine changes, however, scientists and bureaucrats confront the asymmetries that colonial definitions of medicine and healing originally created. Relations between science and governance continue to shape traditional medicine and the bodies and threats to which traditional healers attend. Furthermore, contemporary perspectives on traditional medicine's role in development call into being new forms of expertise.

The Socialist Roots of Traditional Medicine

The consolidation and translation of healing practices into a state-supported and state-monitored Tanzanian traditional medicine was, from the beginning, a product of many international ties and commitments. As the 1968 Symposium on African Medicinal Plants exemplifies, interest in herbal medicine became one arena for cooperation among newly independent African states. Pan-Africanism both fueled and was fueled by interest in the development of herbal treatments in Africa. Funding and expertise to carry out these regionally shared desires, however, tended to come from places outside Africa. Particularly important to the shaping of the postcolonial category of traditional medicine in Tanzania was the country's multiple connections to China[1] (see Figure 3.1).[2]

China's influence and the institutionalization of traditional medicine grew in the context of Tanzania's commitment to non-aligned socialism. In 1967, six years after Tanganyika gained independence from Great Britain and three years after Tanganyika joined with the islands of Zanzibar to form the United Republic of Tanzania, the government outlined its pursuit of self-reliance through the Arusha Declaration, an avowedly socialist construction of policies. Making a concerted effort to avoid the more problematic entanglements of Cold War politics, Tanzania adopted a policy of non-alignment (Gordon 1984). The new nation quickly became a model of socialist development (e.g., Barkan 1984). These commitments to socialism and non-alignment not only affected economic policy but also shaped the growth of medical services. Tanzanian officials studied socialist medical systems elsewhere and were influenced by their observations. In 1967, a delegation to China was particularly impressed (Iliffe 1998). One member of this delegation was quoted as saying:

> We were much impressed by the stage of development of health services, which have been revolutionized and transformed by the new China. In particular the way in which the doctors have to go to the country to serve the broad masses.... The combination of traditional and modern medicine in order to find out what is good in the traditional methods instead of rejecting them is also something which we might follow.[3]

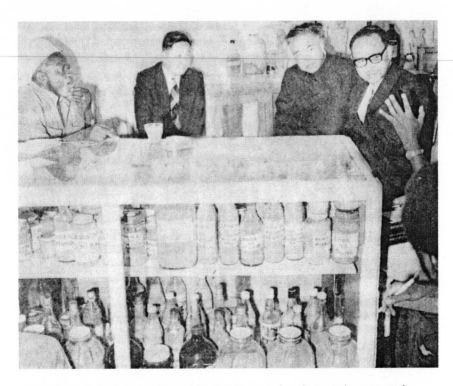

Figure 3.1. A Tanzanian traditional healer sitting in his clinic with a group of doctors of Traditional Chinese Medicine, who are on a research trip to study "local medicine." Photo from the Tanzanian *Sunday News*, February 19, 1984, p. 8. *Reprinted by permission of Sunday News Tanzania and Daily News Tanzania.*

China's effort to integrate Chinese medicine and biomedicine into a simplified therapeutic repertoire for minimally trained "barefoot doctors" came to serve as a model for many Tanzanian officials of a primary health care system that emphasized reaching a large rural population. Moreover, a number of Tanzanians studied biomedicine in China.[4] An unintended effect of this medical training was that while living in China, Tanzanian students of "modern" medicine were exposed to a national system of nonbiomedical therapeutics that operated alongside and within the structure of biomedical practice. Today, some of these practitioners are leading figures in efforts to institutionalize traditional medicine in Tanzania.[5] One particularly central example is Sabina Mnaliwa, who managed the earliest phases of the institutionalization of traditional medicine in the Ministry of Health. She also spent many years working for the formal legalization of traditional medicine.

In the early 1970s, after completing secondary school, Sabina Mnaliwa received a government scholarship for medical training in China. This scholarship carried her through five years of training in China, from 1973 to 1978. After the first year, which was devoted solely to learning Mandarin Chinese, she completed coursework in the basic sciences and clinical practice. Because in China contemporary Chinese medicine is integrated into "Western" medicine, Mnaliwa's biomedical training program included a three-month course in Chinese medicine and visits to hospitals of Chinese medicine. In 1978, upon completion of this five-year course of study, Mnaliwa and her fellow Tanzanian students were granted certificates in medicine and returned to Tanzania. After a two-year clinical internship, Mnaliwa started work as a general practitioner at the Muhimbili University hospital in Dar es Salaam, the primary teaching hospital in the country.

In the mid-1980s, government officials grew concerned that the certificates of medicine that Mnaliwa and her colleagues had received in China were not equivalent to medical degrees. In 1988, they passed a resolution declaring that the five-year training program in China was not a full MD training program. To rectify the discrepancy, the Tanzanian and Chinese governments established a year-long course in China to upgrade individuals who had completed the Chinese certification program in medicine. For personal reasons, however, Mnaliwa could not return to China for further studies at that time. The government offered her two alternatives. She could accept a demotion or she could shift to the administrative side of the Ministry of Health and start the first Office of Traditional Medicine. Even now, she remembers the tumult into which this decision threw her: "I felt as if I was being asked to be an 'advocate of the devil.'" She drew this phrase from a book she found at the time entitled *The Advocate of the Devil*. This book seemed to name her worst fears. As she read it "from the first word to the last," she worried that traditional medicine harbored evil and destructive possibilities. Despite her anxiety, in 1989, she chose to head the ministry's traditional medicine program. Her work, she says, "ended up being very different from the things described in [that] book."

The hiring of Mnaliwa and the establishment of the Office of Traditional Medicine in the Ministry of Health was the culmination of two decades of work to define traditional medicine as a resource for development. Between the late 1960s and the early 1980s, while Mnaliwa was studying in China and working at the Muhimbili hospital, the Tanzanian government as well as the international health community were slowly shifting their positions on herbal medicine. Before considering the Office of Traditional Medicine during Mnaliwa's tenures, I turn to transnational efforts to construct traditional medicine as a strategy for Tanzanian self-reliance and for "Third World" development more broadly during the period 1969 to 1989.

Early Efforts to Institutionalize Traditional Medicine

The earliest initiatives to articulate traditional medicine in Tanzania strove to de-lineate a national body of healing practices by systematically collecting accounts of treatments and samples of *materia medica*. In 1969, the chief medical officer of the Tanzanian Ministry of Health issued a circular to all regional medical of-ficers on the mainland that asked them to collect information on the therapies of herbalists in their area, including the drugs they dispensed.[6] In October 1970, the United Nations Economic Commission for Africa (ECA/UNESCO) convened the Regional Symposium on the Utilization of Science and Technology for the Development of Africa in Addis Ababa. Attendees learned, among other things, of the efforts by Tanzanian scientists in the Botany Department at the University of Dar es Salaam to collaborate with traditional healers. In his country report to the ECA/UNESCO meeting, the Tanzanian representative, Dr. Kasembe (who two years earlier had written the report on the first OAU Symposium on African Medicinal Plants) touted such research as an example of the use of science to promote Tanzanian development.[7]

The 1970s also brought the first attempt by the Tanzanian government to orga-nize traditional healers. As it is remembered now, many healers were immediately suspicious when the government asked them to form a professional association.[8] Only a decade after independence, vivid memories of colonial violence against *waganga* continued to shape healers' relationship with the state. In addition, the establishment of a national association with a leadership structure shaped by the government's priorities immediately institutionalized a hierarchical relationship between healers who had previously worked independently of each other. These factors manifested as accusations of mismanagement and fears of witchcraft almost as soon as the National Union of Indigenous Healers was formed under the Ministry of Culture in 1971. As a result, the government banned the union the same year it was formed.[9]

After this failure, the Tanzanian government temporarily abandoned its efforts to organize healers and directed its attention to the investigation of medicine. In 1974, the Institute of Traditional Medicine was established in the Faculty of Medicine at Muhimbili Medical Center in Dar es Salaam. During its first year, the institute launched the initial phase of its research, which entailed interviewing traditional healers and collecting samples of the plant, mineral, and animal substances that the healers used in their treatments. In 1974 and 1975, the researchers at the institute collected 354 medicinal plants. During this time, a Chinese medical team collected samples of over 1,000 herbs being used by traditional healers in Tanzania through the Joint Tanzania and Chinese Project on Traditional Medicine. Both of these formative research projects enlisted healers as informants—that is, as resources for but not as central organizers of the state's emerging category of traditional medicine. The previous failure of the National Union of Indigenous Healers informed the Tanzanian government's resistance to institutionalizing nonscientific forms of expertise within the state's bureaucratic structure.

Scientists in different segments of the medical community defined the potential of local herbal medicine to contribute more formally to health care in Tanzania.[10] In 1975, Ndugu Madati, the government's chief chemist, presented a paper entitled "Modern versus Traditional Medicine" at the tenth annual session of the Medical Association of Tanzania, arguing that "traditional medicine is an indispensable supplement and not a substitute for modern medicine." He claimed that afflictions "particular to women and children, includ[ing] disease[s] of the mind, asthma, diabetes, bone fractures, cardiac disorders, epilepsy, hypertension, ineffective hepatitis, leprosy, osteomyelitis, small pox, snake bites, and yellow fever could well be cured by traditional medicine."[11] Madati envisioned a (gendered) complementarity between traditional and modern medicine in which herbal treatments addressed biomedical diagnoses.

Scientific research shaped the kind of complementarity and crafted the forms of commensurability that the state considered possible and desirable. The director of Tanzania's Traditional Medicine Research Unit, Dr. Peter A. Kitundu, argued that "good traditional medicine and good traditional practices should be researched, recorded and absorbed in the progressive scientific type of medical practice. . . . I can't see any other way."[12] Plant, animal, and mineral substances used in traditional therapeutic practices gained distinction as scientists defined their botanical, chemical, and pharmacological effects. Laboratory science formed the basis of integration. The first traditional medicine experts within the Tanzanian state privileged scientific over nonscientific knowledge and practice. Their career paths embodied this hierarchical relationship between traditional and modern medicine. For example, Kitundu's childhood familiarity with traditional medicine (learned from his uncle, who practiced as a traditional healer) was recast during his ten years of scientific training in the United States, including his investigation of herbal medicine at the Mayo Clinic in Rochester, New York.

The World Health Organization (WHO) capitalized on the mobility of experts such as Kitundu in initiatives to consider how the "progress" of traditional medicine might be incorporated into broader modernization projects. In 1976, in a series of WHO forums, Tanzania and other nations grappled with how to exploit herbal medicine and traditional therapies in the service of regional as well as national development. African representatives "discuss[ed] ways to bring together the advances of modern medicine and traditional African healing methods"[13] and issued a statement "encouraging African governments to recognize the work of traditional healers"[14] during meetings in Brazzaville in February and March. During the World Health Assembly in May, traditional healers became part of the national health care service plans the WHO had recommended. In August, a three-person WHO delegation toured Tanzania to promote traditional medicine, including WHO assistant director-general Dr. Ch'en Wen Chieh; the secretary of the WHO Working Group on Traditional Medicine, Dr. R. Bannerman; and the chief medical officer of the WHO's Drug Policies and Management Division, Dr. H. Nakajima.

In September, the government-owned newspapers in Tanzania, the *Daily News* and *Sunday News,* were enamored with the topic of traditional medicine.[15] The reports they ran of the twenty-sixth meeting of the World Health Organization's Regional Committee for Africa in Kampala focused almost exclusively on the importance of integrating traditional African healing methods into African health services. This coverage apparently surprised even the director of the Institute of Traditional Medicine at Muhimbili. In an interview with the *Daily News,* he noted:

> Most people thought that the Kampala meeting was purely on traditional medicine. May I correct this impression by saying that the Kampala meeting was the 26th WHO Regional Committee for the African Region. Traditional medicine was just one item on the agenda of 17 items discussed. It is understandable and desirable that the Press was very supportive to the cause of traditional medicine.[16]

Later that month, Tanzania demonstrated a commitment to the development of traditional medicine by hosting the Executive Committee of the OAU's Inter-African Committee on Medicinal Plants and Pharmacopeias in Dar es Salaam.

The attention generated by such public efforts stimulated new kinds of research and collaboration. For instance, in a joint effort with other libraries in East Africa, the Medical Library at Muhimbili in Dar es Salaam embarked on a massive project to document all literature pertaining to traditional medicine since 1900.[17] The next year, the deputy director-general of the WHO, Professor T. A. Lambo, "praised Tanzania's seriousness in developing traditional medicine and said WHO would give funds for traditional medicine research" during a visit to Dar es Salaam.[18]

In the late 1970s, the United Nations also began to consider the role of traditional medicine in development. In 1978, the United Nations Industrial Development Organization (UNIDO) held its first international meeting to look into the technical aspects of the manufacture of plant-based drugs in "Third World countries." At the conference, the director-general of the WHO said that the production of indigenous herbal medicine would enable developing countries to break away from "the imperialism of multinational drug companies."[19] A month later, a WHO-UNICEF conference at Alma Ata about primary health care specifically mentioned the role of traditional medicine and practitioners, and recommended that they be incorporated into health care delivery systems. The agreements and resolutions that came out of this meeting were captured in the conference report, which was titled *The Promotion and Development of Traditional Medicine: Report of a WHO Meeting.*[20] By 1980, the World Bank had not only joined in recognizing traditional medicine but had also begun encouraging initiatives to improve "its efficacy, safety, availability, and wider application at low cost."[21] This recognition of traditional medicine as a resource for development was intimately tied to its inclusion in the work of a variety of institutions, including the Tanzanian Ministry of Health, the University of Dar es Salaam, the Organization for African Unity, the United Nations, and the World Health Organization.

The growing advocacy of the international community bolstered national efforts to develop traditional medicine in Tanzania. In January 1979, the National Museum in collaboration with the Institute of Traditional Medicine at Muhimbili and the Embassy of the Federal Republic of Germany held an exhibition on medicinal herbs and the development of traditional medicine in Tanzania. The Tanzanian government through the Ministry of National Culture and Youth also became more actively involved in research about traditional medicine. In November 1979, the ministry organized a week-long seminar for local herbalists in Tanga Region, northeastern Tanzania, to identify herbal medicine. The regional medical officer and various officials of the Ministry of Health from Dar es Salaam as well as thirty herbalists attended this seminar. Each herbalist invited to the seminar was instructed "to come with a list of herbs he applies in curing various diseases."[22] Before the end of the year, the national legislature had passed an act to establish the National Institute for Medical Research. One of the primary functions of the institute, which continues to this day, is "to carry out, and promote the carrying out of research into various aspects of local traditional medical practices for the purpose of facilitating the development and application of herbal medicine."[23]

Support for the investigation of traditional medicine grew from multiple directions. In 1980, the director general of Tanzania's National Scientific Research Council, Professor Hosea Kayumbo, proposed at the Commonwealth Science Council's eleventh biennial meeting in Nairobi, Kenya, that African countries exploit their national resources and use them to produce drugs and other industrial derivatives. African countries unanimously supported Tanzania's proposal, and the council endorsed it. In February 1981, President Nyerere himself officially opened the Institute of Traditional Medicine at Muhimbili.

The growing acceptance of and interest in *materia medica* contrasted sharply with accusations that traditional healers were exacerbating health care crises. In

December 1978, the minister of health, Dr. Leader Stirling, charged traditional healers with facilitating the spread of cholera during an outbreak by offering "potions purportedly giving protection" that led people to disobey quarantine precautions. Concerns about the spread of cholera also motivated government health officers to investigate a large traditional medicine clinic; they demanded that the clinic comply with the health department's rules for sanitation and hygiene.[24] Such bureaucratic efforts focused on managing activities performed by traditional healers that were seen as dangerous or harmful, while scientific research efforts concentrated on "exploiting the knowledge and experience of traditional healers."[25] In this climate, officials began to reconsider the earlier association of traditional healers. The Institute of Traditional Medicine and a group of Dar es Salaam traditional herbalists drafted a constitution in preparation for the formation of a registered national organization of traditional herbalists.[26] In July 1981, Minister of Health Ndugu Aaron Chiduo told the National Assembly that "regulations and standards to control the dispensing of traditional medicines" were being drafted by the Ministry of Health in collaboration with traditional healers.[27]

These "collaborations" between traditional healers and the Ministry of Health (both government scientists and bureaucrats) were not equal. In fact, the government began to get nervous when the development of traditional medicine moved out of government laboratories. For instance, in November 1981, the Ministry of Health spoke out against a newly established traditional drug company, Madawa ya Asili Company Limited, saying that legislation on pharmacy and poisons prohibited traditional companies and practitioners from commercializing traditional drugs and that they were therefore liable for prosecution.[28] This reprimand illustrates the fairly narrow space the state was trying to delimit for legitimate traditional medicine. Crafting this new category as a solution to the state's development challenges required that healers and their efforts to modernize traditional therapeutics be managed. Usurping healers' relationship with herbal therapies, government scientists emerged as the appropriate experts in this new category of practice. When healers themselves attempted to capitalize on the new approach to traditional medicine promoted by government research and development (by, for instance, mass producing their own remedies), the government cracked down on their "publication." Government officials intended for international and Tanzanian scientists, not healers, to control any economic or cultural development stimulated by traditional medicine.

In June 1985, the minister of health asserted in the National Assembly that "seven types of local herbal drugs being investigated by the Traditional Medicines Research Unit of Muhimbili were expected to be available for use in hospitals soon."[29] A month later, as President Nyerere toured the Institute of Traditional Medicine at Muhimbili, the *Sunday News* suggested that "the[ir] identification

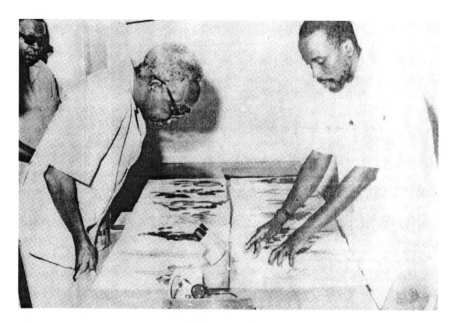

Figure 3.2. President Nyerere looking at botanical samples while touring the Institute of Traditional Medicine. Photo from the Tanzanian *Sunday News,* July 28, 1985, p. 5. *Reprinted by permission of Sunday News Tanzania and Daily News Tanzania.*

is a source of hope and relief as the availability of more local medicines will definitely ease the burden on the government which spends [a] considerable amount of foreign exchange for the import of drugs, and will definitely help improve the country's health services."[30]

During this first phase of institutionalizing traditional medicine, national and international development initiatives established a schizophrenic relationship between the state and traditional healers. On the one hand, efforts to foster new forms of scientific expertise and develop new kinds of biomedical therapies through research into traditional medicine marginalized healers. On the other hand, national and international policies described healers as potential allies of the national health care service who could extend the scarce resources of the relatively new independent nation and enable it to meet its socialist health care goals. National efforts valued healers as local actors who could bring the state into the intimate lives of its citizens to capture their trust and transform their beliefs. Positioning healers as an extension of the biomedical health care system, however, cemented their separation from the social and political basis of healing within their communities. The forms of development and integration officials imagined called healers to attend to biomedical concerns and demanded that the ambiguities created by initiatives to develop traditional medicine through medical science be ignored. In short, efforts to legitimate healers within the national health care system subordinated them to government officials and scientists. As notions of development and the forms through which it was to be achieved changed over time, the relationship between plants and healers as well as their positions in the state structure shifted. Yet state investments in the scientific and bureaucratic development of traditional medicine have continued to demand that healers be marginalized and controlled.

The Changing Politics of Traditional Medicine

The first phase of postcolonial health development policies in Tanzania began with the institution of socialist medicine in 1971;[31] the second phase began with the introduction of policies that promoted economic liberalization in the mid-1980s. By the time that Mnaliwa took up her post, the practical dilemmas of governing a newly independent nation compromised the ideals of Tanzanian socialism (Ibhawoh and Dibua 2003; Scott 1998). In the end, corruption and violence, severe drought in key agricultural areas, the nationalization of major industries, and the war with Uganda against Idi Amin plunged Tanzania into debt. The 1970s oil crisis and the global depression compounded these domestic problems. The reforms the International Monetary Fund (IMF) demanded "emphasized that the role of government was to create a good business climate rather than look to the needs and well-being of the population at large" (Harvey 2005, 48).[32] Under pressure, the Tanzanian government tried to maintain its obligations to the basic needs of a broad citizenry while catering to business. In the early 1980s, Nyerere slowly introduced some "home-grown" structural reforms. The IMF and the World Bank, however, refused loans to Tanzania until Nyerere stepped down in 1985 (Chachage and Mbilinyi 2003). After Ali Hassan Mwinyi took office, Tanzania folded to the pressures of the IMF as the second wave of neoliberalism began to gather momentum (Ong 2007).[33] The structural adjustment programs that the IMF and the World Bank tied to their loans consolidated this neoliberal vision by insisting on the liberalization of the Tanzanian economy through the establishment of a floating currency, the privatization of industries, cuts in social services, and the institution of "cost sharing" measures in hospitals and clinics.[34]

Aaron Chiduo stayed on as minister of health throughout the 1980s. Although private practices began to slowly and subversively reappear in the mid-1980s, his dedication to socialist health care policies lasted until the late 1980s.[35] Medical services at government health clinics remained free until a new minister of health was appointed in 1991. During the 1990s, traditional medicine moved from being a strategy for national and pan-African self-reliance to being part of Tanzania's strategy to manage the impacts of structural adjustment programs while still striving to meet its health development goals. As international scrutiny of the cost effectiveness of national health care increased, the WHO and later the World Bank proposed locally produced herbal medicine as a way to meet the objective of the Global Strategy for Health for All by the year 2000 while still submitting to international economic pressure. In other words, by incorporating the "useful" or "effective" elements of nonbiomedical therapies into the national health care systems (Akerele 1987, 1991, 1998; World Health Organization 1983), Tanzania could potentially "cope with current morbidity and mortality rates" (Sindiga 1995, 1) even while introducing fee-for-service care in public hospitals and clinics.

Outside of state (and statist) discourses, assessments of contemporary transformations in traditional medicine focused less on its potential as a solution to economic challenges and more on the horrors of medicine mobilized for financial and political gain. New notions of modernity promoted through market liberalization drove changes in both "witchcraft" (Geschiere 1995/1997) and anti-witchcraft (Green and Mesaki 2005) practices. In Tanzania, a series of human skinnings of schoolchildren in 1999 and 2000[36] and the more recent attacks on albinos[37] raised great alarm and speculation about body parts as "medicine" for power. These brutal crimes fomented fears of witchcraft, which begot additional assaults that were violent and at times fatal.[38] Attacks on older women who are believed to be witches because of their red or cataract-damaged eyes have occurred frequently enough in northern and central Tanzania to attract the interest of the development community and a nongovernmental organization called HelpAge International.[39]

Within state discourse, however, the gradual privatization of major industries, the institution of cost-sharing measures for social services,[40] and other moves to liberalize the economy turned traditional medicine from an arena for resisting the imperialism of "Western" drugs and multinational drug companies to an arena for engaging in competition with such companies and their teams of experts. Urgent calls rose up from within the national government for the Tanzanian state and its scientists to cooperate with Western researchers.[41] The concern was not socialist equality for the masses but rather a desperate sense that Tanzania was about to be left out of future profits from pharmaceutical research. As one journalist for the *Daily News* wrote:

> Indeed it may soon be too late. Already there is an awareness of a confrontation in the medical field between the developed North, where there are hardly any medicinal plants but where most of the interest is, and the Third World where most of the medicinal plants are but where there is hardly any interest.[42]

Concern about the development of traditional medicine paralleled the state's anxiety about the position of Tanzania within the world economy. Could Tanzania develop the "interest" to participate in the circulation of products and goods that makes up the global economy?

By the late 1990s, when I began my fieldwork, the sense of Tanzania's vulnerability to the exploitation of market forces was palpable in government circles. Traditional medicine now offered not only a site where science could be utilized for development but also a site where Tanzania's wealth could be stripped in ways that profited others. One officer of Tanzania's Commission for Science and Technology angrily told a story of "German researchers" entering Tanzania on tourist visas, calling meetings of traditional healers in a far western town, paying them a pittance for their "roots," and then smuggling these organic materials out of the country in duffle bags and into foreign laboratories. A frustrated official in the National Institute for Medical Research commented on "pharmaceutical companies" who have offered villagers a few Tanzanian shillings for their valuable roots. One researcher, when presenting a paper on the possibilities of cultivating and packaging the bark of the tree *Africanus prunus* for sale as an herbal medicine (Madoffe, Dino, and Mombo 2008), added ominously that Kenyans were already sneaking across the border to strip Tanzanian trees. Rumors about botanical hit-and-runs circulated through state offices, followed by exasperated assertions about the lack of state infrastructure;[43] government officials claimed that non-Tanzanians collecting herbal medicine were slipping past Tanzania's woefully inadequate bureaucratic safeguards. There is no specific permit for which such scientists collecting medicinal products (much less freelance collectors) must apply (Mahunnah and Mshigeni 1996). Under such conditions, it is extremely difficult to prohibit botanical poaching. These sorts of rumors represented Tanzania's natural and national resources as subject to a market with no controls.

The push to keep up and to keep ahead of imperialism through production also emerged in the midst of rising fears about HIV/AIDS. Wildly high and often controversial national and international statistics of deaths attributed to AIDS gave rise to new critiques of healers. Both the government and the public reacted with ambivalence to herbalists' claims that they could treat AIDS.[44] Longstanding accusations—that healers through their fraudulent claims were taking advantage of ignorant individuals—dovetailed with the state's fear that citizens would take advantage of a national crisis and with health officials' claims that certain treatment practices actually facilitated the spread of HIV.[45] In this atmosphere, unexpected alliances began to emerge between healers and hospitals. For example, in the early 1990s, a German physician and his Tanzanian colleagues working at a hospital in northeastern Tanzania began meeting with traditional healers in the area who were treating AIDS patients. In 1994, their collaboration grew into the Tanga AIDS Working Group (TAWG), a nongovernmental organization that currently supports the use of herbal medicine to treat some of the opportunistic infections in people who have been diagnosed with AIDS by biomedical clinicians. Waziri Mrisho, who originally shared with the German physician and the interested Tanzanian hospital staff the herbal therapies he used for people with AIDS, became the first healer to work at TAWG. Mrisho treated patients in the Bombo Hospital in Tanga and made home visits to patients who had been discharged. In addition to administering the three herbs he used and others that were subsequently added to the TAWG repertoire, Mrisho monitored the general health of these patients and provided counseling for them and their relatives. More recently, TAWG appointed Mohamed Kassomo as the organization's new "primary healer" (McMillen 2004). This program has received funding from Oxfam, the World Bank, and USAID.[46] In addition, TAWG treatments have captured the interest of bioprospecting companies such as Shaman Pharmaceuticals, based in California.[47]

In another part of the country, the Faraja Trust Fund, which was established to address the needs of people with HIV/AIDS, started a traditional medicine program in 1995 as part of its home-based care clinic. The Faraja program manager and healers are now negotiating the possibility of forming a relationship with South African researchers. Such collaborations promise more shifts in the meaning of traditional medicine, in the position of healers and medicine within the state, and in the practices the national and international efforts officially sanctioned as healing.

As nongovernmental organizations brought healers and hospitals together under the rubric of AIDS, so did the state. During the 1990s, new funding opportunities facilitated research at the Institute of Traditional Medicine at Muhimbili on some of the herbal medicine that healers claimed helped people with HIV/AIDS. The first social scientist to work at the Institute of Traditional Medicine at Muhimbili completed his dissertation in 1999 on "Traditional Healers and Treatment of HIV/AIDS Patients in Tanzania" (Kayambo 1999). Moreover, government programs have recently provided district-level hospital staff to run training sessions for traditional healers on issues related to AIDS, such as biomedically correct information about how the virus is transmitted, how healers can protect themselves from the HIV virus, how healers can avoid practices that facilitate the transmission of HIV, and when healers should refer patients to the hospital. AIDS even made an appearance in the 2002 parliamentary debates about the Traditional and Alternative Medicines Bill. During the discussion in the National Assembly, the *Daily News* reported that the minister of health had called for "practitioners of traditional medicines to release their medicines including those they claim to cure HIV/AIDS, for clinical studies." The minister said that "potent drugs would be given patent rights and sold in hospitals along with conventional medicines."[48] The Tanzanian Ministry of Health was referring specifically to medication for AIDS that lay health workers—the next generation of "barefoot doctors"—could distribute in the countryside. As the impact of HIV/AIDS refigures economic development strategies as well as health care initiatives, medicinal herbs have become weightier and more elaborate objects of both law and science.

During the 2002 parliamentary debate, the deputy minister of health referred to a recent visit to China, where he witnessed the manufacturing of traditional medicine in pharmaceutical plants as well as the distribution of such medicine in hospitals. Thirty-five years after the first official Tanzanian medical delegation visited the country, China is still the guidepost by which the Tanzanian National Assembly will steer the development of traditional medicine. Much has changed over this time in Tanzania (and China), however. Traditional medicine has become an object in a market-driven economy. A *Daily News* article on the debates concerning legislation about non-biomedical practices in Tanzania concludes with this statement: "The Bill is seeking to enact the Traditional and Alternative Medicine Act, 2002, to put in place provisions for the control and regulations of traditional and alternative health practice against the backdrop of the rapidly emerging demand for such services in the country." Traditional medicine is no longer a site for the establishment of socialist nationhood; now it is an object subjected to the pressures of supply and demand.[49]

Legalizing Traditional Medicine

The path to the 2002 legislation the *Daily News* article mentioned was long. As the sole member of the Office of Traditional Medicine in the Ministry of Health from 1989 to 1995, Sabina Mnaliwa was the person who blazed most of the trail. When she accepted the appointment in 1989, her first and primary task was to move the administrative responsibilities associated with traditional medicine from the Ministry of Culture to the Ministry of Health. The government's efforts of the previous two decades to establish a self-reliant health care service through the redeployment of national resources, including the incorporation of traditional medicine into modern medicine, culminated in this move of traditional medicine from "culture" to "health." Mnaliwa's appointment and the establishment of the Office of Traditional Medicine institutionalized this transition.

Dr. Muhunnah, the director of the Institute of Traditional Medicine from 1996 to 2002, claimed that this move was driven by the institute's efforts to establish a dialogue between the two systems of biomedicine and traditional medicine.[50] Calls for more formal guidelines about administering and exploiting traditional medicine generated the need for such dialogue. The Office of

Traditional Medicine was called into being to advocate for traditional medicine at a governmental level.[51] In addition to assuming responsibility for the tasks previously conducted by the Ministry of Culture—registering traditional healers, organizing a national association, and regulating witchcraft practices—the Office of Traditional Medicine was to help establish regulatory controls for the investigation of herbal medicine and criteria for the safe practice of "alternative medicine."

Mnaliwa describes her first years in the Office of Traditional Medicine as a process of learning "how the government works." To study the bureaucratic functioning of the Ministry of Health, she buried herself "deep in government literature." In addition, she participated in the initial flurry of activity that followed the state's enrollment of traditional medicine in the bureaucratic domains of science and health. In 1990, the South-South Commission sponsored a conference on traditional medicine in Africa through her office. This international conference was held in Arusha, northeastern Tanzania. Part of what conference participants discussed was how traditional medicine could be "introduced in other forums." Mnaliwa credits these discussions for the successful incorporation of traditional medicine into Tanzania's National Pharmaceutical Plan and National Health Policy in 1990.

Mnaliwa remembers the five years following these first steps to define an official traditional medicine through the National Health Policy as very difficult. Although more comprehensive policy guidelines for organizing traditional medicine were under discussion, the legislature could not agree on a concrete policy. In the second half of the 1990s, the Office of Traditional Medicine went through a period of frequent personnel changes and uncertain growth.[52] This flux was accompanied by a broader uncertainty over the status of traditional medicine within the Ministry of Health. Mnaliwa argues that while the Office of Traditional Medicine had the support of high-level government officials, the mid-level employees at the Ministry of Health appeared ignorant of the potential benefits of government intervention into traditional medicine. She spent the 1990s fighting the stigma against traditional medicine within the Ministry of Health.

Mnaliwa attributes her colleagues' skepticism during this period to a lack of imagination. She credits her previous experience of observing and studying within the Chinese medical system for her vision. "Others," she claimed, "not having been in China, could not imagine [traditional medicine] standardized or improved into capsules. They could not imagine that it could come out of *kilenge* [a four-month-old fetus]." Mnaliwa suggests that her colleagues feared that traditional medicine would never emerge as a self-sustaining entity or a truly viable solution to the country's health care problems. A four-month-old fetus shows signs of growth (typically the mother's weight gain becomes visible) and life (the mother begins to feel movement in the womb), but it is not ready to be born or to survive outside of the womb. Traditional medicine, in this analogy, shows scientific promise and movement, as illustrated by a few interesting results in botanical and pharmacological research. Yet scattered laboratory results do not make traditional medicine an independent system. These colleagues were expressing doubt that traditional medicine would ever be "born" as a modern category of practice and knowledge.[53]

Mnaliwa's China-influenced vision not only enabled her to conceive of Tanzanian traditional medicine as integrated into a biomedical health care service but also to have enough faith in this project to carry it to term. In 2000, Mnaliwa shepherded the National Traditional and Birth Attendants Implementation Policy Guidelines through the Ministerial Committee to the President. These policy guidelines finally passed in late 2000. Guidelines, however, unlike acts or laws, are not enforceable by the state. Mnaliwa and Lugakingira, her colleague in the Office of Traditional Medicine, continued to work with the legislature to legally bolster these guidelines. Their advocacy contributed to the Traditional and Alternative Medicines Act, which was included in the 2002 revised edition of *The Laws of Tanzania*.[54]

Mnaliwa claims that the new legal status of traditional medicine removed the stigma from practicing such therapies and from seeking the help of traditional therapists. She argues that legality changes the experience of being treated (patients are now "free," in that they can move without fear of stigma) and the nature of healing practices (they are no longer conducted "underground"). Before the Traditional and Alternative Medicines Act passed, she explains, visiting a healer had been "almost like . . . an illegal thing."

> If you went to a traditional healer, you were not free. Traditional healers were doing most of their work underground. No interaction. In some cases, however, traditional medicine was treating [ailments] very well. But if people went to see a traditional healer, they couldn't say. This was the most important thing about the guidelines and the law. The rest is just additive.

Mnaliwa suggests that legal recognition has redefined traditional medicine. It is no longer a set of occult or hidden practices. The Traditional and Alternative Medicines Act mandates that these practices and practitioners be visible to the eyes of the state.

The elaboration and promotion of traditional medicine as a modern (scientific, legal, and bureaucratic) category of knowledge and practice generates new freedoms and new dominations. While healers are now more "free" to establish a multitude of relationships with the government and to seek support from the ministry, they are also less "free" to operate outside the monitoring and control of the state. Legally established standards for "safe" therapeutic practice and for "effective" treatments apply to both registered and unregistered healers under the Traditional and Alternative Medicines Act. Therefore, the new freedoms being imagined for healers depend on their ability to reshape their practices in relation to state requirements and through government-sponsored training sessions. In contrast, for patients, the new legality imagines the freedom to buy commoditized herbal medicine and to see healers in hospital settings.[55]

The state's focus on integration also brings new connections and new possibilities that dissolve some earlier forms of difference. Perhaps most significantly, the Traditional and Alternative Medicines Act treats "alternative" medical disciplines (rooted in internationally recognized institutions of training and practice)[56] and "traditional" medicine (generated through the histories of local bodies and practices) equally.[57] The new equivalence effected through this conjoining of "alternative" therapies and "traditional" therapies concretized efforts to conceive of disparate and diverse practices in Tanzania as one aspect of a transnational phenomenon. Homeopathy, chiropractic, massage, aromatherapy, acupuncture, and Ayurvedic medicine are no different than herbal medicine, bone setting, or Qur'anic healing in the eyes of the Tanzanian state. The articulation of an internationally applicable catchall category for nonbiomedical healing practices displaced and marginalized previous forms of differentiation and the kinds of authority that made these differentiations salient. The most prominent distinction within the realm of medicine and the primary difference under the law is between biomedicine and traditional/alternative medicine. This contrast creates a hierarchy between two kinds of medicine, establishing biomedical science as the "obligatory passage point" (Callon 1986/1999) in any initiative to develop or integrate traditional medicine.

The Politics of Science and the Materiality of Transparency

Traditional medicine in Tanzania changed between 1973, when Mnaliwa left to study in China, and 2002, when she assisted with the passage of the Traditional and Alternative Medicines Act. Significantly, traditional medicine in postsocialist Tanzania continues to be molded in relation to China and through Chinese networks of practice. While the WHO, the World Bank, and the United Nations helped shape this modern category of traditional medicine through Tanzanian health policy, much of the practical work of articulating these (trans)national directives into a local category of knowledge and practice has happened through refashioned socialist networks.

China's ties with Tanzania did not end with the privatization and liberalization of Tanzania's economy or with the thawing of the Cold War. Although both Tanzania and China have radically changed their ideological stances and their economic strategies between 1970 and today, the countries have remained allies. For decades, Tanzania was China's largest aid recipient in Africa.[58] In return, Tanzania has repeatedly taken strong stands on issues such as China's reunification, publicly supporting the position of mainland China and firmly opposing any separation by Taiwan (Yu 1988).[59] In 2004, I watched the English version of the Central China Network (CCN)—which broadcasts programs on international news, science and nature, and Chinese culture—in Tanzania. The Chinese network competed with the British Broadcasting Corporation for space on Tanzanian public television. Originally drawn together by Cold War politics, Tanzania and China have become entangled in ways that have far outlasted their original shared commitments to the ideological project of non-alignment. As the economic and social ties between China and Tanzania shift and grow, so does the relationship between traditional Chinese medicine and traditional medicine in Tanzania.

Openness

Mnaliwa argues that

> the difference between China . . . and Africa is that, here, there were attempts to close down the system [of traditional healing]; whereas there, there were efforts to make the system open. Now, for example, one of the things that the Office of Traditional Medicine is doing is trying to encourage healers to package their medicine in bottles or boxes with labels that list the ingredients and what the medication treats.[60]

By imagining Chinese medicine as evolving from a process of opening that required no closures and elaboration that did not depend on selection, Mnaliwa distances "Africa" from "China." Her comparison hides the emergence of traditional medicine in Tanzania as a postcolonial category born of Tanzania's ties with China through nonaligned socialism. The distance Mnaliwa produced through this erasure establishes the space for her to imagine new comings together—of China and Tanzania, of the past and the future, and of medicine and the processes through which they are produced. In this light, initiatives to develop traditional medicine in Tanzania move it away from a past marked by colonial repression and toward a future of "openness." This movement through time and stages of development reinvents traditional medicine through the creation of new similarities between Tanzania and China.

Mnaliwa casts China as an example of the links between a particular kind of openness and the development of the forms of accountability that are available through commoditization. For her, "efforts to make the system open" are exemplified through the packaging of herbal medicine.[61] Her colleague, Lugakingira, demonstrated this strategy to me one day in August 1999 in the Office of Traditional Medicine. As I sat wedged between two desks and the wall in the chair designated for guests, Lugakingira proudly showed me medicine he had just received from China—his medicine. He lined up a number of identical small white-and-green boxes. Black lettering on the side of each box described the medicine both in Kiswahili and Chinese, and a haphazardly placed sticker offered a brief English translation. He then took out another neat package. This one contained four-inch vials of a bright red fluid that was also labeled in Chinese and Kiswahili. In order to have his medicine processed and packaged in this way, he had sent to China: instructions, a list of ingredients, and some of the actual plants to be used in processing. He explained that although a few of the plants are available in China, most of the organic matter in this medicine had been collected from his farm north of Dar es Salaam. This particular medicine is used to treat the secondary illnesses of AIDS patients.

The bilateral governmental relationships of the 1960s, 1970s, and early 1980s that supported the training of Tanzanian health experts in China are changing. The educational programs the Chinese government supports now tend to be short courses (ranging from one week to three months) for professionals rather than longer investments in first degrees. After two colleagues who work in the Traditional Medicine Research Unit in National Institute for Medical Research attended a one-month malaria control certificate course in Wuxi, China, in June 2008, they declared that the tours of the factories that process *Artemisia* plants for malaria treatment were the most interesting part of the course. Perhaps even more tellingly, in addition to the connections made through this government-run educational programming, Tanzanian healers are developing private contracts with private manufacturing firms in China.[62] Herbal products and lists of ingredients rather than bright young secondary school graduates are making their way from Tanzania to China. Packaged medicine with labels and lists of active ingredients in multiple languages and well-placed Tanzanian professionals who are knowledgeable about production strategies, rather than young people with freshly printed degrees, are making their way back to Tanzania.

For a moment in time, Lugakingira's medicine embodied the new desires of the post–Cold War transnational relationships that are enacting traditional medicine in Tanzania. They exemplify the move toward the commoditization of medicine of which Mnaliwa dreams. Her immediate turn to the packaging of medicine as an example of "efforts make the system open" belies the forms of closure and kinds of magic that are central to modern forms of exchange. As plants and lists are shipped to China, the production of medicine is moved out of the healer's hands and away from a space that allows for the participation of patients in the preparation of medicine (see chapters 6 and 7). Furthermore, older local names often linked with the historical or situated aspects of a plant are foregone in favor of the wider appeal of regional and international languages. As will become more clear in the chapters that follow, the lines of accountability drawn by the lists of chemically active ingredients on the side of a box of capsules stand in stark contrast to those drawn as healers collect, make, and administer medicine in Tanzania. Packaging does not address public anxieties over "who will be responsible" as much as it articulates who might be scientifically and/or legally held responsible by the state.

This notion of an openness advocated by Mnaliwa and her colleagues in the Office of Traditional Medicine is historically specific and echoes many of the broader contemporary political conversations that assert that transparency is an essential feature of a democratic state and a necessary goal for developing countries. The work of the Office of Traditional Medicine seeks to formulate the kind of openness, transparency, and accountability that is necessary to the fantasy of progress toward health services for scientifically rational publics.[63] Packaging captures these dreams, as it sits at the nexus between regulatory regimes: where actors (human and nonhuman) are to be declared, responsibility is to be taken, and the assemblages necessary for new relations between government and knowledge are to be made visible. The boxes (and what they are to say) link herbal products to the Tanzanian Food and Drug Administration, the patent office, and other regulatory bodies. The box calls on a citizen-subject who desires to make comparisons to optimize his or her choices. It hails one seduced, in Malebo's words, by "ethical herbal products." Imagining the scientific development of traditional medicine, then, serves as one way to chart the transformation of national "tradition" into a very specific kind of national (economic) "health."

Standardizing Medicines

While Lugakingira's medicine augurs the role of commoditization in modern traditional medicine, the activities of one healer are not sufficient to construct a category of knowledge and practice. The Office of Traditional Medicine strives to conceive of governmental policies that would support the large-scale commoditization of herbal medicine. Central to this project is the standardization of medicine.

When Mnaliwa contrasts traditional medicine in Africa unfavorably with its counterpart in China, she blames Africa's failure to modernize unsystematic practices and unstandardized medicine. Most troublesome for Mnaliwa is the fact that "in Africa or at least in Tanzania, power is in the healer." In this statement, she refers to the way in which healers (and the ancestral shades, spirits, and other nonhumans that reside on or within the healer) transform plant, animal, and mineral products into medicine through their engagement with them. Many treatments on the Makonde Plateau are designed to take advantage of the power of the healer's hands (*nguvu ya mikono*). Medicinal baths begin with a healer scooping some of the bath water into her mouth and then spitting it on a child (examples in chapters 6, 7, and 8). Some healers are commanded to gather their plants in particular ways and at certain times of day, having first prepared her or his body in a specific fashion (see chapter 4). Healing is not just a practice of skilled bodies; it is also an effect of relations that simultaneously (re)make the bodies of the healer and the afflicted.

Therapeutic practices localize the power of healers in the body, a fact that leads Mnaliwa to the conclusion that "knowledge [of a particular therapy] is quite limited to that particular person." These forms of healing do not separate healers from their medicine and from their patients. Such separations, however, are critical to the institutionalization of traditional medicine. For this reason, Mnaliwa poses the location of healing knowledge and medicinal efficacy—"in the healer"—as an obstacle to be overcome.

> It is just the way it [therapeutic knowledge] has been inherited. There is no uniformity [in what is learned]. This is one of the biggest obstacles. No two healers' knowledge is the same unless they have been trained by the same healer. . . . Chinese traditional healing is universal. You can pick it from books. A professor can teach it or you can read the book. . . . [In Tanzania there are] no standardized principles. . . . How should you pick from every healer and standardize it? This is where the burden is.

The embodied nature of healing in Tanzania, she argues, confounds attempts to standardize medicine and practices across time, place, and patients. The "power" of the healer becomes a "burden" to the state.

Mnaliwa articulates the deeply situated knowledge of healers as an effect of the way expertise has been generated over time. This analysis shapes her strategy. She calls for the separation of medicinal knowledge from the relations (with plants, patients, ancestral shades, and others) that constitute healers. She frames the work of the Office of Traditional Medicine as an intervention to free medicine from its various entanglements—or stated differently, an intervention to free objects of healing knowledge from the processes through which they have come to be constituted.

By isolating therapeutic knowledge from the processes that generate it, the Office of Traditional Medicine has established a framework that makes it seem as if therapeutic knowledge in the field varies at random. It represents the contingency of experts and medicine as inconsistency. The lack of "uniformity" justifies the practice of the Ministry of Health of selectively recognizing medicinal plant, animal, and mineral products in studies of traditional medicine. As Mnaliwa explains, "some will be missed" in the ministry's efforts to research the diverse nonbiomedical therapies available in Tanzania: "We are going to pick." Not all plant, animal, and mineral products used by healers can or will be equally incorporated into the new scientific order.

The Tanzanian government seeks to standardize traditional medicine in a process that entails the displacement of a variety of therapeutic practices and objects from their various contexts of treatment and then re-emplacing them in a context of scientific investigation. Breaking the ties between healers and medicine make it possible for research to establish new ties, new contrasts, new relationships and hierarchies. Scientific methods enable the selection and ordering of plant materials outside of their relations with particular healers, individual patients, and local histories. Botanical taxonomies and laboratory investigations then produce new relationships among plants, and between plants and research technologies, biomedical diseases, and scientists. Standardizing traditional medicine through scientific work proceeds through this decontextualization of therapeutic knowledge so that therapies can be recontextualized within national health care services and international biomedical agendas.

The series of recontextualizations central to Tanzania's attempt to articulate a national traditional medicine is illustrated in the formal research strategy of the Institute of Traditional Medicine at Muhimbili. The teams of researchers that conduct field investigations under the auspices of the Institute of Traditional Medicine include biomedical doctors as well as botanists, chemists, ethnopharmacologists, and (at times) sociologists. The medical doctor is critical to the framing of the research problem and determining which particular plant, animal, and mineral products are worthy of further investigation. After a selected healer identifies a particular patient but before he or she has administered a treatment, the medical doctor on the team examines the patient in order to make a biomedical diagnosis. The healer then treats the patient as she or he normally would. The research team observes the healer's activities and notes the organic substances he or she uses. When the healer declares that the patient has been cured, the doctor examines the patient once again to assess whether or not the biomedical symptoms have been addressed. In other words, these field teams investigate whether or not a healer's therapy cured the problem as defined by the medical doctor, not the problem as the healer defined it him or herself. If the healer's medicine has addressed the biomedical disease entity, then the research team collects the organic substances the healer used and takes them to the laboratory at Muhimbili for further testing. The institute's scientists work to determine why this substance would have caused the clinically identified problem to disappear. In these scenarios, herbal medicine is translated into the laboratory through a series of displacements. Plant, animal, and mineral products are decontextualized (that is, they are removed from the treatment process and the bodies, times, spaces, and scales that are salient in these treatments) in order to be recontextualized (that is, in order to be incorporated into the laboratory and the bodies, times, spaces, and scales that are salient to the investigations there).

Some therapies and types of therapeutic knowledge lend themselves more easily to the scrutiny of scientists and therefore to the process of standardization. Mnaliwa outlines two kinds of traditional healing knowledge: general or common knowledge and expert or specialized knowledge. The former, she explains, is immediately available for standardization.

> For instance, in many areas there is this thing called *njiri* or *mshipa tumbo*. . . . It is the general knowledge of adults that as soon as the *mshipa* [literally vein or artery, but often translated as a hernia] is seen you pick a certain leaf and chew it. . . . This [kind of knowledge] would be easiest to standardize. Yet if a healer was willing to disclose [his or her specialized knowledge], it would be easy to standardize [as well].

What can be most easily standardized, Mnaliwa claims, is the medicine that is "general knowledge": medicine that is used to address the minor complaints of family members and that can usually be prepared by knowledgeable caretakers. This medicine does not require the assistance of a specialist and can be "picked" by anyone. Mnaliwa distinguishes between general knowledge and specialized knowledge by speaking of a healer's willingness or lack of willingness to disclose the specifics of a therapy. The healer's specialized knowledge is occult in the most mundane sense of the word; it is hidden, out of sight, or secret. Such healing practices are unavailable for scientific study; they cannot be incorporated into processes of standardization. Embedded in a complex set of practices, such "leaves" cannot simply be picked. In noting that "general" or quotidian healing knowledge lends itself to standardization more easily than specialized knowledge, Mnaliwa calls for the disclosure of medicines. She connects the processes of decontextualization critical to scientific investigation with processes of despecialization.

The process of transforming objects of healing from the occult to the quotidian to the scientific is central to the articulation of the postcolonial category of traditional medicine. This transformation is the ground on which roots and leaves become modern medicine. The Office of Traditional Medicine seeks to institutionalize this movement through the policies of the state and the methodologies of scientific research. To illustrate the possibility of fostering these processes of (de- and re-) contextualization and (de- and re-) specialization, Mnaliwa offered a personal example of a childhood incident in which she was taken to a healer for a "dislocated" elbow. She remembers: "This *babu* [grandfather] prepared several sticks" and placed them around her elbow. Then he "crushed some herbs" and put this pulverized mixture around the sticks. Lastly, he "wrapped the whole thing in a cloth." To this day, she claims, her arm is fine. "If this *babu* could say, when a person is injured you can use these herbs," then this knowledge could be standardized, or formalized. Mnaliwa believes that disclosure facilitates standardization.

Standardization requires the willingness of a healer—in Mnaliwa's case, the *babu*—to articulate his treatment in a way that links organic matter to particular complaints. Healers will be useful in terms of the state's project to integrate traditional and modern medicine when they can frame their practice in terms outside of their own involvement. As Mnaliwa argues, the way to "handle traditional healing" is "to expose" treatments and healers, "then you can come up with a few standardized things." Not all things lend themselves to this kind of exposure, however. For example, Mnaliwa confesses that "divination and spiritual issues would be difficult to standardize."[64] While organic medicine, which can be tested in laboratories, can be "picked" and mobilized in the definition of a national traditional medicine, the government's focus on standardization shifts divination and other practices from the domain of *uganga* (healing) to that of "spiritual issues." Old colonial divisions between healing and witchcraft haunt the landscape in new forms.

The articulation of herbal remedies in the spaces, times, and scales of medical science formulates differences between science and spirit, knowledge and belief, the material and the immaterial. The postcolonial state consolidates these shifting claims through the work of standardizing traditional medicine. The scientific research that is fundamental to standardization draws equivalences between traditional and modern medicine that make bureaucratic integration possible. In the laboratory, traditional medicine and modern medicine become two ways of approaching the same objects of knowledge—the same disease entities, the same physiologies, the same chemical processes. They become two perspectives on the same material world.

Such ontological privileging is an effect of power. The cost of this privileging—as the chapters that follow illustrate—can be read in gestures that marginalize therapies that are unavailable to scientific investigation. The process of developing a traditional medicine that speaks to biomedical realities consolidates therapeutic practices around scientifically intelligible bodies and bodily threats; it strives to train attention on a narrower range of matter in the world and to further legitimate those who have authority over it. Scientists speak for herbal medicine; healers gain legitimacy by learning to speak to scientists. The asymmetries this breeds are evidenced in the fact that plant samples move more easily and more frequently than healers between sites of traditional healing and government-sponsored offices and laboratories. The differences in the mobility of medicines and experts within scientific networks of practice has come to shape the progressions of traditional medicine as it moves from ethnobotanical to chemical to pharmacological to clinical studies.

New Forms of Authority and Expertise

Lugakingira, the person who put those colorful, seductively packaged boxes and vials in front of me in 1999, is one example of a modern "traditional healer." While working at the Office of Traditional Medicine in the Ministry of Health, he continued his practice as a healer, growing his own medicine on his farm north of the city as well as seeing patients there. In addition to his years of practice preparing and administering plant-based medicine, he studied basic clinical medicine at a college in Tanga. He has taken further coursework to earn certificates in administration and management. He was particularly proud when he told me that he also completed private distance learning courses in Chinese medicine and basic homeopathy from the Brantridge Forest School in the United States. Lugakingira is an ambitious man who has developed and coordinated multiple forms of expertise. While his example is quite unique, the creativity with which he situates himself between state-recognized categories of healing exemplifies the efforts of many healers in Tanzania. Mnaliwa spoke of a whole "new generation of healers" in the city of Dar es Salaam that is beginning to operate clinics modeled on Chinese medicine clinics. Even more broadly, many healers are weaving together a variety of forms of knowledge and credibility, including hospital-based training sessions about homebirth, prenatal care, malaria, and HIV/AIDS.

In 1991, the minister of health, Professor Philemon Sarungi, publicly advised traditional healers to organize themselves.[65] His call was tied to a continued effort to convince healers to submit their medicine to the government for analysis and approval. This project was conceived of as part of a long-term strategy to manage healers by regulating the production and distribution of the plant, animal, and mineral substances they use. The government envisions that after certain drugs are approved, healers will be permitted to dispense only those approved medications.[66] Because efforts to institutionalize traditional medicine are incomplete and the resources to enforce compliance are scarce, however, healers are responding to the promises and threats of the state in a variety of ways, some of which try to exploit these new potential relationships with science and the state and others of which try to avoid them.[67]

The new forms of difference and diversity spurred by the institutionalization of traditional medicine are fraught with struggles for control. For instance, the organization of traditional healers consolidates control among its representatives. Authority is generated along bureaucratic lines rather than through practices of healing and initiation. Some healers have begun to shape the criteria for including and excluding others. For example, in 1993, the regional representative of the organization in northern Tanzania, "Dr." Dyakyaya, "warned that there was an influx of [unregistered] traditional healers at the central market, bus stand,

and streets in the Arusha Municipality who are just conmen."[68] In the name of cracking down on "cheating," Dyakyaya wrote a letter to the Arusha regional authorities "asking them to revoke all permits that allow traditional healers to practice their profession." Dyakyaya claimed that most of these healers were frauds. In the same letter he appealed to the district medical officers to help *him* evaluate and certify legitimate healers.

Not only new ways of being a healer but also new kinds of desires and new platforms for activism are emerging. In July 1999, the Tanzanian Association of Non-Governmental Organizations in collaboration with a nationally renowned college of the arts in the coastal town of Bagamoyo (north of Dar es Salaam) and a local secondary school convened a meeting about traditional medicine. Idd Msilo, an executive member of the traditional healers' association (Chama cha Waganga na Wakunga wa Asili), used this occasion to argue for the establishment of a traditional healers' college.[69] He exclaimed: "We [healers] are dying, we need to pass on this vital information to the young generation. We must have a college here for herbalists."[70] Over the past forty years, healers in Tanzania have come to craft their identities and cultivate their expertise in the context of the state's efforts to sanction some forms of healing through legal prosecution, scientific research, and bureaucratic institutionalization.

The suggestion of new regulatory norms has catalyzed unexpected initiatives. For example, the Society for the Traditional Healers in Zanzibar has begun to design a laboratory that would be dedicated exclusively to the investigation of traditional medicine. Ideally, after identifying "the contents of traditional medicine and its effectiveness," this medicine will be distributed through the society's clinics.[71] The state's attempt to narrow and homogenize the official trajectories along which healers might fashion themselves and their practices has had multiple effects. Even as some forms of diversity and lines of difference are being erased, others are being created. New forms of organization are developing. New agendas are emerging. Not only is the process of standardization being contested, but also the kinds of universality that might be evoked and the goals that might mobilize it are being negotiated. A wide range of postcolonial desires is breathing life into traditional medicine. New, often surprising and unpredictable therapies and experts are coming into being. Mnaliwa, Lugakingira, and others join Binti Dadi and Kalimaga in illustrating that there are no easy, pure, or authentic positions in the complex negotiation demanded of those interested in traditional medicine— whether they be healers, patients, bureaucrats, scientists, or scholars.

Part 2

~~~~~~

Hailing Traditional Experts

Bring on the traditional medicine men and women—and
their midwives. We have nothing to lose but our ailments!

—"Of Traditional Medicine, HIV/Aids and Marriage,"
Business Times (Dar es Salaam), 5 September 2003

Ah, so you are the one who works with "witchdoctors."

—Medical attendant, Newala District Hospital

4

Healers and Their Intimate Becomings

In 2003, forty-six African countries marked the promise of traditional medicine by declaring the 31st of August to be African Traditional Medicine Day, an annual day of celebration. In Tanzania, this governmental recognition prompted the editorial page of the Tanzanian *Business Times* to issue the daring call to "bring on the traditional medicine men and women—and their midwives." Who are these traditional medicine men and women? How do they conceive of their own healing practices? How do they imagine their relationship with the different substances involved in their treatments? In what ways do these traditional medicine men and women distinguish themselves from one another (and from biomedical doctors and "witches")? Through which processes do they gain expertise and maintain credibility? What categories of knowledge and practice are meaningful to them? This chapter and the next turn to the therapeutic practitioners who have come to be called traditional.

References to tradition in English gloss three different Kiswahili terms: *asili, jadi,* and *keinyeji.* Any connotations of a timeless tradition that represent groups of people as frozen in an exotic past that might linger with the English term begin to dissolve as Kiswahili pluralizes the nature of tradition.[1] The frictions of translation suggest different, more subtle meanings and open up new questions.[2] *Asili* carries with it a sense of that from which things derive, an origin. It is invoked to describe a base or a foundational element. In another context, *asili* is used to refer to a denominator in mathematics. The phrase *kwa asili* ("for the reason"), preempts an explanation for something. In contrast, *jadi* evokes a sense of ancestry, genealogy, descent, and lineage. *Jadi* has some resonance with *mila,* or custom. It speaks most eloquently to the multifarious hybridity of any object as it moves through generations. The third term glossed in English as "traditional" is the place-oriented word *kienyeji.* It implies locality—tradition in the sense of that which has come to distinguish and define an area. Sometimes when *kienyeji* is used in reference to healers or medicine it sits a little sourly in the speaker's mouth. Tone or context can tinge it with the flavor of primitiveness or backwardness. Yet to others, this place-based characterization and the density of connections that it captures is not a problem but a strength. None of these terms (necessarily) define an unchanging past; rather, they evoke transformation over time.[3]

Asili, jadi, and *kienyeji* each suggest different temporalities and spatialities that are critical to healing knowledge.[4] *Asili* suggests derivation—transformation from one state to another, the process of reasoning out, explaining, or following a train of logic. It is most often used in relation to medicine and efforts to scientifically investigate plant, animal, and mineral substances. The Institute of Traditional Medicine at Muhimbili is known as the Taasisi ya Dawa za Asili in Kiswahili. *Jadi* captures development through generations. Government training sessions for lay midwives refer to them as *wakunga wa jadi,* or traditional birth attendants. In official circles, *jadi* has become a respectful way to refer to traditional healers: *waganga wa jadi.* Outside of the official documents of the Ministry of Health in Dar es Salaam, however, this would be an unusual way to refer to healers. Much more common is *waganga wa kienyeji. Kienyeji* implies the growth of (and the growth out of) a place. The word localizes a healer or his or her medicine. This localizing, as illustrated below, is not only a reference to geographic locales or the blunt linking of medicine and linguistic groups of people (such as the Makonde, Sukuma, Shambaa, etc.). *Keinyeji* reflects the importance of specificity and the acts of specifying that lie at the root of some forms of healing. Healing in southern Tanzania enacts an epistemological commitment to temporal and spatial speci-ficities and the forms of contingency such specificity makes necessary.

Biographies of healers reveal the intimacies that shape therapeutic expertise. As healers reflect on the ways they have come to know about specific treatments, they disclose how the ontologies of African therapies emerge in conjunction with social commitments. Healers appear as an assemblage of relations, a site where time, place, medicine, bodies, and threats can be apprehended. Engagements with "the book" and "the bush" evoke different notions of knowledge. Both, however, articulate power in the (re)shaping of temporal and spatial trajectories, the (re) ordering of time and place. Both recognize the danger and promise that healers embody. Probing into the process of how healers come to know treatments raises questions about how knowledge and expertise is constituted. These questions challenge and inspire my own methodological and epistemological practice.

Distinguishing Types of Expertise

Healers defy generalized characterization. As a group, they have been defined more by the discourses from which they are excluded than by any discourse in which they are all included.[5] Contemporary references to traditional healers typically refer to those who mobilize "African" idioms in an effort to transform undesirable states into more desirable ones and who are *not* part of the biomedical system. These may include herbalists, diviners of various sorts, spirit possession mediums, sorcerers, birth attendants, bonesetters, specialists in kinship therapy, and experts in the removal of pollution.[6] Erdtsieck (1997) argues that "no strict differentiation is made by the healers themselves" (7). Indeed, healers have historically traveled to acquire remedies or to learn therapeutic techniques from other healers in other areas, which has resulted in very fluid kinds of practice (Feierman 1986; Rekdal 1999).

In everyday discussions of the treatment of misfortunes and maladies plaguing kin, friends, and neighbors, people categorize types of medicine rather than types of healers. In Newala, the primary distinction between forms of therapy is between medicine of the book (*dawa za kitabu*) and medicine of the bush (*dawa za mitishamba*). Because the skills needed to practice these two kinds of therapies are different, people speak of healers based on whether they use the Qur'an or the bush as their source of knowledge and legitimacy. This does not mean, however, that the practices of *faraki* healers, as those who use the "medicine of the book" are commonly called, neglect the systematic use of plant medicine, nor does it mean that experts of *dawa za mitishamba* ignore all elements of Qur'anic healing. Rather, this distinction recognizes the tendency of each of these types of practitioners to draw on different kinds of authority. The book and the bush connect people, experts, technologies, economies, and a variety of nonhuman things differently.

The material-semiotic worlds of these types of medicine—the words and things through which they move and work—tend to differ. *Faraki* medicine requires knowledge of Arabic. *Faraki* seems to be a transformation of the Arabic word *falaq. Al-Falaq*, "The Daybreak," chapter 113 in the Qur'an, which Muslims often recite for protection against problematic spirits. *Faraki* healers typically draw on one or more thin paperback books to diagnose complaints and to determine which kinds of medicine are useful for a particular client.[7] These books classify physical tendencies according to temporal and spatial histories. Faraki healers assess a patient's constitution and determine treatment based on his or her metaphysical position. A *faraki* healer evaluates the relationships of their patients to stars and to spirits through birthdays, names, and the times of crucial events ranging from the patient's entrance into the world to his or her arrival for treatment. Through a combination of geometry, numerology, and astrology, *faraki* healers produce medicine to wear, drink, and bathe in. These or similar practices of divination by calculation with reference to Arabic books can be found throughout East Africa (Bloch 1968; Swantz 1974; Trimingham 1964; Whyte 1997, see especially p. 64).

In contrast, healers who are effective in their use of *dawa za mitishamba* typically host within their bodies familiars who are knowledgeable about plant, animal, and mineral substances with medicinal qualities. They develop their therapeutic knowledge and expertise through a productive relationship with these bodily inhabitants.[8] By "climbing on the head" of a person, these familiars transform the body of the healer. Plant, mineral, or animal substances then become therapeutically efficacious through their interaction with this transformed body of the healer during collection, preparation, and administration.

The therapies described in the remainder of this book focus on practices that address maternal and child health because this biomedical category of health services has been the most common site of colonial and postcolonial efforts to integrate traditional and modern medicine. In southeastern Tanzania, women and children most often seek help from specialists of *dawa za mitishamba*. Patterns of therapeutic treatment on the Makonde Plateau seem to be consistent with other research that has found that "obstetrics and gynecological conditions" (Kilewo et al. 1987), the protection of infants, and the treatment of the maladies of young children (Reynolds 1996) rank high among the reasons that people seek out traditional healers. I found that many women prefer to seek the assistance of female healers for these problems. Although I did hear one story of a female *faraki* healer on the coast, women rarely have the opportunity to specialize in this type of treatment because it requires the ability to read and write Arabic, skills that are reserved for men who attended Qur'anic schools. Women more often develop expertise in *dawa za mitishamba* through possession (to a greater or lesser degree) by unseen agents. These healers devise treatments by innovating with the materials, forms, and practices that draw on lineages of therapies within Africa.

The differences in how healers acquire therapeutic knowledge derived from the book and how they acquire such knowledge from the bush provide a productive contrast through which to think about pluralism on the plateau. I compare *faraki* healers with specialists in *dawa za mitishamba* for four reasons. First, this contrast is so common on the plateau that it is central not only to any attempt to account for the spectrum of practices that have come to be seen as healing but also to any description of the kinds of pluralism most healers and patients imagine in contemporary southeastern Tanzania. Second, although women do not seek out *faraki* medicine as often as they seek out *dawa za mitishamba*, women do go to and take their children to *faraki* specialists for treatment. These healers prepare many of the amulets that are popularly worn by those who are vulnerable to *uchawi*, particularly pregnant women, nursing mothers, and young children. Third, because the kind of expertise required of a specialist in medicine of the book—and therefore what is considered knowledge—stands in stark contrast to the expertise and knowledge of a specialist in medicine of the bush, comparing the two highlights significant characteristics of both. Fourth, and most important, *faraki* medicine has established a visual lexicon that contributes to the practices of many healers on the plateau. For these reasons, the following account of the ways that women and men develop the ability to heal begins by describing the process of becoming a specialist in *dawa za kitabu* (medicine of the book).

Becoming a Healer: *Faraki*

A brief review of the process through which two of the most widely respected *faraki* healers on the plateau developed their expertise demonstrates what counts as *faraki* knowledge and skill. The training of these healers illustrates the materials of practice and the kinds of skills that are central to the medicine of the book. The first healer, Shehe Awadhi, attended religious and language classes in a mosque as a child and was identified by one of his teachers as a potential healer. The second healer, Chinduli, was born the child of a *faraki* healer. He succeeded in learning Arabic at home and then apprenticed himself to his father. The similarities and dissimilarities of these two men's trajectories highlight some of the features that constitute *faraki* medicine locally.

Central to Awadhi's development as a *faraki* expert was his move from the small rural village of Mchole, where he had been born, to the town of Newala when he was ten years old. Being in Newala afforded him the opportunity to attend a Qur'anic school. He systematically studied both the Qur'an and Islamic practice in a local mosque. During these studies, one of his teachers who knew a great deal about *faraki* medicine identified him as having the potential to learn *faraki*. This elder *shehe* (the title given to a Qur'anic teacher)[9] slowly drew Awadhi into the practice of *faraki* healing. Initially, he sent Awadhi on errands to collect materials to make medicine to cope with a variety of threats or to attract good luck. After the elder *shehe* had made the medicine, he would ask Awadhi to deliver the treatments to those who had requested them. Later he began to introduce Awadhi to the books used in *faraki* healing.[10]

When Awadhi reflects back on his training as both a *shehe* and a *faraki* healer, he asserts a firm distinction between the way religious studies were conducted and the way *faraki* healing was learned. He says that knowledge of *faraki* medicine, unlike knowledge of the Qur'an, is not open to everyone. The power of *faraki* to take or give life makes it too dangerous for such broad teaching. Because *faraki* books manifest the power to harm people as well as help them, to kill them as well as cure them, only people with "wisdom and prudence" can be trusted with the knowledge of reading and applying them. Awadhi warned that the ability to use such medicine would be dangerous in the hands of a person willing to succumb to revenge, arrogance, or greed. To acquire knowledge and expertise in *faraki*, then, one must capture the attention of an accomplished healer and be chosen to be his apprentice. Such selections are said to depend on both intelligence and character. During the long period of assisting and studying with an accomplished *faraki* expert, an apprentice repeatedly proves his worthiness; each of the errands that Awadhi completed for the elder *shehe* demonstrated his trustworthiness, his focus, his loyalty, and his competence.

In addition to practicing *faraki* medicine, Awadhi has worked for one of the government ministries for thirty years. This job and his healing work have enabled him to marry several wives and raise seventeen children. He has succeeded in sending all of these children to school. Such luck (*bahati*) is not viewed by others as coincidental but rather as the result of his use of *faraki* medicine for work, money, love, and health. Throughout the community his success is offered as evidence of his credibility.

Like Awadhi, Chinduli had to demonstrate his worthiness to an elder in order to learn *faraki* medicine. However, Chinduli was not identified by a religious instructor; he learned *faraki* medicine from his father, who was well known in the area as an effective healer. Chinduli still lives in the same small village, Nyambachi (east of Newala on the Makonde Plateau), where he grew up and began studying as a child. Chinduli spent many of his early years learning Arabic. His eventual proficiency in that language led his father to show him the books of *faraki* and to begin instructing him in the ways of this medicine. He was the only child in his family to apprentice with his father and the only one to gain expertise in the use of *faraki* medicine. The books his father shared with him contained descriptions of treatments. Chinduli remembers his instruction as a process of learning how to manipulate the words of the books and other materia medica. His father would repeatedly tell him that "if you meet this type of patient, [first] write this paragraph. Then, get this type of root for treatment according to *faraki*." For many years, Chinduli studied how to treat a variety of maladies through the use of *faraki*. His father began to rely on him to collect herbal ingredients. Chinduli then began to deliver the concoctions, amulets, and other treatments his father had prepared to patients in their homes. Chinduli says that his father was testing him with these tasks—giving him assignments and then checking up on him. After some years of proving his reliability, trustworthiness, and competence to his father, Chinduli began to treat patients on his own. Eventually, his father sent him to Kitangari, Mkunya, and Newala (other larger towns on the plateau) to treat patients. Chinduli remembers traveling to many places during this latter period of his training. His father, he emphasized, would always remain in Nyambachi.

Chinduli's father died in 1985, and Chinduli inherited his father's books. *Faraki* healing books are often passed from father to son. Although he has obtained additional books commercially in Dar es Salaam, Chinduli still uses his father's original *faraki* books frequently. When a patient arrives and mentions his or her name, Chinduli looks in a book or through his handwritten notes to discern the treatment. He explains that a different creature (*mdudu*) controls each day. One whole day may be controlled by a creature who is good, while another day may be ruled by one who is bad. To heal, Chinduli must know the name of the person as well as the day and time that they were born. When people consulting him mention their names and birthdates, Chinduli looks in the book to see who is controlling the corresponding days. Then he prepares a written medicine. The writing may consist of words—quotations from the Qur'an or sentences that (re)structure the patient's experience into a particular set of relationships. Or the writing may consist of a matrix of squares filled with letters and elaborate esoteric symbols that are read through the geomancy of the *faraki* books.[11] Where Chinduli writes depends on the kind of medicine he is making. Some of the medicine is written in the bottom of a shallow bowl or on a piece of paper in red ink. These words are then doused in water to make a pink medicinal solution, which the patient may drink or use to wash an ailing part of the body. Other medicine is written with a ballpoint pen (referred to by its brand name, a Bic), folded, wrapped in leather or some other material, and then sewn into an amulet to be worn.

Although there seems to be some variation among practitioners (see also Swantz 1974), this form of healing is ordered by a fairly discrete set of books. Despite differences in training and sometimes additional diagnostic tools such as a watch or medicinal substances, *faraki* healing is easily recognizable by the use of these geomancy books in Arabic. Healers are constituted through their relationship with these books and the numbers, writing, and prescriptions they employ. Although specific individuals select apprentices and interpret these canonical works, thereby layering their own narratives on those that are written, the books themselves circulate widely, not only tracing but also forging a community of healers who know *faraki*. Furthermore, the practices of *faraki* involve a search for transcendental meanings. The words and squares on paper connect individuals seeking health, love, marriage, money, or luck with deeper structures in the universe. Patients are reestablished in the order of things.

Becoming a Healer: African Genealogies

Unlike *faraki* medicine, the expertise of an *mganga* who works with unseen actors and bush medicine does not make claims to have mastered a certain body of knowledge or a technical skill. As Mnaliwa lamented in chapter 3, *dawa za mitishamba* is not written down in books and she did not find it easy to imagine how one might go about writing it down. The practices of producing and using the medicine of the bush are neither consistent across healers nor easily separable from the body of the healer him or herself. Healers describe their therapies through a complex merging of generative tendencies, human and nonhuman histories, and particular images, objects, and expectations. As healers reflect on their passage into the realm and life of the *mganga*, they do not refer to intelligence or study; rather, they speak of unseen actors called *majini* (pl.; sing. *jini*) and *mashetani* (pl.; sing. *shetani*), of an invisible world, of dreams and visions, of being shown things, of traveling in their sleep, and of seeing in their head rather than with their eyes. This learning process relies on being vulnerable to powerful invisible actors and to the experience of being "climbed on" by these disembodied actors. Perhaps most important, healing implies a kind of reciprocity even more than it implies particular skills. The healer's knowledge resides in his or her ability to build solidarity with both savory and unsavory characters rather than the ability to gain control over them.

Below, I describe the histories of three healers in southeastern Tanzania and one woman who is in the process of becoming a healer. Each of these people is known throughout the area for her abilities. In the main Newala market, people immediately guessed that I was interested in traditional medicine as soon as I mentioned that I was talking to any one of these women. Their names are linked with healing on the plateau. Through the similarities and dissimilarities of their biographies, I explore the practices that have become so characteristic of healing expertise that they serve to broadly identify and establish the credibility of a healer. These practices are similar to what Feierman has called "generative principles."[12] These "principles" are not fixed, abstract values but are they are the very concrete sets of relations that transform a person into a healer. Expertise and credibility emerge as the products of these human and nonhuman relations.

Such defining connections and linkages are made and remade at least partly through the skillful manipulation of the visual and verbal lexicon of therapeutic practice. Fatu Chenga's history demonstrates how falling ill can thrust an individual into therapeutic practice. Seeking treatment and being healed establish a trajectory through which a person can be called into relationship with a variety of actors. Chenga's healing required her to develop the ability to negotiate productive coexistences with other actors. Constituted in this way, therapeutic knowledge means sensitivity to the desires and habits of particular humans and nonhumans and requires finesse and dexterity in order to transform difficult, often threatening relationships into stable coexistences. Binti Dadi and her daughter Mariamu illustrate how such knowledge and expertise can move through generations. What practices produce a genealogy of African medicine? How are particular consistencies developed and maintained over time? Finally, Mama Libongo's description of becoming a healer exemplifies not only the current stability of some generative processes but also their flexibility. What kind of play is there in the hailing of healers?

Relationships with Shades and Familiars

In 1998, when I first interviewed Fatu Chenga, her popularity had already spread well beyond Newala. People from many parts of Tanzania and Mozambique sought her assistance in treating their afflictions. Her home and clinic sat on the western edge of the Makonde Plateau in a residential area of Newala town. Frequently, however, she traveled to Dar es Salaam to offer her services to an even larger population.

Fatu Chenga started treating people very early in her life, only a year after she completed her girlhood initiation (which can happen anywhere between the ages of six and ten). A severe illness initially impelled Chenga to embark on the process of becoming a healer. One day, she grew very ill. Her tongue became so swollen that it hung out of her mouth. Her parents took her to an *mganga* for help. This healer diagnosed her malady as one of *mashetani* (devils) or *mizuka* (ancestors). After she was treated, Chenga began to receive visitations. Nonhuman creatures, which she referred to as *wanyama* (literally "animals," but also used as a colloquial term for *mashetani* and a range of other nonhuman actors), appeared to her and told her of their needs and desires. "The *wanyama* explained [that] *chakula dawa fulani* [a certain medicine is food]." The plant, mineral, and animal products of the bush used to treat affliction are said to be the food of such nonhumans. Their desire for "food" drove Chenga into the bush to collect the medicine the *wanyama* demanded. During these visitations, these nonhumans hailed her, and through her responses she was increasingly included in a complicated set of relations with them and others. The medicine she gathered answered the demands of these nonhumans who "climbed on her head." The sensitivities she developed to their desires were forged through their inhabitation of her body. In this way, the production of the medicine was located in the body of the healer, in the act of being hailed.

Chenga eventually returned to the healer who had initially treated her and asked this specialist to bring her through an initiation (*kualuwa*).[13] This initiation into the healer's therapeutic practice (*ngoma ya shetani*) culminated in an *ngoma*; that is, a drumming ceremony in which the nonhuman actors that have climbed onto an initiate's head are called upon to name themselves. Through the *ngoma*, Chenga consolidated and stabilized her relationship with and commitment to particular nonhuman actors. The ones who hailed her offered their names, and in so doing, opened up the possibility that she could invoke them in the future. Through initiation, Chenga refined her sensitivity to the likes and dislikes of those who had climbed on her head. She came to discern their skills and abilities. She learned how to articulate their character and their substance. When she became adept, she could separate the array of sensations, needs, desires, and demands she felt into distinct groups and attribute each grouping to a different nonhuman actor. In this way, she (sometimes literally) embodied the voices of individual nonhumans. They spoke through her and she crafted subtle and specific responses. This precision has allowed her to cultivate complex relationships based on reciprocity.

Through these *wanyama* (or *mashetani*), Chenga has become attuned to the afflictions of others. During her period of initiation, they began to call patients to her and show her how to address their discomforts or disabilities. She started to treat people for their complaints, particularly people with ailments related to their heads, stomachs, and lower abdomens. Her first clients came to her with swollen stomachs or more widely dispersed swelling throughout their bodies. In southern Tanzania, swelling commonly signals that the condition was provoked by *uchawi*.[14] In addition, women sought her out for help with conceiving. These clients, she asserted, had been trying to get pregnant for years without success. Chenga explained that they "had no uterus (*kizazi*)." Her relationship with the nonhuman actors that had climbed on her head grew beyond her personal struggle to find peace. Their inhabitation became the basis for productive interventions in the human and nonhuman relationships that constituted the lives of others.

For over thirty-five years, *mashetani*, ancestral shades (*babu zetu wazamani waliokufa*), and other nonhumans have continued to come to her through dreams or visions to bring her knowledge of new medicine and to disclose the treatments particular people needed. Sometimes, Chenga says, she may get a vision of someone seeking treatment before that person arrives at her house. When the person finally reaches her, she remembers the vision (*njozi*).

Severe illness can generate the conditions in which it is possible for a person to become a healer. Many expert healers begin their reflections on the path they have traveled to become a healer with a story of a frightening illness that continued even though they tried a variety of therapies. These illnesses exhibited the signs of particularly strong and dangerous *uchawi*. These healers say that when it seemed that no medicine could counter the evil and destruction that had been directed at them, God took pity on them and spared their lives. God sent assistance in the form of *majini* (also referred to colloquially as *mashetani* or *wanyama*), who removed the *uchawi* and then inhabited the space vacated by the *uchawi*. These *majini* "climbed on" the afflicted, thereby saving their lives. In each case, this process was recognized by an experienced healer. Medicine facilitated the replacement of the *uchawi* by the *majini*. In addition, the herbs, incense, and other substances that continued to be offered to the life-saving *majini* to please them were referred to as medicine. When the *majini* were pleased with the gifts they received, they would live peacefully on the person's head. If a person is lucky, the *majini* he or she harbors will know medicine, and when they are content they will share their knowledge. Not all *majini*, as we will see later, have medicinal knowledge to share. Not all of them attract people who need treatment, nor do they all transform the body of the healer into medicine itself.

Like Fatu Chenga, Binti Dadi's career as a healer was forged through an illness. Even before the Newala District Hospital was built in 1959, Binti Dadi was working as a traditional midwife. In addition to catching babies during births, she prepared and administered medicine, in particular remedies that assisted women who were having difficulty getting pregnant, protected the pregnancies of women at risk, and helped move women through difficult birth experiences. At this time Binti Dadi identified as and was considered by others to be a midwife (*mkunga*), not a healer (*mganga*), even though she collected and administered herbal treatments. Then one day when Binti Dadi was already well into her sixties she got sick. She went to the hospital and was given medicine that provoked an allergic reaction. Her tongue swelled until it was too big for her mouth and stuck out between her lips (*ulimi ulivimba na kutoka nje*). Binti Dadi's whole body became swollen. At this time, her youngest child, Mariamu, who was herself a grown woman with two sons, had a vision of the treatment that was needed to cure Binti Dadi. She ran from the hospital to collect leaves and grind them into a paste. She then rubbed the resulting medicine over her mother's entire body. After this, Binti Dadi's swelling decreased and her condition began to improve.

Mariamu said that the plants she collected for the treatment were only partly responsible for Binti Dadi's recovery. She asserted that someone had attacked Binti Dadi with dangerous medicine; she had in other words been "bewitched" (*alilogwa*). The use of *uchawi* against her is what caused the severe swelling. God (Mungu), Mariamu deduced, did not want Binti Dadi to die at this time. Therefore, God sent *majini* to remove the sorcery (*majini yamemwtoka uchawi*) that was causing her malady. The *majini* then took the place of the *uchawi* that was threatening to kill her.

Although Binti Dadi's formal initiation ceremony was not as involved or as long as Fatu Chenga's, she still keeps the red, white, and black clothing and amulets she wore during the period she was an initiate. Like Fatu Chenga, Binti Dadi welcomed the *majini* who climbed on her head through an *ngoma* ceremony. When she allowed them to fully manifest through her, they announced their names. Three relatively distinct *majini*—Mwalimu Mohamedi, Zawadi, and Kiwana—inhabit Binti Dadi. While these *majini* now protect her from further *uchawi*, they are also said to rule her (*walitawala*). Kiwana ruled Binti Dadi during the time when Binti Dadi frequently led *ngoma* ceremonies that involved extensive therapeutic drumming, dancing, and feasting. In the days that I worked with Binti Dadi, Kiwana was quiet, however, and Mwalimu Mohammedi and Zawadi were with her. She attributes to them her knowledge of medicine and her ability to treat others with both *dawa za mitishamba* and a written medicine, referred to as *kombe*.

Binti Dadi's *majini* communicate with her primarily through visions and dreams. Often the figure she sees "in her head" advising her on therapies for particular people and revealing new remedies for afflictions she has not yet treated is that of her maternal grandmother. This grandmother, who was a healer, raised

Binti Dadi for a period of her childhood. Binti Dadi does not speak of dreams of her grandmother as the result of "thinking about" or remembering her grandmother; rather, these dreams are visits to her by her grandmother's *mahoka*. Her *mahoka*, or shade, mediates the interactions between Binti Dadi and her *majini*. As a result, the treatments revealed to Binti Dadi by her grandmother's shade are not limited to the treatments that were in her grandmother's repertoire.

The relationship between the *mahoka* and the *majini* and the healing knowledge that it generates is the result of a series displacements that turn the disorder of *uchawi* into the ground for the development of expertise. Binti Dadi was first displaced by the *uchawi* that was used against her due to jealousy or hatred. The *majini* then displaced the *uchawi*. Their presence offered the possibility of reordering relations between Binti Dadi and the entities that populate the invisible realms so critical to healing knowledge. Binti Dadi apprehended the *majini* through the ancestral shade, who now facilitates her travel in dreams (*ndoto*) and visions (*njozi*). This mobility—and the depths of the nonhuman world it articulates as well as the possibility of negotiating with unseen actors that it raises—is what it means to be a healer.

Binti Dadi's process of learning to write *kombe* illustrates how Binti Dadi's movements condensed realms and relations into therapeutic practices and remedies. Writing *kombe* is a particular practice of diagnosis and treatment similar to the descriptions of *faraki* healing above, but it does not require literacy in Arabic. Nonhumans, which Binti Dadi would often refer to generically as *mashetani*, communicate with a healer by working through her to materialize their analysis as abstract images in red ink on a white plate. The healer reads the plate for the diagnosis and then adds water to the plate, transforming the writing into a healing tonic that may by drunk or used to wash troubled parts of the body. Although Binti Dadi's grandmother never wrote *kombe*, Binti Dadi took up this technology when the *mahoka* of her grandmother came to her.

> She[15] [the ancestral shade of Binti Dadi's grandmother] came herself about this *kombe*. She said, "Let's go." We entered the sea. Having eaten two small creatures [*wadudu*], we came upon a flag there. These creatures [then] sat on this side and that side—the flag in between. My companion told me, "Let's go now." We left our companions there. We returned. We returned to the path. She told me, "Go and write *kombe*." She came again at night. She said to write *kombe*. I went to a person [who specialized in] *majini*. I told him I had been told to write *kombe*. [I asked,] "This *kombe*, what do I write?" The person told me this: "Write [like] this in a plate." The *jini* came again when I returned home. "Don't write [like] this with this ink. Go buy another ink." I went to buy it. I bought ink and put it into a basket. Indeed, sickness was already there [at my home]. After having shown me this medicine, she [the spirit] was bringing me sick people [to treat]. The *majini* gave me this mother with a pregnancy that would not leave [a prolonged labor].

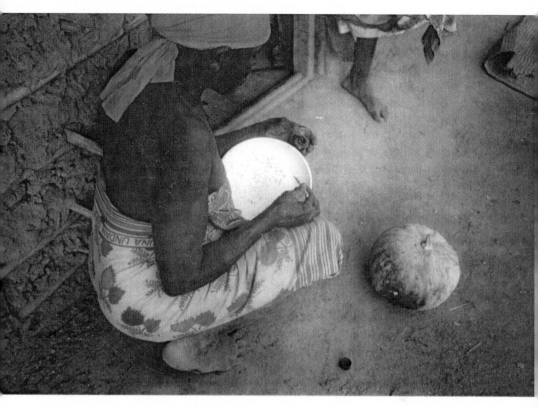

Figure 4.1. Binti Dadi writing *kombe*. *Photo by author, 1999.*

Binti Dadi and the *mahoka* of her grandmother move through the "sea" and back again. Their travel creates the space where they can interact and makes possible the instruction "Go and write *kombe*." Binti Dadi's subsequent visit to another healer stimulated a return visit from the shade. In response to Binti Dadi's trip to the market, the *majini* drew a patient to Binti Dadi's home for treatment. The healer and the *mahoka* moved back and forth in ways that defined and demarcated human and nonhuman realms. Their abilities, skills, and knowledge as well as those of *majini* and other human and nonhumans emerge through these movements.

Learning to heal, then, entails learning how to move between human and nonhuman realms. The healer's encounters express a variety of agencies that constitute the nonhuman realm, and the repetition of the healer's encounters as they travel stabilize the distribution of these nonhuman agencies. The repeated expressions effect the discreteness of individual actors, such as healers, patients, *mahoka* and *majini*. Binti Dadi's writing of *kombe* illustrates this process, for through *kombe* she communicated with *majini*. The *kombe* consists of marks made on the plate, some of which are recognizable figures of objects and others of which are nonfigurative marks. Binti Dadi begins with a simple representation of a crescent moon and a star, which depict the star of the person seeking help. These initial gestures, which reference the astrological heritage of *faraki* medicine from which *kombe* derives, initiate a "conversation" with the *majini*. She then channels the desires of the *majini*, writing what they tell her (*kumwambia*) onto the plate with a sharpened stick and a saffron-based ink. In each case, after completing the *kombe,* Binti Dadi "reads" the plate as a diagnosis of the person who was seeking her help. She then adds water to the ink on the plate and gives the resulting pink solution to the afflicted person as (at least part of) the treatment for whatever malady was divined through the writing. Sometimes she adds other medicine, such as cinnamon, to this solution. She attributes the knowledge that emerges in the process of writing *kombe* to the *majini.*

The matrilineal line running from Binti Dadi's maternal grandmother to herself is central to her process of learning *kombe* and more broadly to her process of becoming a healer. The complex ways in which healing practices and therapeutic knowledge are generated over time and through generations is (at least partly) demonstrated through the relationship of Binti Dadi and her youngest daughter, Mariamu, and the nonhumans that move between them. As was described above, Mariamu participated in the treatment of the illness that led to Binti Dadi's development as a healer. In addition, Binti Dadi and Mariamu say that Mariamu acquired her mother's *majini* through her breast milk as a child (Binti Dadi made no such claims about her other children).

When Mariamu was an infant, her mother's *majini* did not manifest themselves. In her late teen years, Mariamu suddenly fell ill. On that day, it had rained hard for quite some time. After the rain, there was a roll of thunder and then another and another, like it was thundering in her heart. Shaking and in a bad state (*hali yangu ni mbaya sana*), Mariamu went to the house of her neighbors, and they decided to take her to the hospital immediately. In the hospital, her body continued to jerk (*kushtukashtuka*), and she felt very afraid. She received injections that put her to sleep. Each time she woke up, her heart would start racing and she would be given another injection. Mariamu remembers receiving twenty-four injections before Binti Dadi requested that her daughter be discharged from the hospital. She wanted to take Mariamu to see a traditional healer (*waganga wa kienyeji*).

The first healer divined Mariamu's illness through the book (*kwenye kitabu*). He said that she had been the victim of *uchawi* and that the thunder she thought she heard was actually the bomb of the sorcerers (*bomu ya wachawi*). Without telling her who the offending person was, he said that the person who had bewitched Mariamu had come to him previously and that he had given him medicine. Mariamu could not use the medicine of the healer who had produced the *uchawi* with which she was afflicted. He told her that his medicine would not heal her but would instead create an impotent "mixture" (*hataweza kupona sababu itakuwa kuna michanganyiko tu*), and he turned her away. Binti Dadi then took Mariamu to another healer. This second healer insisted that Mariamu stay in his compound while he was treating her. She remained there about two years. Even though she took a great deal of medicine during this time, she grew thinner and thinner. "This medicine did not bear fruit," she explained. The healer said that Mariamu would die if Binti Dadi took her home. Eventually, however, Binti Dadi decided that his therapies were not working. She hired a car and driver to steal Mariamu away from this healer's compound.

Once at home, they sought out a third healer. This time they turned to Namiundu, the father of Chinduli, the *faraki* healer discussed above. Mariamu arrived at his compound weak and thin. She wasn't eating. Very frightened, she refused to enter any rooms by herself and refused to sleep by herself. Her heart (*moyo*) was bothering her a great deal. This third (and final) divination confirmed that the thunder had been a "bomb of the sorcerer." Namiundu reassured them that "the *shetani* will save her. The *jini* of Binti Dadi has saved her. The people of long ago have swallowed the danger and she will be cured." That is, one of the *jini* that had been latent in Mariamu since she was an infant had rid her of the *uchawi* and replaced that *uchawi* with its more active presence. Namiundu gave her a combination of *kombe,* herbal remedies to drink, and medicinal baths. After a month of these treatments, she began to gain weight and her heart calmed. In addition, her *jini,* Hussani, enabled her to see (through a vision or a kind of "second sight") the relative who had bewitched her and to hear him talking about his deed. Seeing that her daughter was growing healthy again, Binti Dadi gathered together a chicken, rice, coconut milk, and spices (the latter are called "medicine of the shops") in order to cook a meal to satisfy (*kuridhisha*) the *jini* that now ruled (*kutawala*) Mariamu. This gift to Hussani officially demarcated the end of Mariamu's treatment and the beginning of a relationship between Mariamu and her *jini.*

Soon after Binti Dadi cooked for Mariamu's *jini* to welcome and recognize his presence in her daughter's life, Mariamu became pregnant with her first son. During this pregnancy, she frequently took Namiundu's medicine. Once when she was not feeling well during this pregnancy she returned to the hospital, but the clinical practitioners there could not treat her fever. When her heart began to bother her again, she decided to leave the hospital and use only traditional medicine. Slowly, her health returned. She gave birth to Abdallah, her first son, without any complications. About six years later, she delivered her second son, Nuru. At one point after this birth, Binti Dadi and Mariamu tried to cook for

Mariamu's *jini* again, but he did not like the food and Mariamu's neck became "twisted." After drinking one bottle of Namiundu's *kombe,* however, her neck returned to normal. Still later, she stopped menstruating. After five months, she went to get another of Namiundu's *kombe.* After drinking it, she began menstruating again. Engaging with and learning to satisfy her *majini* has been a long process for Mariamu that has involved the help of both Binti Dadi and Namiundu.

Through this process Mariamu also began to collect medicine, prepare it, and sometimes administer it. She often advises people about how to deal with familiar maladies. She prepares and sews the medicinal amulets that the patients who consult Binti Dadi are to wear. She has visions and often claims to see sorcerers as they try to go about their evil work in the night. With Binti Dadi's *majini,* Mariamu appears to be cultivating the skills of an effective healer. Yet at this point, Mariamu is not recognized as an *mganga,* a healer, herself. The *majini* bring patients to Binti Dadi. By assisting Binti Dadi, Mariamu continues to strengthen her relationship with the familiars and guides that saved her.

Illness and healing can generate a space for communication between human and nonhumans. The disorder and danger of falling ill and the re-ordering and promise of getting well offer the semiotic and material contexts in which movements between human and nonhuman worlds can be articulated. Yet, while illness is a powerful experience, it is neither sufficient nor necessary to generate healing expertise. As Mariamu's personal history illustrates, affliction may open the possibility of developing expertise in the sense that it creates the opportunity for the called-upon person to mediate between human and nonhuman worlds. But to become a healer that individual must cultivate productive relationships with nonhuman actors. Healing knowledge depends on the development of the potential healer's mediation skills and on the skills of the *majini* and other nonhumans with whom the person comes into relationship. As a result, healing knowledge emerges in unpredictable and unexpected ways through complex sets of relations.

Unlike the analysis in some other ethnographic work in this area, I would like to suggest that while the process of becoming a healer often rests on the experience of an illness crisis (Erdtsieck 1997; Green 1989), it does not necessarily rest on an illness crisis. Rather, becoming a healer rests most fundamentally on the establishment of relationships between the potential healer and their *majini,* ancestral shades, and other nonhuman actors. The story of Mama Libongo demonstrates this distinction most clearly. Her narrative is unusual in that it is a story of possession without illness. Mama Libongo began her narrative of becoming a healer with a description of the resentment and hostility she experienced from others. At times, she could not, she claimed, eat food that anyone else had prepared because it was not offered with an open heart. She could not sit under certain trees or walk certain paths. Typically, such negative feelings—stinginess, jealousy, and greed—are associated with *uchawi*. They are often said to be the motivation for the damaging use of medicine. Yet Mama Libongo did not claim that she had been bewitched. She did not seek out the medicine of another healer as a cure. Her *majini* came and prevented even the initial possibility that *uchawi* could be used against her by dictating her consumption and her movement. Mama Libongo's process of becoming a healer highlights the centrality of access to nonhuman realms. The factors that make a person a healer are the means and ability to engage in an exchange with particular nonhumans, the ability to move between human and nonhuman worlds, and the sensitivities that render visible and animate nonhuman actors.

I noticed Mama Libongo immediately at the first meeting of the national association of traditional healers and birth attendants that I attended in Newala in November 1998. She was a short, thin, strong woman who was full of a tense energy. The meeting was held in a small dark mud-and-wattle room adjacent to the ward office. Long wooden benches were lined up in rows on the uneven dirt floor. At this meeting she was wearing a new turquoise *kanga* with a small black print. As is often done in East Africa, she wore half around her waist, allowing the turquoise cloth to fall to her ankles. She draped the other half of the kanga over her head, enveloping the top half of her body in the bright cloth. At the meeting she was loud and opinionated. She had a sharp wit, and her comments on even the most bureaucratic details created laughter in the room. She frequently let out a high-pitched, open-mouthed laugh herself. By the time of this meeting, she had been a healer for many years. Libongo, she told me, was the name of one of her grandmothers who had also been a well-known healer. Mama Libongo had acquired her grandmother's name during the process of becoming a healer.

Mama Libongo began to "get visions" (*kupata njozi*) after the death of several of her children. All but one of her children who died were over the age of five. By the time I began working with her in 1998, she could not remember exactly when these visions began and could not link them confidently to the death of a particular child. Whereas becoming a *faraki* healer requires long years of memorization and effective practitioners draw explicitly on their powers of recall, healers specializing in *dawa za mitishamba* often "lose" access to their memories. Many healers say that their memories have become scrambled through their intense interaction with nonhuman actors. Events that happened before they hosted *majini* and communicated so often with *mashetani* are difficult for them to place. Life before becoming a healer, as a result, seemed less defining. For Mama Libongo, visions of healing came slowly; her role as a healer evolved gradually in relation to her attempts to treat her afflicted children. As her remaining children fell ill, she was instructed through visions to collect and prepare particular remedies. She remembers that she had to leave her children and go to the valley to collect medicine. At least two more of her children died after she began to be called to the bush. Her medicine, Mama Libongo asserted, came from visions. Healers such as Mama Libongo situate their own ability to heal in their immediate relationships with the nonhuman world, not in their command of a literature, their subtlety in applying *faraki* geomancy tables to individual experience, or their skill in memorizing signs and medicine.

The first person requesting Mama Libongo's help came from Mtwara to Legeza, where she was staying (an approximately 130-kilometer trip over very rough roads). Mama Libongo says that after this first patient came, the *mashetani* told her through a vision that she must move from Legeza to Likuna (a village about three kilometers away). Although she had never lived in Likuna before, she moved. The nonhumans, which she referred to generically as *mashetani*, "ruled" her and compelled her to act through visions. If she was told in a vision to move somewhere, she moved. If she was told not to move, then she didn't. Although one might say that she was plagued by the deaths of her children, she never highlighted this misfortune or made a connection between her children's deaths and her development as a healer. Rather, with each telling she emphasized the seemingly unreasonable demands of her *mashetani* and her submission to her nonhuman guides. During this period, she grew sensitive to their desires and demands and sublimated her own needs so she could meet theirs. At times, she could not do any work. She sat for the entire day, neither cooking nor farming. After waking and bathing, Mama Libongo would sit and wait for the afflicted person whom the *mashetani* had told her or shown her would come. She remembers times when she was forbidden to eat anything for up to five days. During such periods, when she cooked food, a *shetani* would appear in a vision and warn, "Don't eat it." She argued to no avail that she was hungry (*kuchoka*). Then, later, when someone else would cook food and welcome her to join them, a *shetani* would appear and say, "Don't eat it. She is not willing to cook for you (*hakufidhika*)." Her visions revealed that the person who offered Mama Libongo food was not doing so with "an open heart." Libongo confronted this person, asking her why she did not want her to eat. No answer satisfied the *mashetani*, however, and Mama Libongo would not eat the food. She said, "If one calls me openly, if you cook food, then I will eat and eat a lot without any problem." But, she implied, if food is cooked and offered only grudgingly, without an open heart, then she would not eat it.

By sacrificing her needs and subjecting her movements to the desires of nonhuman actors, Mama Libongo began to establish the fundamental relations necessary to working as a healer. She could hear and respond to the commands of nonhumans. In response, her *majini* brought to her people who were seeking treatment for their "hearts." Through these first patients, Mama Libongo cultivated a more sophisticated ability to discern the desires and answer the demands of nonhumans. At first when patients began to come to her compound seeking treatments she did not know what to do. In frustration and desperation, she would start to cry. After crying, she would receive a vision showing her what medicine to use, where to get it, and how to administer it. In these early years of her practice, this pattern was repeated. When a person seeking help arrived at her compound, Mama Libongo would sit or sleep in the small shelter (Kimakonde *lilinge*) that she had built specifically as a place for seeing patients and storing medicine. After a while, she would start to cry, and she would continue until she received a vision telling her how to treat a particular patient. During this time, which she marks as a kind of initiation before her more public *ngoma ya mashetani,* Mama Libongo did not have a set fee for her services. People would leave gifts in appreciation for her medicine. She remembers receiving small amounts such as five or ten shillings (equivalent to less than one cent) for treating someone. Yet when she eventually counted all her money, she found that she had received 80,000 shillings. Her familiars then came to her and told her to buy goats. Thank God, she says, because those goats are now having twins.

Mama Libongo described the process of becoming a healer to me in detail. In addition, because healers often retell their story to patients in order to prove their credentials, I heard Mama Libongo and the other healers discussed in this chapter recount their healing biographies many times. The details of such accounts allowed new or potential clients and their kin to evaluate whether the healer was likely to be helpful. As people listen to a healer's story they judge the strength of her relationship with the nonhuman world and evaluate whether or not she is likely to have the appropriate knowledge of medicine, techniques, treatments, and skills to transform the undesirable states that afflict them into more desirable ones. Mama Libongo, for instance, concludes her story of becoming a healer with a declaration of the wisdom of her familiars in the nonhuman world who instructed her to use her money to buy goats. In following their advice, she has grown wealthier, as these goats bore twins. In telling this story, Mama Libongo offers her own success as evidence of the strength of her familiars and of her relationship with them. By illustrating the relationship she has cultivated with these knowledgeable *majini,* she suggests that she is particularly well situated to mediate conflict and suffering that spans human and nonhuman realms. She makes the case that with these familiars, she is capable of helping others navigate a variety of dangers and grow stronger.

The validity of healers' claims that they communicate with and move through nonhuman realms rests on their success in depicting *majini* and *mashetani* as other; that is, as entities other than the healer. Healers' narratives must prove that the wills and agencies of their *majini,* their *mahoka,* and the range of nonhumans they engage are separate from their own. As I describe in more detail below, the dynamics through which healers come to learn about medicine and receive patients articulate *mashetani* and *majini* as discrete actors rather than as elements of a healer's memory, psyche, or imagination. For healers and patients, *majini* and *mashetani* are not just narrative categories through which pain and inequalities can be made meaningful; these nonhuman actors are also forces that can respond in unpredictable and unexpected ways, and if they are not carefully mediated, they can work against the wills and desires of humans.

In each of these stories, nonhumans appear first as obstacles to be surmounted. For Fatu Chenga, Binti Dadi, and Mariamu, the characteristic discreteness or otherness of these nonhuman actors grew palpable as their illnesses worsened because they refused to accommodate *majini* or the *majini* rejected certain gifts and medicine or the *mashetani* returned to amend their instructions. Mettle and resistance articulated the agency of these others. Mama Libongo's story begins with the challenges she faced in completing the activities of everyday life. She could not eat food, go to the fields, or continue living in her home. As she recounts the process through which she became a healer she provides examples of the ability of her *majini* to make heavy demands on her and control her ability to meet her most basic needs. The sense of challenge, insistence, even oppression that she felt during this early period serve to disaggregate her humanness from their nonhumanness. In all healers, such separations were stabilized through processes of visualization, when they "saw" nonhuman actors (e.g., in visions and dreams) and rendered the presence of nonhumans visible to others (e.g., through possession and writing *kombe*). Sight materialized distinctions between humans and nonhumans, formulating the conditions for communication. Only as separate entities can humans and nonhumans interact in ways that make instruction possible.

Distinctions among Nonhumans

Majini and *mashetani* animate the biographical narratives of healers. Sometimes in casual conversation, I heard these Kiswahili terms used interchangeably to refer to familiars or other nonhuman actors who "rule" therapeutic specialists. When I questioned them directly, however, healers as well as those seeking healing insisted that *majini* and *mashetani* were different aspects of the nonhuman world. They articulated this difference in various ways. For some, distinctions between *majini* and *mashetani* lay in their dissimilar relationships with God (Mungu); for others, they lay in their relationships with a family's genealogy; and for still others, they lay in the kinds of interventions that *majini* and *mashetani* demanded.

The concept of *majini* is sometimes translated as angels (*malika*), although others have heard a *jini* described as something more similar to a soul. Indeed, Feierman (2000) has shown that there are very mixed understandings of (and feelings about) *majini* among the broader population in northeastern Tanzania.

Healers in southeastern Tanzania, however, presented a relatively consistent and resilient, albeit distinct, view of *majini*. To capture this, I sometimes gloss this term as familiar or guide. The healers' narratives above touch upon many of the propositions that define *majini* on the plateau: when a person has grown very ill as a result of being bewitched, *majini* may save him or her by removing and then taking the place of the *uchawi*. They become active when called upon (by God or otherwise) to manifest themselves. *Majini* create deeply intimate relationships: Binti Dadi's *majini* traveled to her youngest daughter through her breast milk, and Mama Libongo inherited her grandmother's *majini*, who then demanded that this intimate connection be marked with a change of name. Yet these intimacies do not always come to matter. *Majini* can lie dormant for a lifetime. In addition, Mariamu pointed out a spatial difference between these types of nonhuman actors by asserting that *majini* "climb on" or "walk in" a person's body, while *mashetani* cannot take up such positions. *Majini* possess a person, transforming them. They can permanently alter the body of their host, whereas *mashetani* merely "bother" or "play with" a person. Often an individual *jini* will establish an identity by assuming a name and endowing the healer with unique characteristics when it is active (a certain voice, a way of walking, certain desires, a sense of humor, songs, and sometimes healing abilities) that distinguish it from other *majini*.

The practical, lived existence of *majini* among healers on the plateau differs from the descriptions of *majini* in the Qur'an or from definitions Frederick Johnson offered in *A Standard Swahili-English Dictionary* (1939/1999). Johnson, for instance, declares that a *jini* is a fairy, a spirit or a genie who is "supernatural and capricious, but not always malignant, like the *shetani*." On the Makonde Plateau, *majini* are not considered supernatural. *Majini* are of the world, and potentially anyone can experience them. Furthermore, *majini* are described positively, as potentially life-saving. If healers or patients hold *majini* responsible for an affliction, they blame the patients' failure to give their *majini* the proper attention and respect rather than the *majini*'s intrinsic maliciousness. Unlike the more detrimental *mashetani*, *majini* do not need to be removed (indeed, they cannot be). Instead, they must be fed, given their due, and generally kept satisfied.

Maladies that result from the activities of *majini* often demand treatments that resolidify or reorder social relations, both through the specifics of the treatment ceremony (*ngoma*) and through the work of organizing the resources to pay for it. For example, the treatment that one woman required—a woman whom Mama Libongo believed to be afflicted by *majini*—called on her straying husband to provide food, clothes, soda, medicine, and drummers. Until he provided for this event (which would redirect his resources toward her), she would continue to be plagued by her *majini*. All Mama Libongo could do in the interval was write *kombe* for her to temporarily calm her heart. Maladies that require a person to accept or welcome *majini* may also renegotiate social relations, in that the afflicted person may evolve into a healer through the treatment process and thereby acquire both a new social status and greater income-earning potential.

The word *mashetani* is often translated as devils, demons, or evil spirits. These entities act more independently than *majini* do. *Mashetani* lack the *majini*'s relationship to God or ancestors and thus are not called to action; they act of their own volition. These devils can suddenly confront, startle, or play with a person. Such torments often manifest as maladies involving convulsions. *Mashetani* are not channeled; they themselves invade. Perhaps it is because of their uncontrollability and the randomness of their actions that they have become less welcome and more feared than *majini*. Although *mashetani* can contribute to both desirable outcomes (visions, healing knowledge, *kombe*) and undesirable outcomes (maladies, disability, death), they are generally considered to be dangerous forces. Fatu Chenga asserted that a *shetani* can bring both sickness and visions that indicate treatment, because both bad things and good things, both maladies and the cure for maladies "are in the company of each other. These things come together. They run parallel to each other." The power to heal and the power over life comes hand in hand with the power to afflict and the power over death. Therefore, *mashetani* are held responsible for a series of maladies and at the same time are credited with making possible some aspects of healing.

During my many conversations with plateau residents that did not focus explicitly on distinctions between these two nonhuman actors, however, people often conflated *majini* and *mashetani*. The word *mashetani* sometimes serves as a generic term to cover all nonhuman actors. The subtlety with which healers discern different elements of the nonhuman world is increasingly masked by the more general use of this term in colloquial speech. *Mashetani* are emerging as a more generic class of nonhuman actor. In some ways, this conflation groups together diverse nonhumans that are evoked in the many languages spoken in southeastern Tanzania as well as in other parts of the country. Furthermore, the use of the word *mashetani* to refer to all nonhuman actors links a general category of nonhumans to (and orders them within) popular idioms of institutionalized religion. Healers use the blurring of distinctions between *mashetani* and other nonhuman actors in everyday speech to draw God into the relations that define treatments. Healers, for instance, pray to Mungu while administering the medicines revealed by *mashetani*. However, because the word *mashetani* still carries the more specific meaning of troublesome demons or devils even as it is expanding to cover references to *majini*, ancestral shades, and other nonhuman actors, these connections are quite ambiguous. The darkness, fear, and danger evoked by more refined definitions of *mashetani* cast a pall over the entire nonhuman realm. For some on the plateau, nonhumans become an undifferentiated threat rather than a critical environment for the constitution of maladies, the play of bodies and spirits, and the mobilization of relationships that can transform undesirable states of being.

Like *mashetani*, *majini* is a Kiswahili word of Arabic derivation. These words translate and transform Kimakonde entities that are known by different names. Therefore, references to *mashetani* as a generic class of nonhuman actor not only conflate more refined definitions of *majini* and *mashetani*, they also further entrench the erasures enacted through the use of Kiswahili on the Makonde Plateau and the growing influence of the coastal life it signals. In many ways, both *majini* and *mashetani* sit uneasily with Kimakonde descriptions of nonhumans that order and disrupt life. But even as explicit references to nonhuman actors in Kimakonde are disappearing, these actors live on, even if relatively silently, in the practices of healers. Below, I will discuss one such set of actors, the *mahoka*[16] (Kimakonde), the existence of which better articulates the practical link between ancestors and visions, death and knowledge in therapeutic practice on the plateau. Whether or not healers in southeastern Tanzania refer explicitly to *mahoka*, they give shape to their visions and dreams.

The Ontics of Dreaming

On the Makonde Plateau, dreaming is an interaction, a meeting, with a *mahoka*. When a person passes away, he or she leaves a *mahoka* who may return to the living through visions or dreams.[17] In Kimakonde, to dream is literally "to make a request of" (*kuvauwa*) *mahoka*. These ancestral shades do not appear only to healers or soon-to-be-healers. When describing *mahoka* to me, one older gentleman, Mr. Mandota, a senior manager in a local transport company, shared a story of the return of his father's shade. One night, many years after his father had died, Mandota had a dream. In this dream, his father told him to make *chai*, so he lit the fire and started to make *chai*. Then, still in the dream, rain poured down in a huge burst. It put the fire out. This happened three times, and then he woke up. That, he said, was his father's *mahoka*. After this dream, he and his wife made *chai* and invited the children to join them, perhaps one could say in the name of his father or for his father or for his father's *mahoka*.

Mahoka play an important role in the life of a healer. One elderly woman in Julia, a village outside Newala, told me that after her father died his *majini* climbed on her. She has been living with them ever since. These *majini* have taught her medicine through visions or through dreams of her father. *Mahoka* make communication possible between a person and the *majini* that inhabit her. The *mahoka* enable the *majini* to appear in dreams; they provide the material for visualization. Dreams and visions are a mechanism through which disembodied actors are seen, "not with the eye, but in the head," as I was told many times.

The presence of such ancestral shades has been found throughout east-central Africa (e.g., Reynolds 1996, 30). In the biographical narratives of healers in southeastern Tanzanian healers I cited above, a particular relative often appeared in the visions of the healer. For both Mama Libongo and Binti Dadi it was their grandmother. For Mariamu, it is an older woman with a lip plug (*ndonya*) whom she believes to be a great-grandmother. These are the *mahoka* of ancestors who were themselves healers. They establish a vehicle through which *majini* channel their demands and desires in ways that are intelligible to their human hosts. As Binti Dadi's recounting of her process of learning to write *kombe* illustrates, *mahoka* come to healers and guide them into nonhuman realms. Through the visitation of *mahoka*, nonhuman actors orchestrate the interpolation of a human into their world.

Mariamu claimed that for traditional healers the *mahoka* and *majini* work together to make possible visions that will reveal therapies. She explained that because the place of *majini* is in the bush, they know medicine and can show a person how to heal by working through the *mahoka*.[18] Moreover, Mariamu said that the *mahoka* and the *shetani* could not work together in the way that the *mahoka* and the *majini* do. These specificities are often lost as many on the plateau today gloss all these entities as *mashetani*. This conflation challenges accurate translations and requires sensitivity to the faint traces of these entities left in the context and connotations of speech. Such subtle distinctions still matter in some of the most compelling accounts of experience. In Mariamu's story of being saved from dangerous *uchawi*, for example, she quoted Namiundu as saying: "The *shetani* will save her. The *jini* of Binti Dadi have saved her. The people of long ago have swallowed the danger and she will be cured." The first reference to *shetani* evokes a generic class of actors. Namiundu, however, continues to refer to the *jini*, and finally referring obliquely to *mahoka* through his comment about the "people from long ago." *Mahoka*, it seems, exist more and more quietly today; they are invoked in roundabout ways. Yet they have remained powerful, if concealed, sites for articulating the links between human and nonhuman worlds.

Teasing apart references to the various nonhuman actors critical to the process of becoming a healer can shed light on the depth and complexity of relationships between humans and nonhumans on the Makonde Plateau. *Mahoka, majini,* and *mashetani* work together to call healers into being through visions and dreams. For this reason, the particular kind of sight available "inside one's head" is central to all of the biographical narratives of healers above. Neither the English phrase "to have a dream or vision" nor the Kiswahili phrase "*kupata ndoto au njozi*" captures what healers do when they dream of medicine as accurately as the Kimakonde phrase "*kuvauwa mahoka*," meaning to make a request of an ancestral shade. Making one's desires known and asking for a response begins to portray the relationship of reciprocity that interpolates healers into the nonhuman world. It describes dreams as a medium of communication.

Mahoka incite healers into existence. They call a person to travel through nonhuman realms. They order a person to apply the knowledge they gather in these travels to human realms. An individual's response to the commands of the *mahoka* determines whether or not she or he becomes a healer. As a person's relationship with a network of nonhuman actors develops, his or her visions gradually become less like sudden and intrusive demands and more like the process of "talking" (*kuongea*). Dreaming changes from being a space of nonhuman imposition and human resistance to being a space for mediation and negotiation. A healer's expertise is both the result of an opportunity to engage with knowledgeable nonhuman actors and the skill and sophistication with which he or she responds to this opportunity. Medicine is the material consequence of these interactions. Or, as Mama Libongo said, "Medicines come from visions."

The Ontics of Treatment

Merely learning about medicine—even collecting it, preparing it, and administering it—does not make one a healer. Many people in southern Tanzania seem to know something about medicine. Even the fifteen-year-old grandson of Binti Dadi helped me by clarifying the names of medicinal trees and plants and telling me some of their therapeutic uses. He was, of course, not a healer by anyone's account. Even those who do not live with a grandmother who is a well-known specialist frequently know how to prepare a few common herbal treatments for minor ailments for kin (Geissler and Prince 2009). Moreover, some people are already familiar with the roots and leaves that the healer they visit uses to treat their affliction. Yet they still go to the specialist. As we will see in subsequent chapters, *majini* render the hands of the healer powerful. Therefore, the application of medicine by the healer herself can be seen as more desirable than the application of the same medicine by a layperson. Roots and leaves become more potent when they are called up for a specific patient and prepared by a specific healer. In this matrix of situated practices and contingent emergences, what does it mean to know medicine?

Knowing Medicines

When I collected the life histories of healers, many revealed a time when they had the opportunity to learn about herbal remedies and other treatments from an elder. For example, during her childhood, Binti Dadi lived in the home of her maternal grandmother, a very capable midwife and healer. She describes her grandmother as her primary caretaker. Their relationship appears to have been similar to that between Binti Dadi and Mariamu's children who live with her, the oldest of whom, as I mentioned above, helped me early in my fieldwork to complete charts of plants and the symptoms they were used to address. Binti Dadi occasionally sends her grandchildren to collect medicine from inside the house or to help her administer remedies when multiple hands or prayers are needed. They are in and out of the compound—playing, eating, relaxing, and half-listening—as Binti Dadi talks to patients each day. Fatu Chenga said that her mother was a healer; in addition, Chenga worked with another specialist when she sought treatment for her own illness. Mama Libongo's grandmother was a well-known healer in the area. The biographies of other healers with whom I worked also illustrated the tendency for healing expertise to move through family lineages. Healers often locate the beginnings of their biography after an elder with such skills has passed away, yet this is not always the case. For instance, Jambili Hamisi, a healer who is the head of the traditional healers association in his area near Chitandi, a village at the western foot of the Makonde Plateau, and his father, who works as a healer in southwestern Tanzania, share knowledge of treatments with each other.

At first glance, the passing on of healing knowledge through generations does not look dissimilar to the process of learning *faraki* medicine. After all, Chinduli's father was a great healer and Awadhi's Qur'anic teacher took him under his wing and taught him *faraki* healing. In contrast to *faraki* healers, however, specialists in *dawa za mitishamba* refrained from highlighting relationships that might imply that they learned their medicine as a set of skills from a parent or guardian or that they simply memorized relationships between materia medica and disease symptoms that had proved efficacious. As Mariamu illustrates above, her process of becoming a healer developed through her own relationship with Binti Dadi's *majini,* not through her experience of working beside Binti Dadi each day. I often only learned of relationships between healers and elders who had knowledge of medicine and a therapeutic practice after detailed conversations with the healers about the broader history of their lives. Healers did not offer descriptions of these relationships in their own narratives of becoming a healer. They did not present these lineages as evidence of their credibility or the efficacy of their medicine.

While healers did not deny their early experience with elders who had therapeutic expertise, they also did not find these previous relationships with living kin particularly salient to their process of becoming a healer. Instead, visions of shades said to be raised by *majini* were central to healers' descriptions of how they learned medicine. In these visions, *mahoka* not only identified medicine but also revealed where it was located, how to use it, and who to treat with it. Practical information about plant, animal, and mineral substances became therapeutic knowledge only when it was displaced through the death of an accomplished elder and re-presented to the next generation by the ancestral shade. Through the *mahoka*, building expertise becomes a process of revealing, not of remembering. The production of therapeutic knowledge depends on a process of the healer forgetting so that expertise can be reconstituted in relation to the need of a particular patient at a particular moment.[19] "Knowing" is not about acquiring a store of information that a healer can draw on in order to address discomforts and disabilities; "knowing" takes place when a healer has cultivated his or her sensitivities to a range of relations with human and nonhuman actors and welcomes useful revelations at critical moments.

These sensitivities are elaborated through the physical and temporal rhythms of a healer's body. In one sense, the body of the healer is transformed through its relationship with the *majini* that climb on it. This makes it possible for the healer to transform plant, animal, and mineral substances into medicine. The efficacy of therapies often depends on the location of the healer's body in time and space as she is collecting and preparing a remedy. Healers articulated this to me through their descriptions of the very specific ways some *dawa za miti-shambaa* needs to be approached. For example, Mama Libongo talked of going on excursions to harvest plants when the moon was in a particular phase and of collecting some medicinal plants at certain times of day. To prepare one of her therapies Binti Dadi had to wrap sticks in a cloth to make a tool to harvest the medicinal plant she required because her *majini* had instructed her not to touch it with her hands. Binti Dadi collected leaves from another type of plant, with her mouth. She chewed the leaves and spit the resulting mash into a white cloth. She would squeeze the juice from the leaves into the red and burning eyes of patients who complained that they were losing the ability to see. This medicine was never to come into contact with her hands, but it had to be mixed with her saliva. Binti Dadi had to be naked when gathering the plants for another medicine that protected infants when their parents had decided to renew sexual relations earlier than tradition would allow. The *majini* of each healer dictated how to gather medicine as well as which plant, minerals and animal substances the healer should gather. The medicine had to be collected exactly as the *majini* prescribed in visions or through dreams.

The specificity of the *majini*'s instructions is why two healers might treat similar symptoms with different leaves and roots. Different *majini* could reveal different medicine for the same symptoms. Indeed, even the same *majini* could insist that a healer use different medicine for the same symptoms in different instances. Most important, even if several healers used the same organic materials, the processes through which they made them into medicine were likely to be different, sometimes dramatically so. In addition, other healers cannot replicate the aspects of a healer's body that transform herbal substances into medicine. Mama Libongo, for instance, could not make use of Binti Dadi's saliva. In the same way, a healer's hands are considered to be a powerful part of a treatment. There were times, for instance, when Binti Dadi insisted that she bathe a child rather than permitting the mother to do so, particularly if the child was very ill.

Majini do not climb on all bodies; all of the persons they do climb on are not capable of building sophisticated, productive relationships with them; and not all *majini* disclose medicine. More often than not, in fact, those who contend with *majini* do not become healers, as Mama Shaibu's story illustrates. *Majini* climbed on her head and removed threatening *uchawi* that had been used against her. Although she now hosts these *majini,* they cannot instruct her in therapies. Alternatively, *majini* that know medicine have climbed on Mariamu, but they are not yet interested in making her into a healer. At times, she receives visions of medicine that she must go out to collect to relieve her own discomforts, but when she begins to feel better, the visions grow less frequent. The *majini* do not show her how to treat others, only how to take care of her own needs, or, more accurately, only what she has to do to please the *majini* that she is hosting.

Mama Shaibu and Mariamu demonstrate the uniqueness of each person's relationships with the *majini* who climb on them. The fact that *majini* inhabit a human only opens up the possibility that transformations occurring in their human host will constitute healing knowledge. Nonhumans, whether described as *majini, mahoka, mashetani, wadudu,* or *wanyama,* orchestrate the realization of this possibility in two ways. First, they reveal medicine to a person through dreams, thus establishing the body of their host as a site for human-nonhuman connections and making it into a therapeutic force through their presence. Second, the nonhumans provoke a moment of healing by bringing together the healer, the medicine, and the person needing treatment.

Receiving Patients

The image of an *mganga* in pursuit of patients produces laughter among people on the Makonde Plateau. Healing expertise, after all, is not a product of human will. Binti Dadi and Mariamu invited me into such laughter as they reflected on our interactions with a man and his story of *majini.* One afternoon in February 1999, a stranger stood outside the fence of Binti Dadi's compound, calling and chanting. When Binti Dadi welcomed him in, he paced up and down through the center of the compound, continuing to sing nonsensically. Occasionally, he spun and skipped in something like a dance. Eventually he put his request to Binti Dadi. *Majini* had climbed on his head. They were playing with him and telling him to treat sick people. He wanted medicine from Binti Dadi in order to treat these people. He asked specifically for *ndonya,* a woman's lip plug. Only very rarely does one see an old woman on the plateau wearing an *ndonya* today, and as they have given way to different fashions, salvaged lip plugs have become a valuable medicine. Binti Dadi obliged this man and shaved off a piece of the *ndonya* she had stored with her other medicine. They agreed that as he got paid for treating people with this medicine he would in turn pay Binti Dadi. His *majini* had supposedly told him to heal, but instead of telling him where and how to find medicine in the bush, they had told him to go to other healers to collect particular medicine. This process of gaining access to therapeutic remedies would be acceptable for someone just beginning to build expertise if his *majini* brought him people that needed to be healed and told him how to use the medicine. However, a month or so later, we heard that this man was selling medicine in the market of a town about seventy kilometers away. Mariamu and Binti Dadi laughed. Mocking him, they told me that a true healer did not have to take medicine from others and go to sell it in a market. A true healer does not have to look for people to treat. A true healer, they said, sits at home and people seek her out for advice and assistance. A healer's *majini* will bring those who need treatment to the healer's home.

Fatu Chenga spoke of a person's arrival in her compound as causing her to "remember" a dream in which she treated this particular person. She said that the *majini* brought her the knowledge of the medicine that the person needed so she would be prepared for the moment when she was called on to heal. Similarly, I have known Binti Dadi to collect particular plants before anyone had arrived with an affliction requiring them. Her *majini*, she said, had told her to collect a particular medicine for someone who would be arriving soon. In these tellings, the agents of healing (e.g., the *majini*), the objects used to heal (e.g., the medicine), and the subject who is healed (e.g., the patient) are brought together, developed in, and transformed by the healer. Therapeutic expertise is not mastery over a particular set of objects or the application of a body of facts; it is the ability to subtly and productively facilitate multiple connections—between humans, between nonhumans, and among humans and nonhumans. The efficacy of any particular medicine is deeply located in time and space. Or stated differently, efficacy is the result of generating the temporalities and spatialities of healing in the process of collecting, rendering, and administering *dawa za mitishamba*.

Making Space

Healers' narratives about the intimacies of becoming a healer illustrate how the process of building therapeutic expertise is entwined with the process of making the spaces and places of healing. While the duration and the specifics of the "initiations" were different for Fatu Chenga, Binti Dadi, Mariamu, and Mama Libongo, all generated the boundaries and borders of healing spaces through their movements. Fatu Chenga's initiation began when she was young and continued over several years as she learned medicine and therapies from the older healer who facilitated her cure. She would stay with this healer for short periods of time, and she returned repeatedly. Mariamu stayed with one healer in his compound for two years before her mother finally stole her away.[20] When she did find a healer who could help her, she returned to his compound again and again as she learned to negotiate her relationship with her *jini*. Mama Libongo's *majini* forced her to move her compound to another village. The command made by Binti Dadi's maternal grandmother's *mahoka* that she "go and write *kombe*" propelled Binti Dadi to travel in ways that constituted the therapeutically meaningful distinctions between human and nonhuman spaces. Likewise, the demands of *majini* that a healer collect or cultivate *dawa za mitishamba* enact spatial distinctions that are critical to treatment. Trips that healers make in dreams show them where and how to collect medicine in their waking travels. All the women I describe in this chapter became healers through the movements, displacements, and emplacements that constitute spaces for healing, places of therapy.

The making of therapeutic space is not incidental; healing power is in significant part an effect of ordering worlds. Relations between humans and nonhumans are most frequently mediated through the demarcation of spaces. As healers travel, their movements establish distinctions between human and nonhuman realms. The most basic distinction marks off the "bush" as the place of nonhumans—spirits, devils, animals, and all others.[21] The category of therapies known as *dawa za mitishamba* holds up the bush as iconic. The colloquial play of words in which people on the plateau call *mashetani, majini,* and a range of nonhuman actors *wanyama* (animals) or *wadudu* (little bugs, insects) emphasizes the bush as the place of nonhuman activity. The search for plant, animal, and mineral substances propel a healer away from her *kinu* (the mortar in which she pounds her medicine) and into the bush. When the healer collects medicinal plants her movements away from her home and back again mark the boundaries between home and bush, between domesticated space and that ruled by nonhumans. Her movements not only describe the layers and depths that constitute human and nonhuman realms but also order them in ways that will, they hope, help sustain life.

One afternoon I found myself implicated in the creation of these generative movements when Binti Dadi asked me to help her harvest old batteries from her garden plot. A woman had arrived with chronic headaches. Binti Dadi used a sharp razor blade to cut small nicks in the skin (*kuchanja*) at her temples and between her eyes, where her head hurt the most. Then, asking the woman to remain in her courtyard for a moment, Binti Dadi took me outside the gate to the nearest of her home-based garden plots. In between the rows of corn she dug up two old AA batteries. Opening the batteries, she took out the sticky black carbon from inside. She brought this substance back to the woman waiting in her courtyard and smeared it into small cuts on her head. The enactment of therapeutic ontologies through movements constituting the bush outside in relation to the home inside are so central to the efficacy of treatments that she insisted on this move even in relation to a synthetic substance.

Being and Time

Initially in my efforts to find evidence of the transformation of therapeutic knowledge over time on the Makonde Plateau, I collected not only the oral narratives of elder healers cited above but also recitations of common folktales. My hope was that folktales might provide information about changes in the patterns of healing practices, the roles of healers, or the meanings of medicine on the plateau. In so doing, however, I still privileged a temporal understanding of the past. I structured my search for history as an investigation of a moment that was separate from the present. I was looking for traces of a previous time. Only when I attended more closely to practices could I see the *majini* and *mahoka* as the radical historians of healing in southeastern Tanzania. Healers' knowledge, their dreams, their power to see those doing evil and to know how to cure their damaging effects, and their ability to transform substances into medicine all come from interactions with those who have passed away. The return of the dead is integral to the production of healing knowledge and to continuity in the practice of medicine over time. Through healing, the past is differentiated not temporally but spatially. The difference between the present and the past is the difference between embodiment and disembodiment.

This engagement with the dead, this reframing of time and telling, casts healers as ambiguous, potentially dangerous actors. They are rarely fully understood and never fully trusted. One of the first things that Jambili Hamisi told me as we were walking through the bush identifying plant medicine outside his village of Chitandi was that "if you know how to cure, then you know how to kill." His truism echoes a Kiswahili proverb, which affirms that one who can cure or protect against *uchawi* can also harm or conduct *uchawi*.[22] Chinduli also cautioned that a person should never pick up a book of *faraki* medicine when angry because he will end up killing someone. You should wait, Chinduli advised, until you cool down to handle such a powerful book. The dangers inherent in the knowledge that healers obtain—and therefore the ambiguous position of healers themselves—are partly a factor of their entanglement with the dead.

For most people, rituals and medicine cultivate a distance between one who has died and the loved ones he or she had left behind. Medicine separates the living from the dead. During funeral rites, for instance, medicine is typically given to the spouse and children of the deceased or, if death has taken a child, to the mother of the deceased. This medicine is used to help loved ones forget or to prevent them from remembering too much (*kukumbuka sana*). The dead are said to want to stay close to those with whom they made their life. The living find such bonds to be dangerous. Medicine, then, protects the living from being plagued by the dead; it prevents the dead from holding on too tightly to their relatives. Although ways of marking death, mourning loved ones, and burying kin have changed over time, particularly through the incorporation of Muslim practices (and, to a much lesser degree on the plateau, the incorporation of Christian traditions), medicine continues to be used during funeral ceremonies on the plateau.

Forty days after a funeral, the family of the deceased holds another gathering called an *arobaini* (meaning forty in Kiswahili) that marks the end of their mourning. Medicine again works to initiate another level of separation between the one who has died and his or her immediate family. They support "forgetting." While *arobaini* ceremonies on the plateau today are conceived of as an Islamic tradition and are framed through Qur'anic study and prayer, their resonance with other traditions in other areas of the country suggests that African practices that mobilize medicine to help the living forget the dead may have merged with Islamic ritual. For instance, *arobaini* on the Makonde Plateau resembles a practice Weiss describes among the (mostly Christian) Haya in northern Tanzania called "finishing death" or "forget[ting] the dead" (1997). *Arobaini* is rather like this celebration that also involves a great deal of food for all who had previously gathered at the funeral. This kind of ritual "forgetting," Weiss (1997) writes, "is an effective and productive means of assuring the dissipation of onerous hierarchical connections, and [the] dismantling [of] the restrictive holds that the dead have on the living" (172). The living use medicine to purposefully interrupt the efforts of the dead to maintain excessively intimate attachments with them.

Although healers help distance others from the hold of the dead, they do not always preserve this distance themselves. Indeed, healers cultivate relationships with the *mahoka* of people from long ago. While ancestral shades may make demands on anyone, healers respond to these demands differently. They use medicine to engage with the dead; they "speak" with *mahoka* and follow them into nonhuman worlds. The *mahoka* that came to Binti Dadi, for instance, first escorted her into the sea to witness other nonhuman creatures (*wadudu*) and the vast worlds beyond the normal capacity of the human eye. The healers described above have developed their sensitivity to the desires of nonhuman actors who "rule" them. Their agency—knowing medicine and receiving patients—is shaped through these relationships. Healers are commonly viewed with ambivalence because their therapeutic practice does not maintain the boundaries between humans and nonhumans that are central to other aspects of their social world. Their power comes from their ability to collapse this distinction; it comes from their ability to mediate this well-purified divide.[23]

For those who are not healers in Tanzania, the separation of humans and nonhumans has been formalized. Medicine, rituals, prayers, and other technologies and techniques close down communication between loved ones and their dead. Distance from the dead enables time to be experienced linearly. For those who have been freed from "remembering too much," the past is accessed through memories, stories, and traditions, not through regular interaction with ancestral shades. Healers take on the task of re-membering, of embodying the ancestors and of housing the *majini* in their effort to heal. In so doing they maintain a more purified, linear experience of time for their patients as they themselves disrupt and reorder that temporal construction. Particularly the *mahoka*—but also the Islamicized *majini* or the more general *mashetani, wanyama,* and *wadudu*—initiate times that come and go as they appear and disappear.

Knowledge Practices

The ability to heal comes from the differently lived spatial temporalities of healers and nonhealers. Healers experience time through their interactions with *mahoka* and *majini*; that is, they experience temporal difference through distinctions between the embodied and the disembodied even while they cultivate an experience of time for others by making distinctions between the past, present, and future. How does one investigate experts who frame their own lives, the development of their expertise, and the efficacy of their practice through spatial temporalities that differ from the linear time they shape for others? How does one follow such actors through what Mol and Law (2002) have called "tidal times"—those that move back and forth, come and go? It is in the back and forth, the trajectories these movements imagine, and the expertise that depends on both the presences and the absences of these nonhuman others, that healers come to understand maladies, know about medicine, and catalyze the transformations that define their care.

As I discussed in Part 1, national and international efforts to craft a modern traditional medicine by transforming the relationship healers have with medicine has thrown into relief questions about what it means to know and to be an expert. The biographical narratives of healers—their stories of becoming—account for some of the ways knowledge and expertise are articulated on the plateau. The healer is located in the web of technologies, economies, religions, desires, and nonhuman histories that constitute healing. Each healer has his or her own repertoire of medicine that is shaped, case by case, in relation to patients, *majini,* and a range of other nonhuman actors. Even if two healers use the same plant, animal, or mineral substances, the conversion of these substances into medicine will depend on the *nguvu ya fundi,* the strength of the healer.

My investigation into healing practices on the Makonde Plateau was shaped by the characteristics of the practices I observed and later participated in. I began my research in 1998 by working with a wide range of healers. After a few months, however, I realized that I would have to study a select group of healers more thoroughly and begin to place them in relation to one another. Although I could not easily study therapeutic knowledge in the aggregate because its production did not generate procedures, protocols, or other ways of seeing from the outside, I could read healers and their therapies against one another. This process involved collecting the histories of particular healers as well as examining how they established themselves, how they gained credibility, and how they evaluated and worked with each other. In addition, by focusing my attention closely on a loose group of healers, I could compare the ways each healer prepared and administered medicine, evaluated treatments, and described patients. As I was increasingly woven into the fabric of healing on the Makonde Plateau, however, I was no longer allowed these multiple assignments. The healers with whom I was working told me in a variety of ways that if I wanted to learn more medicine and more treatments, in essence if I wanted to continue my research, I would have to choose one person with whom to study. In the end, I worked very closely with Binti Dadi and her daughter Mariamu. I came to be known in relation to Binti Dadi. From the market in Newala where I bought supplies to the photo shop in Dar es Salaam where I developed my pictures, people would greet me as Binti Dadi *mdogo,* little Binti Dadi. This locating of me and my research has shaped my exploration of the kinds of locations and positions from which therapeutic knowledge is made on the Makonde Plateau.

This approach was not immune from, or separate from, the politics in which therapies are practiced in contemporary southeastern Tanzania. It seeks to make these politics an explicit object of investigation. One way to situate knowledge practices is to locate them among other knowledge practices—to show their relationship to coexisting efforts to order, structure, and materialize the world—and to reveal the relationships among the multiple orders, structures, and (im) materialities that result.

5

Traditional Birth Attendants
as Institutional Evocations

In the 1980s and 1990s, many developing countries, including Tanzania, trained traditional birth attendants (TBAs) as part of their efforts to meet health development goals.[1] The integration of lay midwives into the national health care service was one response to the challenges of providing "health for all" in countries that did not have enough professionally trained biomedical staff. TBAs extend the reach of the clinic by going to pregnant women in their homes. As part of the outreach and referral services of state-supported medicine, TBAs trouble any easy opposition between biomedical practitioners and traditional practitioners. They embody the complexities of different modes of ordering bodies, times, spaces, and actions.

The Tanzanian Ministry of Health frames the training of TBAs as a process of transferring knowledge from biomedical staff to lay midwives. TBA training workshops raise the awareness of trainees (or what the national health service calls "unskilled hands") by sensitizing them to different threats, dangers, procedures, and responsibilities. Development efforts to "transfer knowledge" to those who assist women birthing at home have a distinct agenda. National and international support for lay midwifery seeks to stabilize a biomedical vision of the of the body of the pregnant woman, the fetus, and those things that threaten them during home births. Training TBAs turns out to be about establishing intimate links between the trainee and biomedically salient objects of knowledge; expertise turns out to be about the relationships trainees successfully establish with these objects. By initiating new forms of therapeutic organization, social relations, ethical commitments, and links with scientific networks, TBA training programs (attempt to) shift both the subjects and objects of "traditional" healing.

In southeastern Tanzania, the way TBA training workshops have been organized contradicts the rhetoric that casts TBAs as a strategy for tapping into indigenous resources for national and regional development. Efforts to train TBAs and incorporate them into the national health care system have called into being a new type of home birthing authority, a practitioner who works under the sign of tradition as an ally of state (biomedical) health care. This chapter examines how the introduction of specific technologies, clinical infrastructure, patterns of interaction, and situated values have shaped one contemporary form of traditional knowledge and expertise.

Training Tradition

The official narratives of governmental and nongovernmental organizations working in Tanzania portray TBAs as features of an indigenous landscape.[2] They are always already there. The Ministry of Health in Tanzania, following the approach of the World Health Organization and other international health development organizations, justify their programming efforts through assertions that TBAs existed in indigenous communities before national and international efforts to ally them with formal biomedically based health care systems.[3] Such rhetoric depicts TBAs as a timeless resource that can be tapped to address newly defined problems. As the principle nursing officer in the Ministry of Health stated: "It is a well known fact that TBAs have been in existence since Adam and Eve."[4] In contrast, a German gynecologist who had worked for six years in Mtwara, located in southeastern Tanzania, told me that "there never were TBAs here!" The UNICEF project and Safe Motherhood Initiative that she had coordinated and implemented at a regional level were supposed to draw on women recognized as experts by their communities, women who had helped to deliver many or all of the babies in a particular village or area, but this doctor's complaint reveals that such women were surprisingly hard to find.[5]

Many of the TBAs with whom I spoke in southeastern Tanzania elegantly articulated the history of their own positioning. They saw themselves as experts created through international public health development projects. Amina, a TBA in Newala District, spoke directly about the making of TBAs as biomedical actors who were distinct from those "old women" who had attended births in the past. Traditional midwives for Amina have historically been linked with the clinic. She discussed this with me in a conversation about the births of her own children. Amina, like many of the TBAs with an active practice on the plateau, bore her children in a clinic. She was born in 1947 and had her children in the 1960s and 1970s. She asserted: "During this period, there were no *wakunga wa jadi* [traditional midwives]—meaning very long ago. During this period, *wakunga wa jadi* were in clinics." While Amina told me that she first learned the ways of attending to a birth from her mother-in-law, who had delivered many children, she asserts that long ago there were no traditional midwives. She framed her own efforts to become a TBA as a process of developing a profession rather than as a response to a call or a continuation of a family tradition.

Similarly, Anna Selemani, another TBA, presented traditional midwifery as something that a person could enter *only* through an official state-recognized TBA training program. Traditional midwifery was not a generic or timeless category of practice that included specialized skill in attending to and caring for women giving birth. Anna alerted me to this distinction when I asked her how many women she had assisted.

> Before the training occurred, I helped three pregnant women, three only; and now that I have entered into traditional midwifery (*ukunga wa jadi*), I have [helped] four pregnant women. And [of the first three] all of them have given birth to children that still have life and of those [four whom I helped after the training] three of their children still have life up to now.

In describing her work, Anna drew a primary distinction between what had happened before she received training and what had happened after she was trained. Only after the TBA training does she refer to her work as "traditional midwifery." Only after instruction by clinical staff working for the Ministry of Health did she enter the field of *ukunga wa jadi*.

Bibi Salum reiterated this point by emphasizing that having experience with attending births does not translate into professional expertise. She learned how to assist women in childbirth by watching her mother. When she began delivering children herself, Bibi Salum would call on her mother if she had problems or questions. Yet she did not see her mother as a TBA. Bibi Salum said her mother "only went around" (*anaendaenda tu*). Although her mother assisted women while they gave birth and was by all accounts quite competent in dealing with a range of complications, Bibi Salum did not consider her mother's work to be *ukunga wa jadi* (traditional midwifery) because she had not received TBA training from nurses or nurse-midwives.

The story of Bibi Salum's mother points to the existence of talented, experienced women who were judged by communities to have gained significant proficiency in delivering babies. Healers on the Makonde Plateau indicated that before the turn of the century some Makonde women specialized in assisting others with unusual or problematic deliveries. Particular therapies for problematic pregnancies and techniques to facilitate difficult births have traveled from generation to generation. Colonial records indicate that in the 1930s mission doctors began to seek out women who attended home births (Langwick 2006). These initial efforts recognized the *wakunga*'s role in addressing complications during births in rural homes. TBAs, however, have emerged in post-independence Tanzania as a new type of health worker who specializes in "normal," uncomplicated home births. In fact, TBA training separates the work of attending births from the work of prescribing or preparing medicine. Only hospital medicine is to be used. Any complication signals TBAs to refer a woman to the health clinic.

The distinctions that Amina, Anna, and Bibi Salum make in describing their training and expertise turn the meaning of "traditional" inside out. The word traditional (*jadi*) as it is used by these TBAs does not refer to long-established practices that have been handed down through the generations. In fact, it erases the history of these older practices in order to facilitate new alliances. When I asked Halima what she learned in TBA training, she told me: "*Ni nilijifunza kuzalisha kitaalamu, tofauti na habari za jadi*" (I learned to cause the birth in an educated way, different from the ways of tradition). As Verran (2002) argues, transferring knowledge "requires and generates possibilities for transformation through encounter" (178). TBAs as such did not exist before they were trained. Transferring knowledge about birth from clinical settings to homes requires a new hybrid actor. The TBA has been called on to fill this position.

Choosing Allies

Although individual health practitioners or hospitals have reached out to local midwives, the post-independence Tanzanian government only developed a national plan to incorporate TBAs into health care education and delivery in response to the WHO's report on the Alma-Ata conference of 1978.[6] In 1983, the new guidelines for primary health care incorporated TBAs into the "expansion of reproductive health" to "marginalized areas" (WHO 1983). When the Safe Motherhood Initiative extended into Tanzania a few years later, the Ministry of Health developed guidelines for TBAs. The first government-sponsored training workshops took place in 1987. The Tanzanian government set the particularly ambitious goal of training two TBAs in every village in the country. Public health planners saw TBAs as locally available resources and imagined that they could also be used to help address health problems beyond labor and delivery. The Ministry of Health envisioned TBAs leading grassroots efforts to teach women what "reproductive health is" and how to take steps that would lead to "good reproductive health."[7] By 1995, 21,467 TBAs had been identified and 6,854 had been trained.[8] Amina, Anna, and Bibi Salum count as three of these trained TBAs. In 1997, the Ministry of Health stated with confidence that "with the support of the formal health system these indigenous practitioners can and will become allies in organizing efforts aimed at improving the health of the community including maternity care."[9]

To date, the training of TBAs within the Ministry of Health has been carried out by the maternal and child health and family planning unit. The original stated goal of this training aligned with that of the Safe Motherhood Initiative: "to reduce child and maternal mortality by half by the year 2000 through increasing the number of supervised deliveries under hygienic conditions from 53% to 80% by the year 2001" (Ministry of Health 1997).[10] Training materials envisioned

TBAs joining doctors, nurses, and health care development workers in an effort to reduce maternal and infant mortality rates. While statistics established the basis for evaluating the ultimate success of TBA training, advocates pointed to the cultural acceptability and localized authority of TBAs as evidence that the new program would be viable. Joyce Safe, the principal nursing officer and head of the Department of Nursing in the Tanzanian Ministry of Health, argued that traditional midwives should be trained and included in national health care plans because "communities like them, trust them, and use them" (1992, 7).

Nurse-trainers identify potential participants for their TBA courses by asking village leaders for the names of local midwives.[11] National guidelines set out the basic criteria for selecting women for TBA training. Because village leaders play a role in choosing appropriate women to become TBAs, trainers hold special sessions for them during TBA courses. The current Ministry of Health training manual for village leaders and implementers defines a *mkunga wa jadi* or traditional midwife as follows:

> A traditional midwife is usually a mature woman with the ability to assess a pregnancy, to give advice and to deliver children [and] who is acceptable to and well known in the community in which she lives. Her skill in delivering babies has either been inherited or is the result of work [as a midwife] for women who are giving birth at home.

In addition, the Ministry of Health asks that *wakunga wa jadi* who are chosen to take the TBA lessons have completed at least Standard 7 education (primary school); they should have basic reading and writing skills. They should also not be too old; the ideal woman is between thirty-five and fifty (Kaluma 1992).[12]

The selection of those who will participate in TBA training workshops is a cause for broad debate and rumor. I have heard healers and midwives as well as nurses and public health professionals complain that village leaders sometimes choose their own mothers, wives, daughters, and other kin rather than other women who have more experience with assisting women in childbirth. Even when village leaders choose women who meet the criteria outlined by the Ministry of Health, the nurse conducting the training may have difficulties. "Mature" women with skill and experience in delivering babies tend to have developed their own ways of practicing. The Ministry of Health officials worry that, "[s]ome of the practices done by TBAs are of no benefit or harm to maternal health but others are downright dangerous."[13] Officials fear that older TBAs will not fully replace their traditional practices with those recommended by their biomedical training program. In particular, older, experienced *wakunga* may continue to use "potentially dangerous herbs, food taboos, or delivery techniques that may cause harm to the woman or foetus" (Safe Motherhood Task Force 1992). National health care reports and plans characterize the activities of untrained *wakunga* as useless at best and fatal at worst. The ministry's programs require trainers to perform a delicate balancing act: they are instructed to capitalize on the theoretical "trust" that "communities" place in *wakunga* while minimizing or eliminating practices that are considered to be dangerous from a biomedical perspective.

Turning when Hailed

Contemporary theories of subjectivity have drawn inspiration from Athusser's (1971) description of interpellation, in particular his popular example of one who turns when hailed by a police officer. Being a subject of and subject to the law, he argues, means that a person instinctively is compelled to turn toward the officer even when confident he or she has done nothing wrong. Below, I account for TBAs as subjects of biomedical discourse. I describe how they have turned when hailed by biomedicine. Yet ethnography complicates the process of subjectification and raises questions about agency. For instance, not all women with skills and experience in attending births respond to an opportunity for biomedical training. Not all *wakunga* felt that it would be desirable or suitable to attend a TBA training course. Those who best match the WHO definition of a traditional midwife appear to be the least likely to be interested in the training workshops. Such instances expose the limits of biomedical discourse and illustrate what I call in the introduction the life of other kinds of power. One popular midwife declined an invitation to attend a TBA training course because she viewed it as "job training." She argued that she already knew her work and suggested that a younger woman should be sent in her stead. She did not see the information shared at TBA training courses or the credentials associated with such trainings as useful. Another older midwife echoed these sentiments, stating she had delivered hundreds of babies and did not need to be lectured by young nurses. She sent the woman who was apprenticing with her in her place. Such reactions may be particularly strong on the plateau; nurses in the maternity wing of the local hospital suggest that women still often give birth to their later children alone or with only the help of a relative. Furthermore, specialized local knowledge about birth grew out of therapies to address complications with conception, pregnancy, labor, and delivery. It involves herbal treatments. It calls on nonhumans. Healers are loath to relinquish their knowledge of herbal remedies and their techniques for addressing problems in childbirth in exchange for an active link with their local dispensary.

Who then are the women who have responded to these internationally funded and nationally implemented calls for trained TBAs? Most women who have become involved with rural dispensaries as TBAs have also chosen to use clinical services at many other times in their lives. More often than not, in negotiations with kin, they advocate for the use of biomedicine over the medicine of an *mganga* (traditional healer) in their personal affairs. These women often preferred, for example, to give birth to many of their own children in clinics. Angela, who had finished her childbearing by the time she was selected to participate in a TBA training program, carried six pregnancies to term and gave birth to six healthy children. The first three of these she delivered in the Luagala mission hospital located in the neighboring district to the east. She bore the last three of her children in the Mnyambe dispensary where she is now learning her practice. When I asked her why she chose to give birth to her children in clinical settings, she told me that this was "during the time before she had been entrusted with being a midwife."

A woman's age does not predict where she will choose to give birth. Halima, a young woman working in her hometown of Lengo, had had three successful pregnancies by 2000. Her first two girls were born at home because the family lived far away from a clinic. Their births were attended by a traditional midwife, *mkunga wa jadi*. Before the last child was born, however, Halima moved. As a result, she chose to deliver her third child in the Lengo dispensary. Bibi Salum, who was originally from Kitangari, moved to the smaller village of Nanyamba "a long time ago"—four children ago. She has been married three times and now has seven living children. Of her ten pregnancies, one ended in miscarriage and two of her children died. She delivered her firstborn at home, although when he became ill, she took him to the hospital for treatment. Unfortunately, he was one of the children who died in infancy. She gave birth to the other eight children in a clinical setting, either at the Ndanda mission, where a German Benedictine order has a hospital, or at the dispensaries at Majeni or Nanyamba.

Georgina was born in Mnyambe. She went to school there and she married there, although her husband is a native of Newala. Georgina married in 1961, "the year of independence," she told me. She has had eight pregnancies. Two of the pregnancies ended in miscarriage (at two and five months, respectively). She does not know why these miscarriages occurred. The two male and four female children who are alive today are all grown and have their own children. She gave birth to her first child at the St. Mary's Mission Hospital in Newala. She delivered the next two children at home, and she delivered her last three children at the Mnyambe dispensary. When I asked her why she delivered some of these children at home and others in clinics, she explained that her husband traveled a lot (*bwana anatembeatembea*). During his sojourns, she and the children would sometimes stay with her in-laws, who live far from any dispensary or hospital, and she would give birth at home. However, if she carried her pregnancy to term in a place close to a clinic, she would deliver her child there. Life circumstances shaped where she gave birth, but her narrative consistently privileged the hospital.

Saidia Dibaki was born in Mikumi. Her parents, who are still alive, live there. She carried ten pregnancies to term and gave birth to all of her children in a clinic setting. In fact, she delivered all but the last child at the Ndanda mission hospital.

She delivered her last child at the Mikumi dispensary. She feels that hospitals are better equipped to deal with complications during birth. She told me: "I like hospitals very much, because of problems of pregnancy and problems of infants when they are born." Six of Saidia's children were alive when I interviewed her in 2000. Four children had died when they were "big" (*wakubwa*). Her first child died when she was three years old. She had taken the little girl to the Ndanda mission hospital when she contracted a fever (*homa tu*), and she died in the hospital. The second one had a troublesome blindness (*kipofu kilisimbua*). She took him to the hospital as well, but "the pills were defeated" (*vidonda vimeshindwa*). This child was one year old when he died. She took the third child to Ndanda when he developed large sores or ulcers. He died when he was only six months old. The fourth child who died was a *vijana* (young adult) with children of her own. This daughter had a sickness of the heart (*mgonjwa moyo*); it pounded hard and quickly (*gonga sana*). She too went to the Ndanda mission hospital seeking treatment and was admitted, but despite treatment, she died.

Amina was born in 1947 in Mkundi, a village in the neighboring district to the west. She has been married three times. Her first two husbands were from Mkundi. Her third husband brought her to Malatu, where I met her and where she is now practicing as a TBA. She has carried eight pregnancies to term. All of her children were girls and seven of them died young. Her first child was stillborn. To deliver it, a nurse in the hospital applied a vacuum. She describes the experience:

> This was my first, she came. She was still heading towards the stomach. Then they were entering by hand. This mama Sister indeed she removed the dirtiness by an electric machine. There, they laid a trap. Still, this child, she came out by herself slowly. She was already dead.

Three of her other children died from measles (*surua*). One had diarrhea. Another "did not have any blood." She received a blood transfusion, but the blood "would not go in." Another fell in a hole. She scrambled out, injured and afraid, and went home and hid. The other children eventually told Amina what had happened. She found her daughter and sought treatment, but the child died. Amina's account of the tragic loss of so many of her children reveals that she frequently sought the help of clinical medicine. She had one fetus removed from her womb through the application of a biomedical technology (a vacuum). She described the deaths of three of her children in terms of a biomedical disease entity—measles. Another received a blood transfusion—a procedure that required the equipment and expertise of clinical staff. She took all of these children to the hospital or clinic when they were ill or hurt. Amina repeatedly used biomedicine for herself and her loved ones. In addition, Amina delivered all eight of her children in the mission hospital at Lulini, Masasi.

I have presented a few birth histories here in some detail to illustrate that these women engaged with institutionalized biomedicine before they entered into the field of traditional midwifery. They demonstrated some faith in clinical staff and their skills by turning to a hospital or dispensary when they were giving birth and when their children and loved ones were in danger. This faith is characteristic of a modern subject. While my sample is not statistically significant, I would like to suggest that the histories of these women nevertheless point to something significant. Those who bore their children between five and thirty years ago delivered their babies in clinical settings more often than they did at home. Given that today half of all births in Tanzania still occur in the home (and this figure is likely a low estimate), it is noteworthy that the women who chose to become TBAs, especially those who maintain an active connection with their local dispensary, are more likely than the general population to have given birth in the clinic. When actors in the biomedical system select and train potential allies, I would like to suggest, they favor women who are interested in and can grow relatively comfortable with the world of biomedicine. The TBA training aims to turn their faith into recognition of and responsiveness to the entities and objects salient to biomedical treatment.

New Ecologies of Traditional Expertise

The Tanzanian government's desire to form an alliance with "indigenous practitioners" in order to facilitate their goals related to reproductive health necessitates a second order of alliance-building. Public health officials as well as the nurses who run the training programs envision their alliance with TBAs as grounded in a common commitment to combating the nonhuman actors that they see as the causes of the infections and hemorrhages that threaten the lives of mothers and newborn children. Training TBAs means positioning them to identify and eliminate things that biomedical practitioners deem dangerous during pregnancy and childbirth. The primary emphasis in these efforts is on preventing infection; that is, on preventing the work of microbes.

The TBA training manuals outline the process through which indigenous practitioners can be transformed from an "untapped resource" to "allies of the health system" in the eyes of the national health care system and its international advisors. In 1998, the Ministry of Health discarded a cumbersome training manual and with the assistance of the World Health Organization and UNICEF designed and printed three new training manuals. The first outlines and organizes the preparation of the people who teach the nurses who will in turn run the training sessions for the TBAs. The second manual includes a series of lessons that structures the training sessions for TBAs. The third manual educates village leaders about the work of TBAs and illustrates how to translate these commitments into broader government goals.[14] Each is designed "to improve the education (*elimu*), knowledge (*ujuzi*), and skills (*stadi*) of traditional midwives (*wakunga wa jadi*) who give reproductive health care for mothers and youths in order to reduce death and preventable diseases to maintain good health." Together, these three manuals map out a strategy for coordinating and aligning traditional and biomedical ways of facilitating birth.

De Laet (2002) argues that "alignments are possible only if new social and technical transformations emerge or, to say it slightly differently: the work of alignment is, in its nature, a feat of socio-technical transformation" (3). The process of refiguring indigenous practitioners within a network of clinical care involves establishing trainees to participate in a set of relations with biomedical objects of practice. For instance, TBAs are taught about germs and bacteria and learn about sterilization procedures, razor blades, and latex gloves. Ideally, those who complete training workshops will use these biomedical implements in home birth settings. In a very practical sense, transferring knowledge requires changing or expanding which things people think about, act on, or mobilize and what kind of relationship they have with these things. The new sociotechnical configurations promoted by the TBA training course establishes a new ecology of expertise, an environment that makes the modern TBA possible.[15]

Below I describe the first seven lessons of the current TBA training manual. They catalogue the objects and entities that TBAs must recognize. The attention to pedagogy in each lesson reveals the kinds of relations the Ministry of Health hopes to forge between TBAs and biomedical objects and entities.

Lessons for the Instruction of Traditional Midwives

1. The Beginning of Pregnancy

The manual begins with a lesson on menstruation and how pregnancy happens. The training manual separates the content of the lesson (on the left side of the page) from instructions for activities the trainer and the TBAs should pursue (on the right side of the page). The left side, for instance, contains explanations about menstruation and describes how a woman's egg and a man's "seed" unite to achieve a pregnancy. The right side directs the trainer to begin talking in the plainest language possible about the organs of reproduction. The trainer is instructed to ask workshop participants what menstruation (*hedhi*) is, then listen to the TBAs' answers in the "words or idioms that are used in their areas about menstruation." Then manual instructs trainers to engage the women trainees in a discussion of what happens when a girl gets her menses for the first time. It tells trainers to ask the TBAs to explain when a woman can get pregnant before they review the biomedical or "correct" account of menstruation and pregnancy. It advises trainers to consistently stress those aspects of the participants' responses that are "accurate" (*sahihi*).

This first lesson demonstrates the importance of biology in any alliance with biomedical practitioners concerned with childbirth. Good allies must not only connect pregnancy with menstruation, they must also know these processes to be a product of specific reproductive organs. Although the manual tells the trainer to solicit other accounts of pregnancy early in the proposed discussion, this is done to establish which "beliefs" need to be corrected. The goal of this lesson is to make assertions about the biological entities involved in pregnancy and childbirth and to establish the biological body of the pregnant woman as foundational to care. Before the training session addresses various birth practices, the trainer must discuss local ideas about conception, correct the misconceptions of participants, and establish the "facts" for trainees.

2. The Care a Pregnant Mother Needs

The second lesson opens by instructing trainers to ask the TBAs how one recognizes a pregnancy. The lesson then guides the nurse-trainers and TBAs through five signs that a woman is pregnant: the woman stops menstruating or skips periods; she may throw up or feel nauseous, especially in the mornings; her stomach and breasts will get larger; a health care provider will be able to feel parts of the "child" (*mtoto*) during a pregnancy examination once it is large; and the child will begin to "play in the stomach" (*kucheza tumboni*) once the pregnancy has reached four or five months. The most often repeated point in this lesson is that a woman needs to go to the clinic if she thinks she is pregnant. This lesson asserts that TBAs must encourage women to go to the clinic during pregnancy, get regular prenatal visits, and know when they need to seek additional treatment. Its explanation of prenatal visits outlines what will be done at the clinic: the pregnant woman's weight and height will be measured, her urine will be examined, and her blood pressure will be checked. Additionally, her body will be scrutinized to see if there are any problems: her eyes, tongue, and fingernails will be observed for signs of a reduction of blood (anemia), her stomach will be examined to assess the uterus and position of the child, and a nurse will listen to the heartbeat of the child in the mother's stomach. In other words, things are done in the clinic that TBAs cannot do in their own homes. They do not have the scales, rulers, stethoscopes, blood pressure meters, and urine test kits needed to complete these tasks. At this point, the manual stresses how important it is that pregnant women get vaccinated against tetanus, obtain medicine from the Maternal and Child Health clinic to increase their blood (iron), and get protection against malaria (e.g., antimalarial drugs and mosquito netting). This lesson distinguishes the activities and abilities of the TBA from those of the nurse-midwife in a prenatal clinic. It depicts the TBA as someone who can crudely recognize pregnancy but is incapable of knowing much about that pregnancy. It emphasizes that the health centers are full of equipment that make clinical practitioners sensitive to variations between different pregnancies. In this scenario, TBAs are encouraged to take on the responsibility of ensuring that all women go to the clinic regularly during their pregnancy to seek out practitioners with greater expertise than the TBA herself has.

In addition to the routine activities of a prenatal visit, the manual identifies certain "clues of danger" (*vidokezo vya hatari*) that should indicate that a pregnant woman is to be sent to a clinic immediately. Clues that can be seen during pregnancy are fever, vomiting in the mornings more than once a week, vaginal bleeding, swelling of the legs and hands, convulsions, bad-smelling green vaginal discharge, bad pains in the stomach, pale skin under the eyelids, severe pain when urinating a little, and severe headaches. These lessons do not encourage TBAs to administer any sort of therapy. For all of these problems, the manual instructs trainers to emphasize that a woman needs the help available at the local clinic. TBAs are taught the clues that there is a problem with a pregnancy and the signs that indicate that a woman might have a dangerous birth later and therefore should plan on giving birth in the clinic or a hospital. Such an approach teaches TBAs to be outreach workers and troubleshooters for the biomedical health care system, but it does not teach them to be healers. The Ministry of Health envisions TBAs as an educated, alert, on-the-ground referral service.

3. The Hygiene of the Mother and Child

The objectives of the third lesson are to "debate" (*kujadili*) the importance of cleanliness during pregnancy and birth and after birth; to "debate" how infections occur; to explain the kinds of illnesses that are contagious during a delivery; to explain how to prevent contagions from being transmitted to the TBAs, the parent, or the child; and, finally, to demonstrate the hygienic activities that will be necessary during a delivery. This lesson is also an introduction to microbes. This is the first lesson that addresses the practices of TBAs. The TBA needs to understand the importance of cleanliness so thoroughly that she can teach pregnant mothers about contagions and hygiene. The lesson stresses the need for a clean body, clean clothes, a clean environment, and the frequent use of soap. At this time, trainers are guided to warn TBAs against delivering a child while lying on the ground. The mother should ideally be lying on a bed or a cot. If neither of these is available, then a clean grass mat is better than the bare ground. The manual also warns that the newborn should not be washed with water and soap immediately after its birth, although a cloth can be used to reduce the oil that covers its body and to remove the "dirtiness." Focusing also on the bodies of the TBAs themselves, this lesson emphasizes that a midwife's nails should be cut and clean when she is assisting with a birth. Her hands must be washed in boiled water and the instruments must be sterilized in boiling water. Trainers encourage TBAs to wear clean and new disposable gloves, particularly if she has a wound. A previously unopened razor blade is also required to cut the umbilical cord of the newborn child. Nothing at all should be put on the umbilical cord. The manual stresses that any local practices involving the smearing of ashes or cow dung on the cord after it is tied are to be discouraged. Trainers review diseases that might be transmitted (*kuambukiza*) during pregnancy: tetanus, AIDS, syphilis, illnesses of the vagina or uterus, infections of the umbilical cord, and diseases in the eyes.

One wonders if the women in the training sessions see a connection between these insistences or if they seem like a random, even an overwhelming, list. Whether or not the TBAs can see this material as coherent would hinge on whether or not they understand how bacteria work in the body: the manual introduces TBAs to the existence of microbes through instructions on how to control them. It enlists TBAs in the fight against bacteria, parasites, and viruses, but it gives them minimal biomedical information about how these entities operate in the body or what the consequences of their presence can mean for a mother and her baby.

4. Feeding the Mother and Child

The fourth lesson instructs trainers to emphasize the importance of a varied diet and sufficient food for women who are pregnant or breast-feeding and for children who are weaning. It associates the lack of certain vitamins and minerals in a woman's body with particular problems or dangers. For instance, a decrease of blood (anemia) can cause death or low-birth-weight children. A deficiency of Vitamin A affects the development of the child in utero and leaves both the mother and the newborn vulnerable to diseases. Insufficient iodine can cause a stillbirth or a miscarriage or it can slow the development of the fetal brain. The manual presents a lesson organized to teach women to eat enough food, to eat three times a day, to eat lots of protein, and to eat a mixture of foods that includes fruits and vegetables. It says that women should eat more food than usual while breastfeeding and advises TBAs to tell pregnant women to eat salt with iodine. It emphasizes that pregnant women should take "medicine to increase blood."

The manual instructs TBAs to encourage women to give newborns the first milk right after the birth and then to continue breastfeeding for at least two years. Trainers are to state emphatically that children should drink breast milk and only breast milk until they are four months old. After that, children should be weaned

slowly. The manual states that new foods should be introduced in small qualities and one at a time. In the workshop, TBAs learn the importance of vitamins,
minerals, and breast milk and take on the responsibility of promoting them.

5. Danger Signs during and after the Birth Process
That Require Immediate Action

This lesson guides trainers through a discussion of eleven different potentially
dangerous situations during and after a birth. The manual presents the signs
and symptoms of each and explains the immediate first aid the TBA should
administer. Each of these crisis situations ends in a referral to the hospital.
Building on lessons one and two, a particular biological body compatible with
biomedicine is further elaborated through illustrations of emergencies during
and after birth. The TBAs' obligations to women in a medical crisis are determined in relation to the obligations of the clinic. Good allies know where they
fit into the operation and they know when to move people and things along. The
manual stresses how important it is for TBAs to know the limits of their powers
and their proper roles.

6. Giving Birth

This chapter organizes and lists the things that are needed during a birth: ten
pieces of clean cloth, soap, *dodoki* (a natural fiber or a corn cob from which the
kernels have been removed), boiled water with salt, a new razor blade that is not
unwrapped until it is needed, clean string, clean clothes for the newborn, a large
vessel filled with boiled water, a vessel in which to clean the newborn, clean sheets
or cloth for the bed, a plastic or paper bag, hot and cold water, a clean grass mat
or bed, sugar or honey to make a hot drink during the birth, and a separate clean
space for the birthing process. This lesson discusses the importance of arranging
for these items to be available during the birth and of caring for them and using
them. The manual instructs the nurse-trainers to emphasize the need for cleanliness throughout the birth. The narrative divides childbearing into three steps:
(1) the beginning of labor until the neck of the uterus has opened completely;
(2) pushing until birth; and (3) delivering the placenta. The manual guides the
TBA to put the newborn on the mother's breast after the placenta has been delivered. It stresses the importance of this first milk in helping the child grow well
and build immunity to diseases. It notes that if step three does not follow closely
on the heels of step 2, this initial feeding may also help the woman expel the af-
terbirth. In addition, the manual makes the point that the TBA must record each
birth and each death of a mother or newborn during childbirth. It also stresses
the responsibility of TBAs to persuade the mother to send her children to the

clinic for vaccinations and checkups. The mother, too, should go to the clinic to have her health assessed and to receive family planning information.

Good allies are not merely a referral service. They must also recognize, care for, and know how to use the tools that allow them to contribute to the fight against microbes. This pivotal lesson presents the elements of the clinic—the pieces of the clinical network—that must be moved into the home in order to ensure "hygienic," "safe," and "healthy" deliveries.

7. Care of the Mother after She Gives Birth

This lesson draws on the concept of *arobaini* (literally, forty) to distinguish a period of time (about forty days) during which mothers and infants are due special care. The manual lists things that should be kept clean: the body of the mother and infant, the breasts and genitals of the mother, the clothes and cloth used during birth, the mother's hands and nipples when she is breastfeeding. The lesson introduces the need for a series of vaccinations for the child in the first years of life and postnatal examinations for the mother. In the language of the manual, the clinic becomes a resource for women and children with any problem. TBAs are agents who will hasten (*kuhimiza*) the mother's use of the clinic. They are expected to move women and children toward clinics, biomedical practitioners, and pharmaceuticals.

The importance of tracking births and deaths is also impressed upon TBAs in this section of the manual. A notebook with the express purpose of registering births and deaths enters the narrative in this section. TBAs are taught how to construct a chart that includes the name of each child in whose birth they assisted, his or her sex, whether he or she is alive or dead, and any problems that may have occurred during birth. Trained TBAs are instructed to take these notebooks to the nurse at their local dispensary at least once a month. In this way, the manual prioritizes information and demonstrates how TBAs can collect data about home births that could assist in the compilation of national statistics.

The lessons that follow these seven units instruct TBAs about particular actions they should take during the delivery of a child and the care of a mother and a newborn. Each of these lessons further articulates the ideal relationships TBAs should have with the biomedically relevant actors, both human and nonhuman, that have been introduced. Cleanliness, soap, and boiled water play a prominent role in many of the scenarios the manual depicts. Lesson eight focuses on infant care. TBAs are told to direct mothers and newborns to a local dispensary or maternal and child health clinic for antenatal care and they are prepared to promote vaccines. Lesson nine guides trainers through the details of immunizations: the disease entities they fight, the tools used to administer the vaccines, where on the body they are administered, the immunization schedule. Lesson ten introduces various methods of birth control: the Pill, Depo-Provera, condoms, and sterilization. Lessons eleven, twelve, and thirteen introduce TBAs to topics that are likely to seem even more tangentially related to birth: AIDS, venereal diseases, adolescence, and statistics.

Scholars of science and technology studies insist that knowledge is tied up in natures and cultures of things-in-themselves. The act of transferring knowledge cannot be captured through descriptions of ideal cognitive processes; transferring knowledge necessitates structuring encounters between human and nonhuman actors. The training manual attempts to structure such encounters. Birth attendants are repeatedly instructed to use soap, to wear gloves, and to sterilize the string they use to tie off the umbilical cord. The instruction nurses provide encourages new relations between the trainees and the microbes, gloves, standardized progressions, and other technologies that are critical to healthy births.

The Manual Performed

The Ministry of Health incorporated the revised TBA training manual into an initiative designed to educate 32,000 TBAs during the period 1997 to 2001 and integrate them into the formal health care system. Public health care policymakers intended the manual to be an active partner in the transfer of knowledge, the building of alliances, and the making of TBAs. The central office of the Ministry of Health sent copies of this training manual to every provincial and district hospital and health center. The TBA manual and its companion pieces are used in all governmental and some nongovernmental TBA training workshops.

Two things dramatically affect the way that training proceeds and the effect of the manual: (1) who attends the training and (2) how many days are allotted for the training. The TBAs I met in training workshops or to whom dispensary staff directed me differed in important ways. Most significantly, some were elderly women in their seventies or eighties who had been helping other women give birth for many years. Others were younger, in their late thirties or early forties. This latter group typically had not assisted with very many births—perhaps they had helped a relative or two. Workshops proceeded differently depending on which of these cohorts dominated the particular gathering. The training officers commented repeatedly on their struggles with the older women, emphasizing how slowly they learned and how they resisted change.

Perhaps the most significant sticking point in relations between these older women who had been assisting women in childbirth for many years and the nurse-trainers was the use of remedies made from plant, mineral, or animal products. Historically, on the plateau, family members called *wakunga* to births only when problems arose. Medicinal treatments were a critical part of *wakunga* attending to women who had complications during labor. In the Newala District Hospital, nurses complained of midwives who used herbs to stimulate or speed up contractions. Some had seen pregnant women arrive hemorrhaging as a result (they believed) of these herbal remedies. In the training workshops, nurses might describe these experiences to illustrate their conviction that TBAs should not administer herbal therapies to pregnant women or newborn children.

During one training I attended—which was co-conducted by the maternal and child health coordinator for Newala District and the assistant coordinator for the Rural Health Center in Kitangari, a village about thirty kilometers north across the Makonde Plateau from Newala town—a trainee ventured to initiate a discussion about medicine. It was after a fairly long and rather unexciting exchange about healthy food that she seized the opportunity to change the subject to this issue that was more central to her practice. The TBAs were crowded on a set of grass mats on the floor and the trainers were seated in wooden chairs behind a table in front of them. The trainers had divided the topics to be covered between themselves, and whoever was responsible for a given section rose as she began talking. When one of the speakers was emphasizing an issue she would at times pace back and forth in front of the trainees sitting on the floor. A toothless *bibi* with a delightfully mischievous grin nudged me secretly and then asked the nurse-trainer in an innocent voice, "How about the use of medicine (*dawa*)?" The sense of boredom in the group vanished, and the TBAs grew more animated. Medicine, the nurse answered, is not bad. However, a woman should always go to the hospital to get safe, clean (*safi*) medicine. She should not use the medicine of *wakunga wa jadi* (traditional midwives). The nurse-trainer told the TBA trainees that medicine was good, but only modern hospital medicine. Then she resumed her lecture on nutrition. The trainee did not follow up on her concerns, but the women on the floor whispered jokes to one another. The older woman had made her point. She had introduced the topic that most divided people in that room. Each had her own feeling about the use of medicine and her own set of skills. All of them knew, though, that a TBA's commitment to use hospital medicine brought her into a network of biomedical actors that included doctors and nurses who discouraged the development of relationships with *majini, mashetani,* and ancestral shades. Younger women tended to look at this prospect favorably. Older women tended to have a stake in these other relationships.

Stacy Leigh Pigg (1997b) has critiqued similar TBA trainings as promoting "a biomedical ideology not simply through the theory of physiology and disease causation they teach but also through the insistence in the format of the trainings themselves that the physiological be clearly separated from social, moral, and religious concerns" (247). Although some nurse-trainers may know a great deal about practices in the areas where they are conducting training sessions, "the structure of the training plan restricts them to emphasizing the medical message of the formal curriculum over local ideas, practices, and conditions" (243). These restrictions and marginalizations emerge as the trainers perform the manual. There is no room in this training for an extended or subtle discussion of lay midwives' use of medicine. Even if some nurse-trainers have used herbal remedies themselves and even if they privately harbor more complex and ambiguous critiques of nonbiomedical medicine (Langwick 2008a), in the space of the training their responses prevent any meaningful exchange. This foreclosure is perhaps most dramatic when the length of the training has been shortened and the nurse-trainers feel the pressure of time.

While the manual's intent is demonstrated through its layout, dialogue, description, and illustrations, its effects cannot be too easily assumed. For instance, although the manual was designed to be taught over a course of thirty days (ideally spread over two months), in my research, I found that most TBAs had participated in training workshops that lasted for only one (or perhaps two) weeks. Some were only two days long. District staff complained about the difficulty of finding the staff time, transportation, and necessary funds to implement even these shorter training workshops. While the manual remained the primary source for trainers, on-the-ground dynamics meant that the trainers often had to combine several lessons and even skip some lessons.

In some areas, district officials felt that the time and expense of training could not be justified year after year. Local dispensary staff in these areas sometimes chose to develop ad hoc and improvisational methods of training TBAs. In such cases, they still used the manual as a reference book. Nurses might select particularly evocative pictures from the manuals to catalyze discussions. The manual still prioritized the most important forms of relation, but it played a more minor role in structuring interactions. In order to examine the sociotechnical communities the manual not only envisions but also helps enact, I turn to the histories of TBAs in the district of Newala and examine their experience of training and their current practice.

Becoming a TBA

The relationships of individual TBAs with their local dispensaries and dispensary staff vary greatly. Yet it is the specifics of these dynamics that define what constitutes TBAs in practice. In the remainder of this chapter, I draw on interviews with eleven TBAs drawn from over half of the wards with rural dispensaries in the Newala District. Their accounts begin to situate the official vision of TBA training workshops articulated in the training manual with the broader range of encounters that generate TBAs.

Saidia Dibaki began to practice through an apprenticeship with her mother. She had assisted many women in childbirth before she ever attended an official TBA training course. In fact, she has lost track of the number of babies she has helped deliver (*nilifanya kazi hiyo hata hesabu sijui*). Saidia (whose name means "help" or "assistance") started this work in 1960. In her tracing of the development of her expertise, she claims to have learned in "all places" (*mahali popote*). The most significant influence, however, was her mother, whom she describes as an exceptionally intelligent woman and a skilled midwife. Saidia learned to attend births and to assist with complicated births by observing her mother and by following her careful instructions. Saidia's mother, in turn, had learned these skills from her own mother, Saidia's grandmother. Saidia expressed her intention to teach these midwifery skills to one of her children, Somoyo. Of all the TBAs I met who continued a close relationship with clinical staff, Saidia was by far the most skilled. In addition to being familiar with salient traditional remedies, she knows techniques for determining the position of a fetus in the womb and how to turn it if it is "sitting badly." In fact, her husband bragged to me that the Ndanda mission hospital (widely regarded as the best hospital in the southeastern part of the country and one of the best in Tanzania) asked her to demonstrate how to turn a fetus inside the mother and position it for birth. He added that during this demonstration she managed to turn a breeched fetus in three minutes.

Saidia remembers that after she had her children, someone came to her and asked her to do the business of the government (*mambo ya serikali*).

> When I arrived here [at the Mikumi dispensary], the village leadership had decided that it was not necessary for me to continue my work outside the affairs of the government. Therefore, it was preferable [that] I become a lay midwife in order to improve traditional care.

Strikingly, Saidia explicitly advocated that all women give birth in the hospital. She claimed that when she is attending a birth, if she sees that the woman will not deliver for at least two hours, then she encourages her to go to the clinic to deliver. Perhaps her advanced skills made her overstate her attachments to the clinic, for she did still work as a midwife. TBAs, unlike healers, read me as part of the clinic and as a representative of development and modernity. Their statements to me reflected their own ambitions about their relationship to the forms of professionalism and modes of authority that attachments to biomedicine could offer. Saidia's claims countered any suspicions that her knowledge of medicine and other "traditional" skills might generate among her biomedical counterparts.

Angela Mnichalewa's story is very different. When the Mnyambe village leadership selected her to become a TBA, she did not know why. When I talked to her four years later, she told me only that "they have their committee." She was pleased with this opportunity, however. Angela had no previous formal or informal experience. She never knew her grandmother, and her mother died when she was very young, so Angela does not know if they ever did such work. In 1996, at forty-five years old, she started going to the Mnyamba dispensary to meet with the nurse-midwife and to learn the skill of delivering babies. As far as she knew, there was no formal plan of instruction or any set curriculum. Four years later she had delivered approximately fourteen babies. She had not yet attended an official training, but for two years she had gone to the dispensary in her village every Monday, Wednesday, and Friday to receive lessons from the clinic staff. She considers herself—and the clinical staff considers her—a TBA. The other TBAs in Mnyambe and the surrounding villages (six in all) were also supposed to come to the clinic for additional instruction. However, they did not make it as regularly as Angela did. The environmental health officer commented that "none of the *wakunga* have shown up. Each for their own reasons has not come to [the] meet[ing]. They are going their own way one by one." Angela, in contrast, has not gone "her own way." She is maintaining a very consistent and involved relationship with the dispensary and the clinical staff there. The dispensary staff praises her as someone who takes her work seriously (*kutilia*) and who has shown the heart to get down to work and become involved (*alionyesha moyo wa kujituma*).

Somoye, a young woman, is an extreme example of this new cadre of health practitioners. Before attending a training workshop for TBAs, she had never assisted a woman giving birth. Indeed, even at the time of my interview with her, she had not attended a home birth. Instead, she accompanies women to the clinic, where they give birth. Sometimes the nurse-midwife calls her when a woman is in labor in the dispensary. Unlike the other TBAs with whom I spoke, Somoye explains her job as assisting the nurse-midwife, not as assisting the mother. Somoye's only professional interaction with older women who have attended home births for many years was to visit one of them in order to tell her about the benefits of hospital birth.

Each of these women has been trained in a different way. Saidia, who knew a great deal about assisting birthing women before attending a TBA training workshop, was quickly regarded as an expert after this training. Even hospital staff sought her out. Angela did not have the opportunity to attend an officially organized training workshop but has "studied" for several years with the nurses who work at the dispensary in her village. Somoye attended a TBA training workshop without having any prior experience. After this training, she has continued to assist nurses in her local dispensary and to learn about midwifery from them. Although only one of these women neatly fits the ideal description portrayed in the documents and training manual discussed above, each of them is known throughout her village and by local dispensary staff as a TBA. This professional distinction owes more to the woman's commitment to recognizing and responding to salient biomedical agents (described in the TBA training manual) when attending births than to the extent of her experience in assisting with home births.

General Practice

Despite the claims by (or hopes of) the international community, TBAs on the Makonde Plateau still do not systematically attend to women during pregnancy or after the birth. They focus their work on labor and delivery. When labor begins, the husband or a relative goes to the *mkunga*'s house and accompanies her to the birth. TBAs reported that they only assisted women within their own villages. Rarely, if ever, do they walk for more than half an hour to assist with a birth. Women on the plateau do not gather a large number of people around them while they are giving birth. In addition to the TBA, only the pregnant woman's mother or mother-in-law is likely to attend the birth, especially of a first child. Occasionally a sister may join this small group. The husband sits outside. The TBA leaves the new mother and her infant child a few hours after the birth. Whether or not a TBA has attended a full, official training or participated in a more improvisational exchange with clinical staff, three activities enact their allegiance with biomedicine: (1) mobilizing tools; (2) marking time; and (3) recording births. Woven together tightly with normative statements, TBAs' accounts depicted the forms of gathering, talking, and writing that good "traditional" allies engaged in.

Tools of the Trade

TBAs began descriptions of how they work with the process of producing a rough-and-ready home clinic. Their explanations of the work required to prepare the birthing space centered on the things that linked them with modern medicine: soap, gloves, razor blades, beds, and prenatal cards. A strong focus on hygiene and the objects and procedures used to ensure hygienic conditions framed TBAs' reports of their midwifery practice. Water, soap, and the requisite hand washing play a prominent role in preparing the TBA and the home for a birth. When they talked about cutting the cord, many trained TBAs asserted that a clean, unused razor blade should be used. Each detail in their narratives reflected the TBAs' understanding of what makes a good ally in the eyes of the biomedical community.

The bed or rope cot on which a woman delivers emerged repeatedly as a significant detail, the mark of a trained TBA. Anna emphasized the importance of preparing the bed.

When I arrive there [at the house of the woman in labor] I ask her about the state of the labor. After some time, well, I know that right then she is ready to give birth. At this time, I examine her again. I use the method of lying down. Well, indeed, I look for and bring a bed; I carry other heavy cloth; I make up the bed. I lie her down there in the bed. We are telling her to start to do work. Then after we tell her to do work, we tell her if you feel [that] the pains have calmed down, [then] don't try to push [because] you will finish your strength [too] early.

The mothers and grandmothers of the women living on the plateau today would have given birth sitting on a mat, holding on to both of their ankles, their backs leaning against a wall of their home.[16] In the TBA training manuals, sitting this way on a mat is discouraged "for reasons of hygiene." The idea of sitting on a dirt floor while giving birth represents the antithesis of modern, hygienic, safe births to many biomedical practitioners.

Cloth and coverings appeared in TBAs' descriptions of births in other ways as well. As Halima explained:

Eeh! After we tie the child then we preserve this part of the child well, then I dress the child in good clothes, then we put her/him in a good place. Then we take care of ourselves. I finish removing the placenta, then afterwards the mother goes and washes herself well. Then I protect her well with clothes which are necessary for the mother to be protected.

Halima's colleagues also stressed their attention to changing their own clothes, using freshly washed cloth during the birth, and dressing the newborn in clean cloth.

Clinical records as well as birth kits shape the TBAs' practice and explicitly mediate their relationship to the clinic. Angela claimed that when she enters the home of a laboring mother, she first asks to see the card on which the nurse-midwives at the clinic have recorded the pregnant woman's status during her monthly prenatal visits.

SL: What treatment do you use or what steps do you follow to help a pregnant woman?

Angela: When I arrive there, I start first by reading the hospital card. If I read the card in the place where they have written that [she must go to] the big hospital, well then I do not play [around]. I only insist that "You should now already [be at] the big hospital because my midwife, together with all of the government, has [said so]." If they disagree, I explain more to them. I explain to them [the consequences of] not going to the place where each thing is done that you know you want. You may feel bad, but there, she [the nurse] gives an exam in order that she does not fail [to cure you]. Because first . . . the first part of the care when we give each other these explanations, it is of use when a person has given birth to six or five children. Indeed those are the ones who need [the explanations]. They go to the big hospital. Therefore, after being there, indeed, we have a way to help her.

SL: Then . . . ?

Angela: Then for others who are typically there when I arrive, first we discuss with each other. After discussing they [the mother and her family] instruct me and I tell them that I will arrive after a certain number of hours. After this I start to examine her. If I examine her, I wear gloves, which I have instructed the family to buy.

SL: Therefore, it is necessary to have gloves?

Angela: Eeh! This is necessary.

Both of the objects that Angela describes—the prenatal card and the gloves— establish her as an actor allied with clinical care. While the gloves indicate efforts by TBAs to protect themselves and the mothers and newborns they are assisting from "new" threats such as AIDS, the prenatal card works to place her within the hierarchy of institutionalized health care. Angela articulates this most explicitly when she refers to the nurses' aide at the dispensary to whom she reports as "her midwife." The relationship became even more evident when Angela described how she instructs pregnant women who belong to one of the state's high-risk categories to deliver in the hospital, where "we have a way to help." This "we" includes Angela and the nurses' aide.

Tools situate cooperating TBAs in relation to their clinical colleagues. Both TBAs and biomedical staff argued that ideally, the only difference between a home birth supervised by a trained TBA and a clinic birth supervised by a nurse-midwife is the range of technological options with which they can respond to complicated cases. All the TBAs I spoke with asserted that there was no difference between giving birth in the hospital and giving birth at home in instances where no complications arise. While a mother might go to the hospital if she is bothered (*usumbufu*) or if she simply prefers the hospital, the critical difference in her delivery will be visible only if there are problems, for in the clinic there is more equipment. Tests can be run, blood can be given, operations can be performed, and vacuum pumps can be used to help babies through the birth canal.

Marking Time, Facilitating Experience

After establishing the setting for their midwifery practice, TBAs examine the laboring woman, looking for signs they can use to interpret and describe her condition. Their assessments of the labor require a careful marking of time as well as visual and tactile investigations of the woman's body. TBAs evaluate the state of a woman in labor by examining the patterns of her contractions. To

facilitate a "proper" birth experience, they coax a woman's body to adhere to
a "standard" pattern of contractions. To this end, TBAs decide when a woman
should lie on her side versus when she should lie on her back, when the mother
is "ready," and when she should push.

Bibi Salum moves smoothly in her narrative from the objects used to facilitate a safe birth to her authoritative role in dictating the actions of the laboring
mother.

> In order to help a pregnant woman, if there is soap there, I wash my hands. I put
> on gloves. If the birth is near, then I tell her, "Lie here. Not yet, mama." I go for
> water and soap. I watch and watch her. I probe inside [with my fingers]. I watch.
> [*Ninaingiza. Natazama.*] Then, I say, "Push hard mama, you are ready." [*Sukuma
> sana mama uko tayari.*] I sit until it calms down, until the child comes out well,
> or does not come out well.

All of the TBAs with whom I spoke stressed their role in determining when the
child is about to be born—that is, when the mother "is ready." Halima notes:

> I sit here [in front of the woman]. What I will do is I watch how she is lying there
> and I examine how she is. I watch her there lying on her side. Then I examine
> her. I explain the stage at which she has arrived. . . . After delivering this child,
> I cut the cord well.

TBAs organize their observations and the laboring women's experience into a
productive progression through stages of birth.

The skills and sensitivities that the training workshops cultivate aim to increase the TBAs' ability to interpret the experience of the laboring mother. Amina
mentioned checking the lower eyelids of a laboring woman to determine if she
is anemic. Clinical staff members encourage TBAs to refer "a woman without
blood" to the hospital for delivery.

> The treatment that I use: when I go there, first I wash my hands to remove all the
> dirt, then there I find the place that she is lying. I inform her of the news. I tell
> her, "I am sorry, mama." And I examine her eyes. In the examining of her eyes,
> if they are very white, I tell this mama that there is no blood. Then if I find sud-
> denly the child wants to come out, well then, I help her. I carry a *kanga* [cloth]
> and place it on her origin/beginning. When the child wants to leave, "O.K.,
> mama, do your work." She opens herself [gives birth] there. My *nyuzi* I cut five
> times; another I leave the mother; two I shake for the child. Now, I cut the cord
> here. Well then if the placenta is there, work has come. Indeed this mama helped
> herself by herself. She bends down. She does this [and] slowly it comes out. I
> carry clean clothes that have been washed by guests. I give the child these and
> put him/her aside. I do not wash him/her with water. This is the treatment that I
> do during this time.

A primary role of the TBA is to mark time. The TBA seems to regulate actions through a process of negotiating the desires of various actors, which in Kiswahili are depicted as the child "wanting to be born," the mother "opening herself," and the health professionals "causing the birth." The TBA is the one who tells the mother when to "do your work." She may also hold up time, as we will see below, by instructing a mother not to push until other assistance has arrived.

Auditing for Development

National health care programs included TBAs in an effort to reduce the number of unhygienic births and reduce the maternal mortality rate. This alliance is bound by numbers. As a result, counting and record keeping have become prominent features of TBAs' descriptions of their practice. Even TBAs who have not yet had the opportunity to attend a full training have learned from the nurse-midwife in their local dispensary how to keep track of the births they have assisted and the problems they have experienced. Bibi Salum, for instance, started writing the names of the children she delivered as well as their date of birth, sex, and any complications during the birth in a notebook a long time ago. She exclaimed that the nurses at the health facility in her village "gave me happiness here. They said it was necessary, if you have worked as a midwife causing a person to give birth well, you must write them down. If you assist in a troublesome birth, write it down." These nurses at the Nanyamba dispensary instructed Bibi Salum after the training workshop she was supposed to attend was cancelled. They deemed record keeping the most immediately useful if not also the most critical skill for TBAs to learn, and they instructed her privately. Their concern with the accuracy of birth and death statistics and their hope that TBAs such as Bibi Salum might help in the collection of data has a longer history supported both by the WHO and other international health development organizations (Langwick forthcoming a).

Causing Births, Changing Skills

Of course, there is more to midwifery than moving objects around, talking, and writing down the names of babies born. Indeed, in Kiswahili, the work of a midwife is articulated with the causative form of the verb "to give birth" (*ku-zaa*). The midwife is said to cause the child to be born (*kumzalisha mtoto*). This form of expression highlights the transformative skills of a midwife. Through massage, herbs, and a range of therapies, midwives co-generate the actively birthing body. Biomedical training of TBAs appears to be moving midwives away from the role of a catalyst and toward a role in which they "catch babies." This is a broad shift away from practices that involve the midwife in labor and toward a lay midwifery that is limited to protecting an already active, basically self-sufficient, body from germs.

This transition is illustrated in the different skill levels of older and younger birth attendants and in the effect of training on the practices of TBAs. For instance, only rarely did a trained TBA such as Halima mention that massage might be used to enable a mother to deliver a large child. She noted:

> Most of all if I am delivering a very large child then I help her there in the path to the uterus [vagina]. I help her [Halima starts massaging the air demonstrating how she coaxes the vagina to stretch] . . . I help her . . . I help her until I help her again, a little not a lot. A little only.

Halima described how she massages the vaginal opening of a woman who is having difficulty delivering a large child. She uses massage before deciding to rush the woman to the local dispensary, where an episiotomy would likely be performed. The practical effects of training can sometime be best assessed at these critical moments that demand immediate action. When the birth of a healthy child and the survival and health of the mother are at stake, what expertise do TBAs draw on?

The most common problem TBAs faced was delivering a child who was "not sitting well." Older TBAs indicated that they had learned from their mothers or grandmothers how to determine the position of a fetus and how to turn a child in the womb. Younger TBAs who gained most or all of their midwifery knowledge from training by clinical nurse-midwives asserted that such complications must be referred to the health center. They often not only lacked these skills but were unaware that such a feat was even possible. Officially, biomedical guidelines indicate that TBAs only assist with "normal" births. To ensure that more complicated births occur in the clinic under the supervision of biomedical practitioners, clinical staff used their time in prenatal visits to advise women considered to be "at risk" for complications to arrange to deliver their babies in the hospital. As I discussed above, TBAs are also taught these "clues of danger" and are instructed to refer such women to the clinic. Regardless of these precautions, however, TBAs did sometimes assist at complicated births. Their training and their relationships with the local dispensary staff shaped their reactions.

Angela described two challenging incidents, both of which compelled her to call for help from health center staff. In the first situation, the baby was presenting in a posterior position—that is, face up rather than face down.

> **Angela:** The first problem, the first day, after examining the child [in the womb] this child was not sitting well as a child sits. For s/he had been putting his face forward first. Looking [around]; looking down. . . . While being born, we were looking at each other.

SL: Eeh. You saw the face first?

Angela: Eeh! Well, I said here I do not have the ability because this state is bad. It is not usual. It was necessary that I ask for help from the doctor, and truthfully, they examined her and they saw this child having put herself forward. Eeh, as a result there [in the clinic] she gave birth well.

The second incident she described had a number of complicating factors. Not only was the child "sitting badly" but also the mother was young and very short. Angela remembered that mothers who are fifteen years of age or younger and are under 150cm (five feet) tall are considered to be at risk of complications. In addition, Angela identified another clue of danger, and she articulated it in terms of a biomedical disease entity, asthma.

Angela: Well, I sat. Again another mother came. This one was having her first pregnancy. Therefore, first before preparing themselves to go to the hospital, she and her husband had to come to know [if it was time]. When I arrived, I judged that it was necessary to see the doctor because [she was suffering from] asthma which cannot be reduced by this work. [Also] I did not have the ability to help such a small child.

SL: Mmh. The mother was a small child?

Angela: Eeh! She was short, too.

SL: How old was she?

Angela: Eeh! She was sixteen, and she was short. For this, I said I needed additional help. But by then she had already begun labor. I thought it necessary that first the doctor arrive to help me. Before the doctor arrived the fetus was already pushing himself. The child was pushing in order to get out. This child was putting forward his hips. Eeh. Therefore, I told her [the mother] to leave it first. "Do not push." She stopped. When the doctor arrived he gave instructions.

The practical response to complicated births in which fetuses are not "sitting well" illustrates what it means on the ground to be a part of the medical system, to have been called up through the technological, economic, political, and ethical regimes of biomedicine. In such situations, TBAs call for clinical help.

Part 3

~~~~~~

Healing Matters

Why is matter the way it is?

—Exhibit in the museum of the Organisation Européenne
pour la Recherche Nucléaire (CERN), Switzerland

Method needs to be sensitive to the complex and the elusive.
It needs to find ways of knowing the slipperiness or "units
that are not" as they move in and beyond old categories.

—John Law and John Urry, *Enacting the Social*

6

Alternative Materialities

Beginnings are especially dangerous. Both traditional and biomedical practitioners consider the first years of life to be particularly vulnerable. *Mashetani* love to play with young children. *Wachawi,* those who wish misfortune, favor attacks on infants who promise to extend the lineage and bring wealth. High infant mortality statistics justify this special attention and biomedical care in the first years of life. People in southern Tanzania engage in a wide range of activities to protect the lives and ensure the strength of their children.[1] Kin rally medicine of the bush and medicine of the book around newborns to protect them from harm. Regular checkups and hospital treatment are free in government hospitals for children under five. How do these efforts distinguish forms of care, types of expertise, and kinds of threats? At what point do vulnerabilities come to be seen as dangerous, and by whom? How do practices of prevention and protection shape what is being threatened as well as what threatens?

Answers to these questions vary, of course—not only across cultures and over time, but also among healing practices. Driven by national and international goals to lower morbidity and mortality rates, biomedical institutions in Tanzania have tended to establish both administrative and practical divisions between the maternal and child health clinic and the rest of the hospital (the laboratory, the wards, the X-ray rooms, the consultation rooms, and the administrative offices). Routine practice in the maternal and child health clinic is clearly focused on specific threats to the well-being of young children. Steps that parents and healers take outside the hospital are more varied because these protective practices have not been institutionalized.

Medicine for protection is referred to as *dawa za kukinga,* literally "intercepting" medicine or "obstructing" medicine. Tanzanians distinguish substances that establish a medicinal screen to protect people from the effects of *mashetani* and *uchawi* from substances that remove devils or the filth of sorcery (*uchafu wa uchawi*) in the bodies of those who have already been afflicted. In Kiswahili, the verb *kutoa* (to make come out or go out) is used to describe the activity of a treatment designed to heal by removing the malady that is afflicting a patient. However, some *dawa za kukinga* intervenes before a person falls ill; this protective medicine is interposed between the person and the threat. As a result, this group of therapies is a particularly productive place from which to pose the questions: What is dangerous and to whom is it dangerous? The answers elaborate that which is on either side of the medicine. Like all boundaries, these medicines constitute that which they divide. They have the power to produce by demarcating, differentiating, and separating.

Throughout Part 3, I develop an argument that *mashetani* and other entities central to healing on the plateau become comprehensible—that is, are enacted—through a series of interactions that are structured through therapeutic practice. Entities that are active in and objects that are critical to healing develop as trajectories of events; that is, they emerge over time in the process of resisting and reacting to others (e.g., instruments, medicine, other objects and entities). Healers mobilize objects and enlist other entities to create occasions for interaction. Or, as Bruno Latour illustrated in his studies of laboratory experiments, aspects of the world that are invisible to the naked eye and unadorned senses take shape as they are put through the trials of experimental practice (Latour 1988; see also Latour and Woolgar 1979). These trials bring the things, the substances, the matter of the world into being. This insight, I argue, is not limited to scientific forms of knowledge. Therapeutic practice on the plateau can also be seen as making the body and threats to the body visible, tangible, and knowable through a series of trials. Each introduction of a medicine or shift in the therapeutic landscape offers the possibility that particular bodies and bodily threats will become better articulated; that is, that more characteristics will be attributed to them and more distinctions will be made to differentiate them. *Mashetani,* for instance, are growing more multifaceted on the plateau as they face the trials of newly emerging diseases. In contrast, Kimakonde entities such as *nadenga* and the *mahoka* have become less well articulated, and as a result they may be said to be growing less articulate.

This chapter describes objects of therapeutic attention as they are molded, shaped, targeted, defined, and circulated through both nationally mandated preventive procedures in the Newala maternal and child health clinic and through the protective treatments healers use to ensure the well-being of pregnant women and young children. My approach does not try to differentiate natural and social maladies by translating "natural" or "naturally caused" maladies as biomedical. Rather, it focuses on ways that semiotic-material practices produce objects for intervention and discussion in clinics and in the homes of healers. By empirically investigating how therapeutic objects are generated, I illustrate the ontological natures of entities that are central to healing in southeastern Tanzania and argue for the importance of pluralizing our conceptions of materiality. "If," as Margaret

Lock has urged, "we are to give materiality its due,"[2] then we must allow it the diversity we allow such concepts as agency, history, body, and modernity. The range of preventive and protective medicine typically available in contemporary southeastern Tanzania renders three primary objects of therapeutic practice—devils, jealousies, and future patients. The practices through which each of these epistemic objects is generated, elaborated, and maintained evoke different kinds of materiality and enact specific sorts of objecthood.

Distinguishing Maladies in Southern Tanzania

In southern Tanzania, as in other parts of East Africa, healers (and often those seeking treatment from them) express complaints about and changes in states of being through distinctions between maladies of God, maladies of Person, and maladies of Mashetani (Abrahams 1994; Feierman 2000; Janzen 1982, 1992; Livingston 2005; Reynolds 1996).[3] These distinctions are not rigid categories of complaints as much as they are narrative technologies through which stories may be created and experienced, and conditions may be described and engaged. They shape the trajectories along which unwanted transformations may be further altered, changed bodies further changed, and undesirable states converted into desirable ones. Implicit comparisons with biomedicine have led to ethnographic and historical descriptions of African cosmologies in which a division between the natural and the social is mapped over distinctions between God, persons, and *mashetani*. This section outlines the ways that these three categories are articulated in Newala and examines the effects of such mappings.

Maladies of God

Janzen (1982) translates part of this local triad through the dualism supported by scientific rationality. He equates "naturally caused" diseases with maladies of God.

> A crucial cosmological notion . . . is the distinction drawn in many Bantu so-cieties between "naturally-caused" (God-caused) diseases or misfortunes and those attributed to "human cause." The former misfortunes "just happen" or are "in the order of things" as, for example, in the death of a very old person or in an affliction with readily recognized symptoms and signs which respond to treatment as expected. (13)

For many years, Janzen's interpretation has been broadly accepted by those study-ing healing in Sub-Saharan Africa.[4] As this book focuses on the ways that the substance of the body and bodily threats (that is, the matter of nature) comes to be differently articulated and experienced, I am interested in the quotes in which

Janzen place his reference to "naturally-caused." Feierman (2000) has recently questioned the similarity between maladies of God and scientifically described diseases, arguing that efforts to draw such connections lead us away from the concerns of those who seek treatment from healers. His account, which includes the perspectives of both healers and those being healed, is an important step in an effort to narrate the subtleties of lives filled with both biomedical and non-biomedical therapies and scientific and nonscientific entities. In his rethinking of biomedical notions of the efficacy of medicines, however, he maintains that some maladies[5] are events "in the world of material objects" that can "be cured with medicines that work just because they worked, and not because of moral, religious, or social forces" (320). My analysis picks up where Feierman's work leaves off by continuing his poststructuralist critique and subjecting scientific understandings of matter (particularly in relation to disease entities) and the category of "diagnosis" to cultural and historical analysis.

On the Makonde Plateau, claims that maladies of God "just happen" have much less to do with an attribution to "natural causes" than with the practical understanding that they cannot be prevented or, more accurately, that a person cannot use medicine to protect him or herself against them. The only exception might be the protection immunizations offer for a few maladies. I would suggest that maladies of God share part of their history of emergence with the expansion of biomedicine in Africa. In colonial Tanganyika, the church made significant contributions to biomedical development, particularly in rural areas, through a range of missionary societies. When maladies are viewed as encounters, the ability to transform undesirable bodily states into more desirable ones indicates a relationship with the offending agent and therefore an ability to negotiate with it. Missionaries throughout Tanzania and in many parts of Africa understood this well and offered effective medical treatment as a way to win converts to Christianity (Comaroff and Comaroff 1997; Ranger 1992; Vaughan 1991). The phrase "malady of God" may suggest that certain discomforts and unpleasant situations were first systematically addressed by mission hospitals or are now best addressed by hospital medicine. The subtle workings of the category of maladies of God on the plateau have lead me to hypothesize that these maladies carry the categorization as being "of God" because at one critical point in the history of biomedicine in the region mission doctors were best able to negotiate with the threats that produced these maladies.

Much has changed, of course, since the days when missions ran the only hospitals on the Makonde Plateau. There are different distributions of maladies as well as different maladies to be healed and a population that is more familiar with the workings and diagnostic techniques of clinics and hospitals. It may also be that because maladies "of God" are the effects of inevitable, unintentional, or even random encounters with other entities in the world, they have been analytically conflated at times with "real" or "natural" biomedical diseases. For example, Tanzanians consider a number of complaints about red, swollen, painful eyes and the sudden loss of vision as well as worms in the stomach or other discomforts associated with water-borne agents to be maladies of God. However, on the plateau, people do not use maladies of God to refer simply to scientifically explainable ailments. The distinguishing characteristic of maladies of God is that there is no protection, no defense, and no way to avoid them if they come your way.

Healers seem less certain in their treatments of these maladies than they are in other cases. Their medicine cannot necessarily cure them. Fatu Chenga claimed that if a person plagued by a malady of God comes to her, she prays by using many different kinds of medicines. That is, she addresses the patients' complaints by trying different types of treatment and also by praising God. Chenga claimed that she found it easier to address maladies of Person (*uchawi*) than maladies of God. If a patient is sick by the will of God, she argued, one cannot be sure of the treatment. She can only try (*kujaribu*). She strives to "cause good luck" (*kubahatisha*) by praying to God. Although a dean at the nursing school in Newala who heard this assertion interpreted it as meaning that Chenga simply does not know how to treat these maladies, I would like to posit a different interpretation. Healers with whom I worked were willing to admit when they did not know how to treat a particular problem. In such cases, they would send a patient on to another healer.[6] Chenga was not suggesting here that maladies of God are not her specialty. Rather, she was saying that human beings cannot claim to reverse the will of God. A healer cannot "know" how to cure a person with such a malady; he or she can only "try." Medicine may be able to facilitate a cure in one person and not another. There is greater uncertainty and greater ambiguity with these maladies, not because they are more complicated or debilitating but rather because the healer is in a very weak negotiating position with God.

Throughout this chapter, I explore some of the vulnerabilities that can be treated by medicine in southern Tanzania. Obviously, one vulnerability is to the things of God. But the world in southern Tanzania is made up of many other things as well. Agents "of God" are the ones that the church acknowledges and accepts as threats. It recognizes their existence. The church—and on the plateau today, the mosque—have discredited other threats. Healers often classify these discredited threats as maladies of Person (*uchawi*) or maladies of Mashetani. As I suggested in the introduction, the latter might also be translated as maladies of devils, which perhaps captures the more derogatory and dangerous implications these maladies hold for those in religious circles. Tanzanians feel compelled to take precautions against both maladies of Person and maladies of Mashetani. While some turn exclusively to prayer for protection, few on the plateau find that sufficient. The vulnerabilities of the first years of life occasion the widespread use of protective medicines against maladies of Person and Mashetani.

Maladies of Person

Maladies of Person are undesirable states that have been visited upon one person by another. In Kiswahili, these maladies are the result of *uchawi*. Therapies to address such maladies have changed. Healers claim that they rarely, if ever, divine (*kupiga ramli*) these days. Such practices were used in the past to reveal which individual was the cause of another's problems, but healers today argue such revelations might cause anger and catalyze acts of revenge. In Newala, the two people who were identified to me by name as *wachawi* were men, and while one of them did stumble drunkenly into a well and die during my period of fieldwork, there were no public attempts to harm them.

Maladies of Person are most often dealt with in two ways. First, healers treat afflicted persons individually with medicines that remove the filth of the *uchawi* from their bodies. Second, many people protect themselves against the jealousies of others. Men, women, and children seek out medicinal assurances that the attempts of others to direct violence toward them will not be successful. People living throughout the Makonde Plateau use these protective practices. The vast majority of pregnant women and mothers wear, bathe in, rub on, or bury such medicine to protect themselves and their children.

Wachawi use medicine to destroy, damage, or disable others. These substances might be directed toward individual bodies, relatives, families, farms, or businesses. In other words, maladies of Person are the effect of the intentional disruption of the relations that sustain another person's life. Maladies of Person are not simply maladies perpetrated by other people; they are most precisely maladies that afflict the bonds between people, objects, and entities that determine personhood. Healers on the plateau strive to intervene in these relations in ways that will cultivate the life of the individual seeking their assistance. Their work supports Maia Green's (1996) notion of personhood as "an attribute of the living, constituted through the performance of appropriate acts and the incorporation of substances classified as medicines" (488). Therapies for maladies of Person remake or refigure the bonds that enact personhood. Changes in the way that Tanzanians address maladies of Person are part and parcel of historical changes in the notion of personhood. Both the decline of divination and the rise of treatments that address afflicted individuals' physical ailments without addressing the person who wished them reflect a world in which life is increasingly conceived of through modern notions of persons and bodies that are self-contained units rather than relational.

The evolution of the transition of therapies for maladies of Person deserves more detailed research. Here, I would simply like to note that like the category of maladies of God, the category of maladies of Person has proven to be both resilient and flexible, changing in relation to the material conditions and the series of relationships in which it is mobilized.

Maladies of Mashetani

The third common classification of maladies on the plateau is maladies of Mashetani, a range of complaints that are the result of run-ins with devilish nonhuman actors.[7] A *shetani* may startle a person, causing extreme fright, or it may bring cold (*baridi ya shetani*). Although the symptoms differ, similar medicines are used to treat these two different states. Being startled usually brings on convulsions (as in the case of the *degedege* discussed in chapter 7) and/or fevers (as in the case of the *makanje* discussed in chapter 8). The coolness of the *mashetani*, however, is illustrated in a variety of concerns and discomforts that are often characterized by swelling. In children, for example, a swollen stomach and bitter-tasting hands are taken as a sign of the coolness of devils. When one licks the palms of a child being bothered by these devils, they taste strong (*mikono mikali*) like the medicine that is used to cure such coolness. Another sign (*dalili*) that indicates that a child has the coolness of the *mashetani* is that they are pale. Such a child is said to look white.

My discussion of healers' visions in chapter 4 examined the contemporary conflation of *mashetani* with ancestral shades known as *mahoka* (Kimakonde). The term *mashetani* not only masks the distinctions around this ancestral figure but also blurs together various disturbing and unwelcome entities that instigate maladies. Although the broad Kiswahili category of *mashetani* used in southern Tanzania has absorbed many of former Kimakonde distinctions between unseen actors, the activities of *mashetani* continue to hold at least some of the conflicting and diverse energies of their ever-more-distant ancestors.

Many of the details of these specific actors are elusive. Yet distinctions among the ways that *mashetani* act and differences in the therapies used to address them may point to the fault lines where once-separate types of entities have now been collapsed into one type. The most common Kimakonde translation for *shetani* (or *mashetani*) is *nandenga*.[8] When Binti Dadi explained why people have sought treatment for maladies of Mashetani more often in recent years, she referred obliquely to *nandenga* through their location and their preference for inhabiting specific trees.

> Eeh, people often get maladies of Mashetani. Nowadays, they get these things very often. So today I will tell you [why this is]. Long ago, this *shetani* was there in the big trees. They sat in these big trees—the creatures (*wadudu*), these *mashetani*. Now, though, at this point, they [people] have cut down all the big trees. They left only cashew trees and this tree [points to tall *nyonyo* shrubs]. Now the *shetani* comes to sit on the bodies of people. It comes to sit on the bodies of people. The *mashetani* come to build even on me here . . . eeh.

Nandenga are these nonhuman agents, glossed more generically by Binti Dadi as *mashetani* but specified as those who previously sat in large trees such as baobabs, *mbuyu,* and trees known as *ntanga* and *mkongo.* As discussed in chapter 1, only a very few such trees or remaining stumps could be found on the plateau around Newala at the end of the millennium. They have disappeared over time as the population has grown, as land ownership practices have changed, and as the state—first through villagization policies and now through the distribution of social services—have compelled people to settle and cultivate the same plots indefinitely. Although healers now have to travel farther to obtain pieces of these large trees, they are still used in medicine to treat the maladies that result from being climbed on by one of these roaming, homeless devils.

The uses of different substances to treat maladies of Mashetani may actually hint at what were previously distinctions between unseen actors. A unique set of remedies is used to address *mashetani* that are bothering a child whose mother has previously lost a child. In such cases, the *shetani* is a shadow (*kivuli*) of a dead child, which is "calling" its living sibling. If a woman has many consecutive miscarriages, specific medicine is used to address a *shetani* who likes to remove pregnancies. *Nyoka,*[9] as this unseen abortionist is recognized, likes to drink the blood of mothers. Similar plant-based treatments are used to address maladies that result from raucous devils that commit adultery with women, although the method of delivery is different. In the most colorful of these stories a devil assumes the form of a woman's husband and then after kicking the "real" husband onto the floor proceeds to have sex with the woman. This violation can manifest itself in a variety of different symptoms. (This is discussed in greater detail in chapter 8.)

Mashetani are not simply a class with many members that includes *mahoka, nandenga, kivuli, nyoka,* and others. *Shetani,* as I discussed in the introduction, is a historically specific Kiswahili word that has come to refer to many distinct Kimakonde entities as a more generic form of devil or demon or spirit. This shift has been so successful that many people incorporate the Kiswahili term *mashetani* into conversations that are otherwise spoken in Kimakonde. The sharpness with which distinctions in Kimakonde can be made concerning the realm of the unseen is dissolving. At the same time, this linguistic shift has tinged these nonhuman actors with connotations of the occult, sacrilege, and evil.

The Threats and the Threatened

To illustrate how different therapies generate and maintain the objects in which they intervene, the remainder of this chapter accounts for the three primary objects of preventative and protective therapies: devils, jealousies, and future patients. The practices that render objects of protective therapies substantial and therefore actionable are examined with the same ethnographic eye as the practices that render the objects of preventive medical care in the Newala maternal and child health clinic substantial and therefore actionable. On one hand, protective practices, such as wearing amulets, taking herbal baths, and drinking the dissolved ink of passages from the Qur'an, objectify the agents of future maladies. Those things in the world that may lead to affliction—devils, ancestors, and witchcraft—take form and are attributed sensitivities through the use of protective medicines. Below I examine how devils and jealousies emerge as objects into which healers may intervene. On the other hand, through clinic-based preventive care practices and the many inscriptions they produce (e.g., images, charts, and numbers), a biomedical body emerges as an object into which clinic practitioners may intervene. Bureaucratic interventions creating a predictable and comprehensible population are combined with medical interventions to produce a more predictable and resistant body (as a unit of that population). In the end, protective practices evoke the agents of future afflictions, while preventive practices evoke the entities that may later be afflicted.

The boundaries and distinctions that constitute objects of therapeutic practices—whether those objects are mischievous Makonde devils, potent jealousies, or future patients—are not self-evident or universal. Rather, they emerge through particular processes of objectification. As discussed in the introduction, this analysis complicates more pejorative understandings of objectification (see also Good 1994; Mol 2002; Prentice forthcoming). It refers to the processes through which diverse knowledge-production practices produce their objects of knowledge, and in the case of therapeutic knowledge, which is implicitly interventionist, it refers to the practices through which therapies produce the objects in which they intervene. A comparison of the processes of objectification that generate substantially different therapeutic objects calls on descriptions of medical pluralism to account for more than just the coexistence of different healing practices. It also reveals that different therapeutic practices are distinguished by more than the different cultural shapes they offer to humans' interactions with a universal biological body. Accounting for diverse processes of objectification draws attention to the different ways that the materiality of the body and the materiality of various agents of affliction emerge. Juxtaposing processes of objectification in clinical medicine and traditional medicine demonstrates how distinct forms of "objecticity" (Rheinberger 2000) are conferred on biomedical and nonbiomedical objects and raises the possibility of alternative materialities—that is, simultaneously occurring different versions of the matter of the body and bodily threats.

During my fieldwork, I interviewed many women who were hoping to conceive, working to protect their pregnancies, and tending to their newborns. I also watched healers at work and helped them collect and make different kinds of protective medicine for these women. The uses of these therapies are not institutionalized, recorded, or enforced through any sort of state-sanctioned program.[10] It was not possible for me to track large groups of patients through government statistics. Yet, my in-depth ethnographic work reveals a detailed understanding of the interventions that parents and healers make to protect children during the first years of life. Below, I focus my attention on one child with whom I had close sustained contact: Yanini, Binti Dadi's grandchild, a little girl who was born to Mariamu early in my research. I watched, heard about, and participated in many of the therapies initiated to protect her, including burying her umbilical cord, shaving her head, washing her daily with medicinal substances, acquiring medicine to protect her from people who were jealous of my affection for her, and even accompanying her and her mother to the maternal and child health clinic for some of her monthly under-five visits. While Yanini's conception, birth, and early childhood care were not particularly unique, Mariamu's articulateness about the practices in which she engaged and the ease with which she engaged in them may be a little less common. The rhythm and variety of treatments used to protect children in southern Tanzania came into particularly sharp focus around Yanini's treatments.

Rendering Devils

Two days after Yanini's birth, Mariamu wrapped a small bundle of medicine that included frankincense, hemp seeds, pieces of the strong-smelling *mvuje* tree, and slivers of roots from the *nandenga* and *numokamungo* trees in a piece of black cloth around Yanini's left wrist. Typically small children in southeastern Tanzania wear such medicine to protect them from "getting the fever of *mashetani* before growing up." *Mashetani* can startle, dirty, climb on, or otherwise harm a child. The medicine in the small black bundles varies. Those who are wary of traditional healers (this group often includes the few Christians who live in an area that is 95 percent Muslim) make the simplest bundles at home from a little incense and *numbati,* a kind of red earth purchased in the market in cylindrically shaped chunks. Others take their child to a healer, who tends to prepare more elaborate combinations of medicine such as Yanini's. Children wear these black bundles on their left wrist from infancy until they "are able to walk well." Their early medicinal protection is only the first (and for the untrained eye the most visible) step in separating the child from the *mashetani* that threaten him or her.

Despite the fact that Yanini wore this medicine, her mother reasoned that she was being bothered by *mashetani* when she started to cry a great deal two weeks later. As a result, Mariamu gathered other medicine to further protect her child from these familiar devils. She began to incorporate herbal and mineral treatments into her everyday routine of caring for Yanini. Mariamu gave Yanini regular medicinal baths of *lipande,* a mixture of plant medicines soaked in cool water for days or even weeks. These baths protected her against maladies of *Mashetani* as well as maladies of Person, which are discussed more extensively in the next section. Moreover, she bought Johnson's Baby Oil from the local market and infused it with *numbati*. Each day after Mariamu bathed Yanini she rubbed this medicinal oil into her joints to guard against the effects of harmful nonhumans. Occasionally she preventatively washed Yanini in the remnants of medicinal baths that Binti Dadi had prepared for other children with *degedege*, a malady of Mashetani. Yanini did not have *degedege*, but the leaves that had been crushed and mixed with water to treat *degedege* served to keep *mashetani* from attempting to play with her.

Protective medicine as it is used on the Makonde Plateau "works" by driving off or chasing away (*kufukuza*) *mashetani*, those devilish nonhuman threats. In the process, a person or a body grows less sensitive to *mashetani* (that is, less vulnerable), while the *mashetani* become more sensitive (that is, more vulnerable). They come to recognize bodily boundaries. As they encounter the medicine used to protect Yanini (and the other children in the area), *mashetani* acquire the qualities of objecthood and become actionable. *Mashetani* come into being as that which may be scared off (*kuogopesha*) by strategically worn medicines, forced away (*kufukuza*) by particular medicinal baths, or flushed out (*kurutubisha*) by herbal medicines that are given to acutely ill children to induce diarrhea. In these ways, the medicine prevents *mashetani* from conversing with (*kuongea*) or playing with (*kuchezea*) a person.

In a very practical sense, therapies to protect children objectify *mashetani*. They make the *mashetani* into an object for discussion and intervention. Purposeful encounters with medicine provoke interactions that give *mashetani* an empirical existence. In this process of objectification, *mashetani* become entities with distinctive characteristics. Their contours become clear through their responses to medicine. They come to be known as active: they converse, play, fear, and leave. Such devils do not circulate in scientific networks. However, *mashetani* are central to nonscientific ways of addressing discomforts, disabilities, and afflictions in southeastern Tanzania. The coexistence of diverse therapies can be accounted for and compared, without solidifying differences in descriptions of systems or paradigms of knowledge, by attending to diverse practices of objectification. I continue to unfold this argument in the next two sections by turning first to practices that confer objecthood on jealousies and then turning to practices revealing the specific form of objecthood that medicine confers on biomedically standardized bodies.

Rendering Jealousies

Mashetani are only one kind of entity rendered through protective therapies available in southeastern Tanzania. Therapeutic practices that protect against the effects of *uchawi*—the use of medicines to do harm—also render jealousies material. A set of treatments administered to Yanini when she was one month old illustrates how "protection" requires articulating the materiality of jealousy (*wivu*). During the first month of Yanini's life, Mariamu had not been able to attend community events such as funerals because she was "nursing a child that had not yet been shaved." This process of shaving the child's head is part of a series of treatments that prepare a child to participate in a wider circle of relationships, to be exposed to and held by people other than the very closest of her kin and, therefore, to be opened up to potential dangers. Medicine that protects a child from *uchawi* not only enables that child to resist the effects of deliberately harmful actions, but also establishes the bodily boundaries that make it possible for healers or others to discern and intervene in any future destructive use of medicine.

On January 13, 1999, I accompanied Mariamu, Yanini, and Yanini's father as they traveled across the Makonde Plateau to see Chinduli, a *faraki* healer, one who knows "medicine of the book." Mariamu's relationship with Chinduli's family had begun many years earlier when his father had saved her life when it was acutely threatened by *uchawi* (see chapter 4). After introductions, Chinduli asked Yanini's full name as well as the day and time she was born. These were critical pieces of information for each of the four medicines that Chinduli would prepare for us that day, which included medicine for Yanini to wear, two kinds of medicine that Chinduli rubbed onto and washed over the bodies of both Yanini and Mariamu, and medicine to protect their home.

Reiterating that each day is "held" by a particular unseen agent (*mdudu ambaye anatawala*), Chinduli identified the ruler of the day of Yanini's birth. He then planned treatments that addressed the characteristics of that ruler. On half of a piece of notebook paper, Chinduli wrote in red ink with a sharpened stick. Looking at me, he noted that saffron ink "is the food of the Arabs" (*ni chakula waarabu*) and for this reason it is used to write *kombe*.[11] As Chinduli was writing in his small neat Arabic script, Mariamu told him about a certain old woman and her grown daughter who lived behind them and who "saw or felt" jealousy (*kuona wivu*). They said "bad words" (*maneno mabaya*) about Yanini, Mariamu, and Binti Dadi. In addition, these neighbors questioned why it was that I went to see Binti Dadi so often but did not visit them as regularly.

Mariamu continued her complaints as Chinduli studied a handwritten notebook and a thin paperback book in Arabic. He then took up the other half of the piece of notebook paper and continued writing, this time with a blue ballpoint pen. This next medicine, he asserted, provides protection from fights. "If there is a fight, it will turn to water." Later, he elaborated, saying that the protection works by transforming harmful substances. "For example if a gun is shot [towards the wearer of this medicine] then the bullet will come out as water."[12] When he was done with this writing, he ripped the paper to the exact size of the portion on which the words were written. He folded inside the blue writing a sliver of a fallen star, Yanini's shadow, a small piece of Yanini's hair, and a piece of an animal that had been shot.

Next, Chinduli took the remaining strip of paper and began to write words of protection that specifically named Yanini's enemies. He placed these words with some black powder in a section of *nchunju* wood with a split in it. This wood is a powerful medicine that can only be collected in certain places with the permission of those who steward the land on which it grows. Healers who collect the medicine must first make a request to the head of the area who will in turn pray to the ancestors, assuring them that the piece of the tree that is to be taken will be used to heal, not to do harm. If permission is not granted before a person digs up the medicinal root, Chinduli asserted, the thief is likely to be found dead and dried up at the foot of the tree. As he finished stuffing the script inside the *nchunju*, he instructed that Binti Dadi should bury this medicine at the entrance to her compound, just inside the door. She was to do this secretly at night. This medicine was meant to extinguish the strength of the words of those who wished harm. If anyone attempted to enter with bad intentions carrying *uchawi* to be used against a member of Binti Dadi's household, then this medicine would cause the person to fall down. Chinduli assured us that their legs and arms would break before they crossed the threshold. If one of these enemies tried to cause harm to Binti Dadi or Yanini, he continued, their throat would get stuck, they would not be able to swallow, and they would die.

Finally, he poured a little medicine called *ndumba* from a bottle onto his finger and dabbed it on both Yanini and Mariamu. As he rubbed it into Yanini's wrists, the top of her head, the tops of her hands and feet and her ankles, he prayed for her protection from bad people. He continued this prayer as he marked Mariamu's throat, hands, and feet with the same medicine. Then we returned home.

The next day, three final steps completed Chinduli's therapies and closed this particular stage of Yanini's young life. First, Mariamu sewed Chinduli's medicine into an amulet using a piece of vinyl she had collected from scraps in a furniture shop. Second, she ripped the paper holding the red ink of the *faraki* medicine into pieces and stuffed the fragments into an empty Coke bottle. She added water to the words in the bottle and shook it. She used the resulting solution to bathe Yanini and herself. In addition, they both drank some of this light pink medicine. Third, because, as Chinduli cautioned, "many people wanted her hair," she shaved Yanini's head. In addition, she buried Yanini's umbilical cord on that day. Mariamu had been carrying the knot of Yanini's umbilical cord with her since it had fallen off. She had kept it safe by tucking the small, shriveled knot into a cloth that she wore tightly wrapped around her waist in order to help her stomach shrink back to its pre-pregnancy size. Breast milk and special oils from local plants and other things would also be brought into this collective of objects and agents needed to render the jealousies of others incompatible with Yanini—to render them as objects for discussion and intervention.

In June of the next year, when Yanini was approximately a year and a half old and the medicine described above had been working for about the same time period, I went with Yanini and Mariamu to see Chinduli again. Chinduli confirmed Mariamu's concern that the medicines Yanini was wearing could be losing strength. He prepared fresh, potent medicines to add to those he had given her earlier. Mariamu attached a second amulet to the black string that Yanini already wore around her neck. The same neighbors remained a particular threat. At one point when I had left Newala for a period, they had used an axe to chop down a tree outside of Binti Dadi's compound that we had often sat under to talk in the afternoon while waiting for those needing treatment to come. The neighbor claimed that she had felled the tree so that Binti Dadi would no longer have a place to sit and talk to me, so that I would no longer visit.

Through Chinduli's medicine, the jealousies of others come to be articulated as an object of therapeutic intervention. Treatments to protect Yanini and others in Binti Dadi's household against their neighbors' jealousy, or *wivu*, do not refer only to disturbing or unsettling emotions. While jealousy is a reason for someone to use *uchawi*, it is also much more. Words, looks, and harmful intentions can kill in and of themselves. Jealousy in English is a thin translation of the Kiswahili notion of *wivu*. *Wivu* is not merely an abstract emotion in Tanzania. It is a material force that threatens life and wellness. The matter of this threat is articulated through protective treatments. Treatments such as Chinduli's both formulate their objects of intervention and intervene in them.

Mariamu engaged in many actions to protect Yanini from those who might wish her harm. As discussed above, she removed her hair and buried her umbilical cord; these are things that in the wrong hands could be used in powerful concoctions designed to weaken, injure or murder her daughter.[13] Mariamu also obtained medicines from Chinduli for Yanini to wear in an amulet around her neck. The amulet worked by establishing compatibility and incompatibility between different entities. First, Chinduli included medicine that would inspire love in family members, friends, neighbors, and all who would meet her. The fallen star in the amulet, which is worn at all times, attracts people, motivating feelings of affection and generosity. Second, several substances in the amulet were designed to scare off anyone who might be tempted to make a concoction that would cause injury to the child. Two items, the shadow and the hair, are frequently used in mixtures designed to cause harm. As substances that could be used in damaging ways, they served here as a sort of "anti-serum" protecting the child and warning any evildoers that the child was already fortified by medicine. Third, he included a piece of an animal that was harmed by being shot.[14] These three kinds of medicines are designed to startle anyone with evil intentions and strike fear into them. If, however, they should overcome this fear, there is another set of medicines: the Arabic words. Both Qur'anic verse and the naming of the child's enemies will turn any "fight into water." They will render any remaining aggression impotent. After Chinduli prepared the items for the amulet, he marked the spots on Yanini and Mariamu's bodies that were particularly vulnerable to *uchawi* with a medicinal paste. In this way, he isolated the places where jealousies could intervene in the body and protected them.

Then, lastly, Mariamu received medicine from Chinduli that Binti Dadi buried at the entrance to her compound to prevent anyone from entering the home with harmful intentions. This medicine trips up anyone with such intentions. Sometimes people say that such medicine reflects the greedy, jealous, and hurtful intentions of a person back onto him or her. This medicine is not directed at the individuals themselves, however; it is directed at their aggression. A person without jealousy may cross the threshold and enter safely. However, if the same person tries to enter with the desire to harm, then he or she will be injured.

The renderings of jealousy and certain things (such as hair, a shadow, the Qur'an, and medicine) incompatible—and the child and other things (such as family, community members, other medicines) compatible—are at the core of therapeutic interventions. As more relations of compatibility and incompatibility are established with each treatment, jealousy and other agents of affliction grow more substantive. Their characteristics become more clearly articulated. In this way, protective practices constitute those threats that are likely to be the targets of healing interventions throughout the child's life. These medicines, then, are not only "protective" in the obvious sense; they also make later healing possible by defining things that can be held responsible for discomfort, disability, or other undesirable states of being. Protective medicines serve to (partly) define that which is dangerous and that which is in danger.

Generations of ethnographies—whether they be structuralist analyses attuned to the function of ritual elements in therapies or hermeneutic analyses uncovering the deep meaning of circulating symbols or phenomenological analyses interested in the processes through which subjects create and invest meaning—have neglected the authority of such therapies to (en)act, and to have material effects by ignoring or denying the existence of the entity or entities mobilized. Arguing against the heavy weight of social scientific analyses that often locate the efficacy of African therapies solely in the realm of the social, Maia Green (1996) has insisted that people consume medicine "for their power, not for their symbolic qualities." Understanding *wivu* as an object produced through sustained therapeutic attention begins to imagine the power of greed and the aggression of envy. *Wivu* is not merely an emotion that is trapped inside an autonomous individual. Jealousy in the context I have described on the Makonde Plateau is a circulating material force with the power to act. A look can bring sickness, and words can kill.

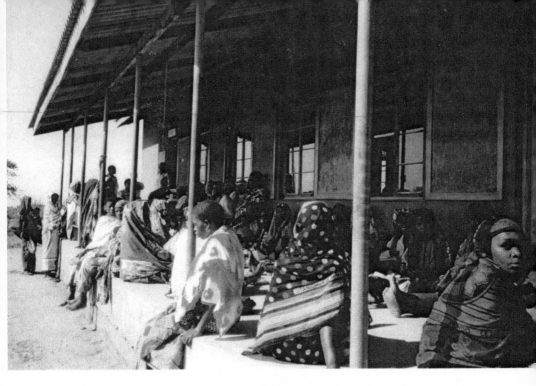

Figure 6.1. Mothers and children on the verandah of the maternal and child health clinic in the Newala District Hospital. *Photo by author, 2003.*

Rendering Future Patients

In addition to all these efforts to protect Yanini from maladies of Mashetani and maladies of Person, Mariamu took her each month to the local public health clinic for preventive care. In contrast to Chinduli's protective medicine, the preventive practices of the maternal and child health clinic did not articulate future threats, but rather these biomedical practices generated a body for future therapeutic intervention. In this section, I describe some of the most routine elements of these wellness visits to the maternal and child health clinic at the Newala District Hospital. The Tanzanian Ministry of Health, through its network of hospitals, clinics, and dispensaries, requires that all children visit the clinic to be weighed every month for the first five years of their lives and receive vaccinations according to a schedule. These routine postnatal and childhood visits have been designed to enable medical practitioners to assess individual children's risk and to limit the vulnerability of both individuals and larger populations. The monthly requirements establish mechanisms through which the clinic attempts to foresee problems and recommend action. Like most other children in the area, Yanini was washed, dressed in her best clothes, and taken to the Newala maternal and

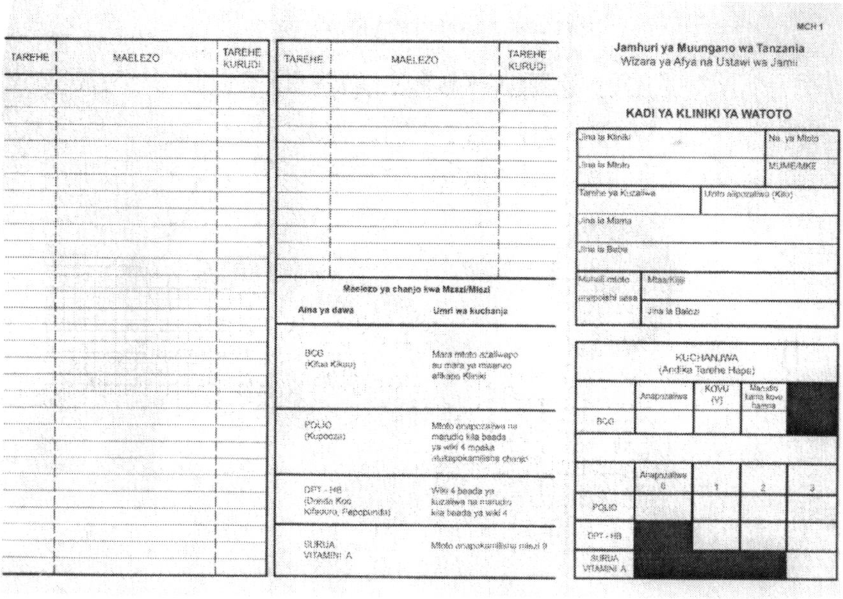

Figure 6.2a. Front of the under-five card used in Newala District Hospital in 2003.

child health clinic each month. This last section explores the objects of therapeutic intervention that health care practitioners enacted during these visits.

At 9:00 AM each weekday morning, nurses or nurse-midwifery students conducted a health education class on the veranda of the maternal and child health clinic. Mothers of young children gathered outside under the long roof. The nurses stood at one end of the veranda behind a desk. The mothers placed their child's notebooks and cards on the desk and then sat with their children on the benches that line both sides of the veranda if they could find space. Otherwise, they sat on the concrete floor.

First, one of the nurses gave a health education lecture. Then, the nurses identified and registered the sick children and referred them to the main hospital to see a doctor. After these tasks had been completed, one of the nurses looked at the under-five cards and called the children to the front one by one. When Yanini's name was called, Mariamu walked to the center of the verandah where a scale had been hung and allowed a nurse to weigh her baby. This nurse called out Yanini's weight and the first nurse wrote it down in the appropriate box on her card. In addition, she marked the weight on a graph on this card, which recorded Yanini's weight in kilograms (on the y-axis) and by age in months (on the x-axis). The nurse connected this data point to the line from the previous

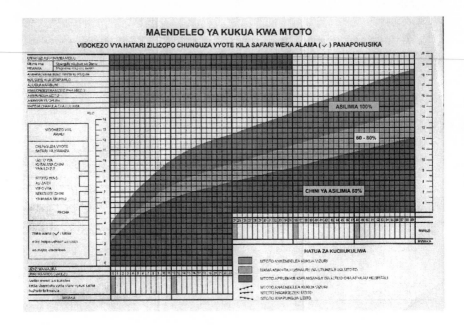

Figure 6.2b. Back of the under-five card used in Newala District Hospital in 2003.

month on a graph over a tricolor background. The lower block of color represented severe malnutrition, the middle color illustrated the range for average weight, and the top block of color represented weight that is over the average. The drawing of this line immediately created an image of Yanini's growth—one that Mariamu grew extremely proud of and was eager to show to friends because Yanini consistently measured above her cohort. Each month, the nurse would consult Yanini's immunization table on the card to make sure that all her shots were up to date. When she was scheduled for an immunization, the nurse would instruct Mariamu to take her to the other side of the clinic, where still another nurse would administer an oral polio vaccine or an injection for tuberculosis, DPT (diphtheria, pertussis, and tetanus), or measles. After administering the required treatment, the nurse would write the date in the vaccination table on Yanini's card. In addition, the nurse would mark a line in a clinic register that records the number of vaccinations given out on that day.

Nurses' narratives of their work were replete with explanations about registration books, patient's notebooks, under-five cards, and the processes of measuring and recording. This is not surprising. The cards for each child attending the clinic have become especially productive actors in Tanzanian clinics. They organize activities, elicit numbers, demand regular visits, determine next steps,

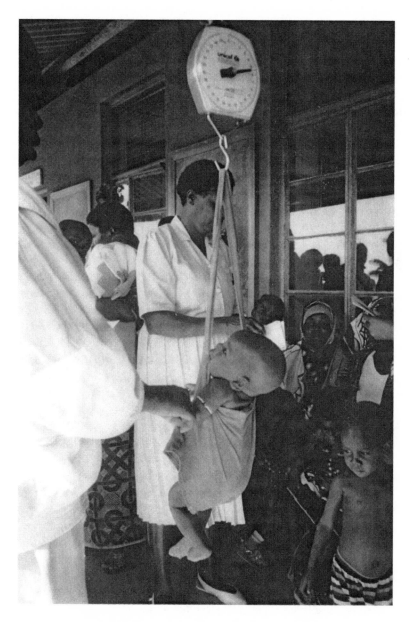

Figure 6.3. Nurses weighing a child at Newala District Hospital.
Photo by author, 2000.

and even imagine the child's growth in relation to a population of his or her peers. These cards structure interaction and make significant the succession of numbers that are produced during each visit. They draw together a range of tools and gestures—including scales, counting procedures, lines, registration books, examination rooms—and make the routine of the clinic intelligible. Through training and education, practitioners learn a range for each measurement that is "normal," and in the process also learn what falls outside the range and is therefore considered dangerous. The most colorful of these practices visualizes the body of each child under the age of five as a line that rises and falls with the number representing the weight of the child during his or her monthly visits. The line climbs or dips into different-colored areas, charting a child's course through wellness and malnutrition. Often the job of a public health nurse is to make bodies conform to these standards of mathematical percentages. Clinical practitioners justify interventions based on information that demonstrates that a patient falls outside the range of acceptability or "safety."

Charis Cussins (1998) argues that in the clinic, the "mundane steps that render the body and the instruments compatible are at the heart of objectification" (180). These simple under-five cards play an active role in arranging those "mundane steps" that are required to make a patient discrete, predictable, and intelligible. In so doing, they make concrete a relationship between a fictive average child of World Health Organization growth charts and the child in the clinic.[15] By making children in southeastern Tanzania compatible with this fictive global child, such monitoring and supervision turns children into patients-to-be. In other words, these efforts render children's bodies biomedically comprehensible and formulate them as objects in which clinical therapies might later intervene. These routine practices—measuring, comparing, graphing—not only establish wellness and illness, but are also one way that clinically intelligible bodies are enacted.

The spacing and timing facilitated by these cards are not separate from but are critical to the efficacy of the vaccines the clinic administers. Without their discrete paper accomplices or some other way of organizing immunizations, vaccines would not produce the wanted effects. Only the careful organization of stimuli in the clinic have been found to elicit the bodily "memory" and the "herd immunity" that are the goals of immunization (concepts I discuss in more detail below). For instance, the carefully choreographed encounter with a vaccine in the clinic should take place before an uncontrolled (or "natural") exposure occurs. The cards issued by the government at birth immediately initiate a newborn into the postnatal routine. The desired effect of vaccination, as will be discussed below, is the faster and greater proliferation of particular cells as a result of their second exposure to a malady. The cards elicit the necessary exposures by planning immunizations through the administration of a series of each vaccine. Furthermore, exposure to specific maladies in combination could inhibit or complicate the desired effects. The cards record an individual child's personal schedule for different series of vaccines and thereby compel particular vaccines to be administered at particular times. Desirably predictable bodies and discrete populations emerge only as a result of the combined work of medicine and bureaucracy.

The efficacy of vaccines is conceptualized through the actions and reactions initiated by the introduction of a threat into the body. The reactions to this threat create a physical "memory" that allows a body to respond more quickly and with more force when it is exposed to that particular threat in the future. Claims as to what immunizations do—that is, how they work—have evolved over time.[16] Most recently, medical science's articulation of the immune system, and therefore of the things that immunizations are said to effect, have changed as a result of studies of HIV/AIDS.[17] Through their own distinct processes of objectification that are too involved to attend to in detail here, molecular scientists now attribute the effects of immunization to a range of agents, most notably antigens and antibodies. Through immunizations, nurses introduce antigens (in the form of attenuated, spun-off, or otherwise altered material of viruses and bacteria) to children. Scientists believe that antigens select for the particular antibodies whose physical shape complements theirs. More specifically, each B-lymphocyte cell produces antibodies that have one specific shape. The antibodies coat the surface of the lymphocytes establishing themselves as the antigen recognition sites for the lymphocytes. An "invading" antigen meets an array of lymphocytes. Each lymphocyte bears its own individual antigen recognition site. If the antigen and the antibody "recognize" each other—if their shapes complement each other—then they will bind together. This binding triggers the production of plasma cells, which in turn produce more of the antibody needed to bind with the antigen that is present (this process is known as clonal expansion).[18] The second time this sequence of actions and reactions takes place (for instance, because of a second vaccination in a series), the speed with which lymphocytes "recognize" an antigen and reproduce antibodies increases. This increased response is what medical scientists call "memory."

The successful enactment of this standardized memory, particularly in young children, relies on carefully timed exposures. Children's cells "forget" too easily. The first time an antigen is introduced through a vaccine it stimulates a short-term production of antibodies. After about two months there is a sharp decrease in antibody production. However, the second (or third, etc.) time this antigen is introduced it stimulates longer-lasting, higher-affinity antibodies. Repeated exposure coaxes a body into "remembering." Or, more precisely, after repeated exposures, measurements of the production of antibodies remain high. Therefore, the efficacy of a vaccine rests on a series of exposures. The under-five card mediates the activity of populations of lymphocytes, the production of specific antibodies, and the creation of bodily memory (as it regulates the comings and goings of well-dressed children and their mothers that we saw above). Vaccines and cards work to produce biomedically predictable objects of therapeutic practice: bodies with a similar range of specifically shaped antibodies and with similarly speedy cellular reactions to these specific antigens—a type of standardized body.

In addition to establishing bodies that tend to react more predictably, controlled exposure to specific threats through immunization is also a process of producing "herd immunity." Epidemiological literature defines herd immunity as the decreased likelihood that an epidemic will be found in a population in which most of the people have been previously exposed (Nelson, Williams, and Graham 2001, 268). In other words, if most people are immunized against a certain disease, even those who are not immunized are less likely to contract this disease because they are less likely to get exposed to it. Immunizations not only restrict the maladies likely to manifest in individuals, they also restrict the maladies likely to manifest in populations.

On one hand, vaccines are evaluated on their success in equalizing the varying abilities that bodies have to attend to maladies. By stimulating "acquired immune responses," vaccines alter bodies in an effort to standardize their reaction to particular maladies, thereby, creating a more predicable patient-to-be. On the other hand, vaccines work at the level of the population, delineating the area in which exposure to particular maladies is more or less likely. Early childhood care, then, produces and maintains both the "population" central to public health initiatives and the "body" demanded in clinical treatments. Unlike the protective medicines of healers in the area, these objects of therapeutic practice are not those things that might later be accused of afflicting, but rather they are those things that might later become afflicted.

Materializing Difference

In gathering together these accounts of rendering devils, jealousies, standardized bodies, and herd immunity, I am arguing for an expansion of which processes we see as a means of objectification. By objectification, I mean the way a range of entities and gestures are brought together in an effort to shape a vague mass of threats into manageable trajectories, to identify stable actors, and to establish objects of therapeutic intervention. Processes of objectification materialize practical, usable objects of therapeutic attention and care. The use of protective and preventive medicine in southeastern Tanzania—both of which generally precede acute discomfort, disability, or misfortune—illustrate most clearly how particular objects come to establish "the patterns of reality" for which people are held accountable (Haraway 1991). Nurses, healers, patients, communities, and institutions become engaged in and are held responsible for specific realities through the evocation of objects in various treatments.

These different patterns of objectification are critical to different ideas about relationships and justice within various collectivities in Tanzania. In a postcolonial context such as southeastern Tanzania, however, whether or not alternative materialities are deemed legitimate is not just a theoretical issue. Whose processes of objectification, whose knowledge, are communities, health services, international development programs, and anthropologists accountable to? In the dramatically unequal relations between the First World and the Third World, what metaphors and practices will be used to pattern engagement in the world? Which objects of practice will have the right to exist in our studies? How the lines between the material and immaterial are drawn and reinforced changes who is held responsible to whom and for what. After all, as Donna Haraway (1988) writes, "what counts as an object is precisely what world history turns out to be about" (588). Which objects of therapeutic practice are allowed to exist is not an esoteric question; it means, quite simply, what things really matter.

The ontological politics of therapeutic objects is at a critical juncture in Tanzania as "traditional and alternative medicine" are claiming new institutional status in the law and within the Ministry of Health and the National Institute for Medical Research. The postcolonial reification and institutionalization of diverse healing practices (made homogeneous only in their distinction from biomedicine and witchcraft) into a category of knowledge and practice is occurring in the interstices of transnational and national desires. These include international efforts (most notably those of the World Health Organization) to promote and elaborate a transnational category of traditional medicine through policy and scientific research, state initiatives to meet the needs of the Tanzanian population as structural adjustment programs create increasingly severe class differentiation, and the work of pharmaceutical companies to develop new drugs that are economically viable. Tanzania is attempting to coordinate traditional medicine within its national health care system by disciplining therapies through science. As we saw in chapter 3, national labs strive to make the matter of therapies—that which grounds their efficacy—intelligible through practices that identify the active ingredients in herbal therapies. In these efforts, the lines of demarcation between what is science and what is not science are falling once again along the old lines of nature and culture (not to mention the lines of rural/urban, formally educated/not formally educated, less cash wealthy/more cash wealthy, etc.). This is not the only way that the relationship between traditional medicine and modern medicine might be elaborated, however.

In this chapter I have argued that healers assert alternative notions of nature, alternative ideas of what makes up the world, as they articulate that to which they must attend. This praxiological approach to bodies and bodily threats suggests that traditional medicine holds out the possibility of democratizing material worlds by coordinating practices of objectification, that is by coordinating the events that establish practical alternative materialities. The next chapter describes the work that such coordination involves. Differences in medicine become even more salient and their coordination more urgent in the context of curative practices. As traditional and modern medical practitioners battle over the same afflicted bodies, they fight both for the right to treat certain individuals and for the rights of particular social differences to matter. As practitioners jockey for the upper hand in their encounters with each other, they also strive to articulate the relationship between traditional and modern medical therapies. In these everyday struggles, there is the potential to re-envision the differences that make up the lived world. The politics of object formation lies at the heart of these efforts. Nothing, however, guarantees that the results of these struggles will be democratic.

7

Interferences and Inclusions

In southern Tanzania, *degedege* and malaria are considered two of the most common threats to the well-being of pregnant women and young children. Responding to international and national concerns that malaria contributes significantly to poverty and to high rates of maternal and child mortality in Africa, the Tanzanian Ministry of Health has implemented programs to motivate stricter adherence to malaria prevention and treatment protocols. These programs include local public health education initiatives that aim to impress upon people the importance of recognizing certain physical symptoms as malarial and the urgency of the need to go to the health clinic at the first sign of these symptoms. In these efforts, the "traditional" malady known in Kiswahili as *degedege* has come to be translated as the "modern" malady of malaria. By tracing the processes involved in treating *degedege* and the processes involved in treating malaria, this chapter examines what is at stake in assertions that *degedege* is malaria.

Public health narratives draw an equivalence between *degedege* and malaria by insisting that these maladies refer to the same physical condition caused by the same biomedically recognized entity. This understanding makes it possible for health care professionals to see *degedege* as the Kiswahili interpretation of a biological reality. From this perspective, healing practices that treat *degedege* threaten to interrupt, delay, or interfere with life-saving malaria treatments. Individuals who accept this model feel that those who pursue therapies other than those supported by the hospital are the victims of a dangerous form of ignorance. The translation of *degedege* as malaria masks the possibility that there is another set of relationships, another network of actors, institutions, and propositions in which to locate experience. There are, however, other translations. Healers, for instance, argue that the needles of malaria treatments will kill a person if he or she has not been treated for *degedege* first. These multiple and layered translations connect and separate *degedege* and malaria.

Any focused attention on the work to make *degedege* into malaria (by and) for southern Tanzanians reveals that these maladies are identified, shaped, and

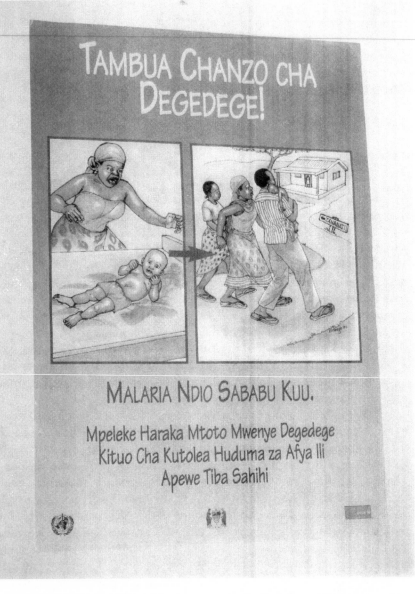

Figure 7.1. A poster placed in pharmacies in Newala. Translation: "Recognize the Origin of Degedege. Malaria is the main reason. Quickly take your child with degedege to the health care clinic in order that s/he gets proper treatment." *Photo by author, 2008.*

elaborated in relation to each other. For example, nurses diagnose *degedege* when hospital medicine for malaria does not appear to be "working" and refer patients to healers outside of the clinic. Family members slip herbal medicine into the nasal-gastric tubes of loved ones whose diagnoses of malaria have confined them to hospital beds. *Degedege* and malaria are both propositions constituted through the encounters of healers, doctors, nurses, needles, medicinal baths, and innumerable other objects and agents. The analysis below examines the making of these collectivities and the ways that therapeutic practices formulate objects of therapeutic intervention and care such as bodies, parasites, and disease entities. In this way, the contours and materialities of *degedege* and malaria are seen to be less dependent on their membership in mutually distinct alternative systems of healing and more profoundly defined by the objects of therapeutic care that emerge through practices conducted in their names. In southern Tanzania, *degedege* practices are primarily focused on the articulation of a body—something that is being afflicted—while curative malaria practices are primarily focused on the articulation of a parasite—something that is afflicting the body.

This chapter considers the ways that similarities and dissimilarities between *degedege* and malaria are articulated, and by whom. Focusing on the details of therapeutic practices challenges facile translations of indigenous categories of healing into biomedical ones. As discussed in the introductory chapter, I do not mean just linguistic translation but rather how we come to explain—sometimes to explain away—one cultural concept with another. Some voices and agendas seek to explain *degedege* away, to see it as encompassed in explanations of "malaria." More than language is at stake in these descriptions and translations. When hot, convulsing bodies become a ground for ontological struggles between healers and biomedical practitioners over devils and parasites, they illustrate the stakes implicit in descriptions of affliction—most acutely because these descriptions circumscribe the sorts of interventions that are conceivable. As biomedical and nonbiomedical practitioners work to maintain the salience of their forms of expertise, they also articulate the separations and connections that structure life (and death) in southern Tanzania.

Locating the Comparison

In southeastern Tanzania, *degedege* is considered an old problem, a common malady that is most frequent when the corn is in bloom. *Degedege* always begins with a jerk or a start. In Kiswahili, one says *anashtuka*. He or she is startled. A person's arms and legs grow suddenly stiff and he or she jerks repeatedly. Shortly afterward, the person's body may get very hot, foam may come from the mouth, and the eyes may roll to the back of the head (or "empty out"). *Degedege* may strike anyone, but children are the most vulnerable to these attacks, that is most vulnerable to being startled. *Degedege* is for many the manifestation of a run-in with a mischievous devil. A child with *degedege* is being played with by a *shetani*.

In contrast, almost everyone in Tanzania agrees that malaria is caused by mosquitoes (Winch 1999). While the first signs of malaria may be felt as a fever, terrible headaches, and an exhausted, aching body, the actual presence of the illness is determined through a count of the parasites in the patient's blood.

Yet in the daily public health education classes on the verandah of the maternal and child health clinic at the Newala District Hospital, nurses say that "*degedege* is malaria." In private or to other medical personnel, they will say that *degedege* is a symptom that may be caused by malaria, meningitis, epilepsy, or any infection that results in a very high fever. This assertion that *degedege* is a symptom resonates with the typical Swahili-English dictionary translation of *degedege* as "convulsions" or "fits."[1] In the context of the estimated 16 million cases of malaria that occur in Tanzania each year, nurses feel comfortable telling lay audiences that all convulsions are the result of malarial fevers. Their goal is to reduce the impact of this disease, which is the primary cause of mortality and morbidity and the most common reason people use health services in Tanzania.[2]

Below I do not deal with questions of comparative efficacy between treatments in and outside of the hospital. Such evaluations remain difficult to address in this setting, where affliction and death are not yet sufficiently dealt with by any form of healing and everyday obstacles to treatment can be life-threatening. Given the scarcity of resources, people (the afflicted, their family members, nurses, doctors, and healers) do the best they can to negotiate meaningful lives and, if necessary, deaths that are as comfortable as possible. In this setting, much is at stake in struggles over where hot convulsing bodies should go and how maladies are understood. The historical contingencies that motivate public health comparisons of *degedege* and malaria as well as the particular health concerns that compel such intellectual work can be understood only in the context of the concrete and empirical realities through which they come to be thought together. Why are smart, dedicated, and savvy doctors, nurses, government officials, and laypeople investing valuable time and energy arguing against healers and convincing people to go to a hospital with undertrained staff, little medicine, and at times no water? To situate the relationship between *degedege* and malaria, this section considers who is accounting for what sorts of similarities and dissimilarities between *degedege* and malaria. How and why have *degedege* and malaria come to be seen in relation to one another? On what grounds are these translations made, and by whom are they made? I describe the multilayered field of comparison and the unequal power between differently composed descriptions of the similarities and differences between *degedege* and malaria.

Any attention to these questions of comparison and translation must acknowledge that the boundary between *degedege* and malaria shifts from one person to the next and from one conversation to the next. While for some people at some times *degedege* may "be" malaria, for other people at other times, it is not. These two maladies do not map neatly on top of one another. Nor does making a distinction between particular signs and symptoms lead to an effective and clinically practical (and therefore stable) distinction between these maladies. Indeed, as mentioned above, many hospital nurses confessed confidentially that the best way to diagnose *degedege* is to observe a patient's response to regular hospital treatment (Langwick 2008a). If a person fails to respond to hospital medicine, then she or he may have *degedege*. Even among biomedical practitioners in the hospital, the distinction between *degedege* and malaria is not self-evident but rather emerges through practice.

For nonbiomedical healers, these maladies are often differentiated through treatment as well. Binti Dadi and Mariamu, who, as *degedege* specialists, see many people with this affliction, explained that distinctions between *degedege* and malaria hinge on commitments to particular practices, treatments, and experts. Mariamu argues:

> *Degedege* according to hospital research is malaria. According to the research of traditional healers, [however] malaria is *degedege*. . . . In the home *degedege* can be cured by a healer who uses traditional medicines. Now, for a person who does not believe (*kujiamini*) and who does not have faith, well s/he will get [treatment] from both sides. In the hospital, s/he will get the needle for malaria and the medicine of malaria and here s/he will get traditional leaves.

As Mariamu dissolves public health assertions of the ontological equivalence between *degedege* and malaria in a description of practices, she also diplomatically resists the control such assertions attempt to exert. What Mariamu calls "getting from both sides" is a problem in the eyes of biomedical practitioners in Tanzania. They are concerned that children are dying unnecessarily of malaria because their parents are bringing them to the hospital "too late." Doctors and nurses at all levels of the national health care system acknowledged that the reasons for this tardiness may be the difficulty of travel to the hospital as well as the complicated arrangements mentioned earlier that family members must make to care for a child in a hospital if he or she is admitted. Clinical practitioners in southern Tanzania and in the capital repeatedly asserted, however, that one of the most significant factors for this tardiness is that people see *degedege* as a "traditional" disease. Tanzanians take children exhibiting certain "malarial" symptoms to a traditional healer first. According to these clinic-based practitioners, by the time the parents and other kin are convinced that the traditional healer cannot help their child and they manage to get the child to the hospital, it is often "too late." They complained that these children are in critical condition when they arrive at the hospital and often die within hours. The drugs and procedures at the disposal of these biomedical doctors and nurses cannot prevent these deaths, though these practitioners feel that their treatments might have been effective during earlier stages of the disease. Dr. Mwita, the coordinator of the National Malaria Control Program for the Tanzania Ministry of Health, said that the goal should be to "enlighten the people on malaria. So that the people can discover the symptoms. They can realize that malaria is treatable. They can take their children with fever [to a clinic]. They can know what convulsions are, that those are not evil spirits."

The struggle to control how the convulsions of children are interpreted and to have the opportunity to change the state of such children is laden with a great urgency not only for biomedical practitioners but also for traditional practitioners. Healers argue that if a child is taken to the hospital first and diagnosed with malaria, the shot (*sindano*) given as malarial treatment will bring on *degedege*.[3] The result may be that the child loses her strength (*nguvu*) or her intelligence (*akili*) or her life (*hai*). Mariamu explained:

> Yes, the needles are very fierce, because when you give a child a shot then [comes the] sickness of *degedege*. The child dries up a great deal. The veins of blood and the veins of consciousness stand still. This child dries up a lot because of the needle for malaria. This "injection" of "chloroquine" [brings on *degedege*]. Then the sicknesses compete.[4]

The needle, healers state, is fierce (*kali*). They argue that children must go to a traditional healer first and begin treatment there before going to the hospital. According to all healers with whom I spoke, after the initial *degedege* treatments, the child may go to the hospital, be diagnosed, and receive treatment for malaria. They asserted, however, that a child must receive medication from a traditional healer first or the hospital medicine is likely to do more harm than good.

Parents seeking help for their child often take the child to see a healer and to the hospital. During my fieldwork, I met with healers who were treating *degedege* and with those they treated nearly every day. I encountered a greater number of people suffering from this malady in the rainy season, when the incidence was higher. In the more than 100 cases I saw, each family wove together various ways of treating their child. Only rarely did a family seek treatment for one of these maladies and not for the other. In Ward 5, the children's ward in the Newala District Hospital, where there were often two or even three children to a bed during malaria season, almost every child wore medicine made by a traditional healer.

Biomedical and traditional practitioners as well as many Tanzanians draw a comparison between *degedege* and malaria. The controversy over claims to bodies at a critical moment and the sense of urgency the illnesses involve compel this comparison. Hence, the question becomes: Where are children taken *first*?

Because of the institutionalization of biomedical knowledge and the links such institutionalization has with development projects, the politics of this comparison often drive health care professionals to explain *degedege* in terms of malaria. In other words, they position malaria as the more fundamental concept. Not only does the Tanzanian Ministry of Health (whether at the level of Mr. Mwita, whom I quoted above, or the Newala nurses whom I observed during their early morning public health education classes) privilege malaria in its analyses, some anthropologists concerned with developing more effective public health education programs in Tanzania do so as well.[5] Furthermore, this move to position malaria as more fundamental can be seen in the claims of many mothers who told me that "*degedege* is malaria that has gone to the head." The head is the place of spirits and familiars: where they climb on a person, where they sit, and where they live. Such translations are not merely abstract or formally linguistic. The translations of *degedege* as malaria and vice versa are embodied and material as well as cultural. Such translations demand that people move back and forth between healing settings, that they take a variety of kinds of medication, and that they subject themselves to different therapeutic tools and procedures. They also open up the possibility that novel versions of the body and bodily threats will emerge through efforts to coordinate a variety of biomedical procedures and nonbiomedical therapies.

Case Studies in Newala

The following three case studies emphasize the concrete details of identifying and treating *degedege*. While each healing moment is constructed by a unique confluence of actors, the stories of Juma, Jamia, and Musa illustrate some of the differences (and similarities) in one healer's series of encounters with three patients over defined periods of time. Even with this focus on *degedege* treatments, these case studies are also necessarily stories of how traditional and biomedical therapies are woven together in the range of treatments typically received by those with hot bodies, who are alternately weak and then convulsive in southern Tanzania. They are in some senses familiar stories to those who study medical pluralism.[6] In these narratives, however, *degedege* and malaria are not self-evident entities that are destabilized by the movement of people and medicine; rather, these maladies are constituted as objects of therapeutic practice through such movements (and a multitude of others). After presenting the case studies below, I will draw on them to describe how *degedege* and malaria are enacted in therapeutic practice and the narration of this practice.

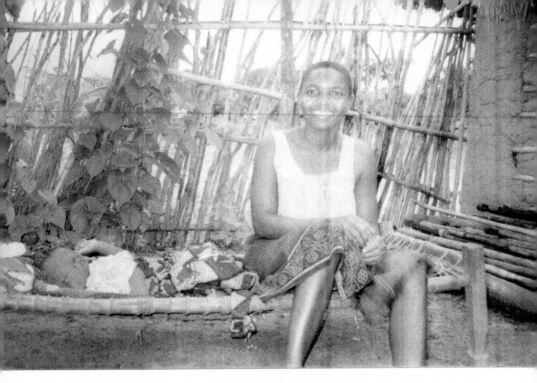

Figure 7.2. Juma and his mother in Binti Dadi's compound. *Photo by author, 1999.*

The Story of Juma

Juma was about two and a half years old in February 1999 when he arrived at Binti Dadi's compound. The day before his arrival, Juma had been taken to the hospital by his mother. There he had been diagnosed with malaria and prescribed chloroquine syrup. Afraid that these treatments would bring on *degedege*, Mama Juma (mothers are most often referred to by their child's name) came to ask Binti Dadi, the local *degedege* specialist, for preventive medicine. Binti Dadi made a very small cut on the end of Juma's nose with a razor blade and smeared a black powder called *kitamango* (Kimakonde) into it. She had made the medicine from *chitamango* (Kimakonde) roots by roasting and grinding them. Sometimes she would add roasted and pounded medicine from *nanamavele* (Kimakonde) roots. After Juma received this treatment, he and his mother returned to their home.

When Juma started to convulse that same night at about eight PM, his mother decided that the preventive medicine had not been strong enough. She and Juma's father rushed him back to Binti Dadi's home. When Juma arrived in the middle of this fit, Binti Dadi bathed him.

She pounded nine different kinds of leaves together in a mortar.[7] She added water and one hot coal to the mashed leaves. Because Juma was in such a dangerous state and it was the first time that he was receiving this treatment, Binti Dadi bathed him herself in an effort to capitalize on the strength attributed to the hands of healers. Binti Dadi scooped water into her mouth and spat it out, once onto the child's head and once onto his buttocks. Then she washed his entire body with the medicinal water, including the bottoms of his feet. Afterward, she ground up root medicine and prepared a thick drink for Juma.

Following his initial treatment, Juma's mother returned to Binti Dadi's home twice a day. Binti Dadi did not generally administer these additional treatments to Juma, but she and Mariamu always personally collected all the medicine, sorted and arranged it, and prepared the medicinal baths. When Juma's mother brought her son to Binti Dadi's home, she would bathe Juma herself and grind the root medicine for him to drink.

Several days later, Juma's parents took him back to the hospital. The hospital staff tested him again, and this time they admitted him for treatment for both malaria and severe anemia. According to his mother, Juma received twelve shots for this bout of malaria before he was released from the hospital. In addition, he was given a blood transfusion. Juma did not start to convulse again when any of these needles were administered.

When Juma left the hospital, his parents brought him back to Binti Dadi. Upon her recommendation, they decided to "cook for" him. This entailed preparing a special meal with Binti Dadi, a meal that would remove the dirty froth (*uchafu povu*) from his stomach. This final treatment, she argued, would prevent him from frothing at the mouth the next time he was startled and began to convulse.

On the chosen day, Juma's parents brought rice and a chicken to Binti Dadi's house. Juma's father slaughtered and cleaned the chicken, which he then cut in half. Binti Dadi stuffed the bottom half of the chicken with a bundle of *mmala* root cut up like matchsticks (the bundle was referred to as *lihungo*). She then cooked this half of the chicken in a pot outside with oil from the seeds of the *nyonyo* bush (*mafuta ya nyonyo*). As soon as the chicken had browned, she then added root medicine (Kimakonde, *mnkun'gulu, mnuvi, mkulanga, mbwabalawa*) that she had pounded into a fine powder. Inside the kitchen, Mama Juma cooked a large pot of rice. Juma and his family sat together to eat from one large plate. After eating, Juma defecated soft green feces. Mariamu commented that the *dawa* cooked with the chicken makes a child run to the latrine. Meanwhile, Binti Dadi wrapped the leftover parts of the chicken in a large *nyonyo* leaf for Mama Juma to carry home. She would boil them again to make a soup for Juma to drink later.

On the day of being "cooked for," the child also receives medicine to wear. This medicine includes a piece of the heart of the chicken and pieces of other organs of the chicken that are considered "dirty" as well as the shadow of the threatened child and a bit of *mmala* root (the same medicine that was cooked inside the chicken). Mariamu wrapped this mixture in a black cloth and tied it

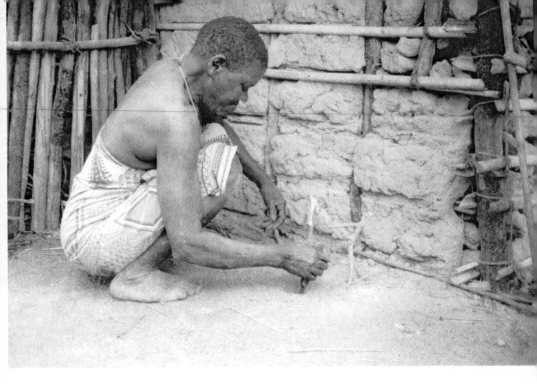

Figure 7.3. Binti Dadi building a fire to cook medicine for Juma.
Photo by author, 1999.

around Juma's neck. Even after Juma was cured, he continued to return to Binti Dadi to get medicinal baths for some time.

The Story of Jamia

In a more striking case in December 1998, a little girl about five years old named Jamia Muhammad was brought to Binti Dadi with fairly severe mental and physical disabilities. She could not stand, walk, talk, or feed herself. Jamia's parents said that three years earlier, after Jamia had learned to walk, she was in the fields with her mother one day. Unexpectedly, she jerked and then began to convulse. Her parents took her to the hospital, where she was diagnosed with malaria and treated. After these therapies, she could no longer walk (*ameshindwa kutembea*). Frustrated that the hospital staff deemed their daughter to be "cured" while she remained debilitated, her parents sought assistance for what they came to see as the continued effects of *degedege*.

Between the time that Jamia was rid of her bout of malaria and the time that she was carried into Binti Dadi's compound, her parents took her to a number of government and mission hospitals in the region. None of the doctors she saw or the medicine they prescribed stimulated her to regain physical basic skills. Binti

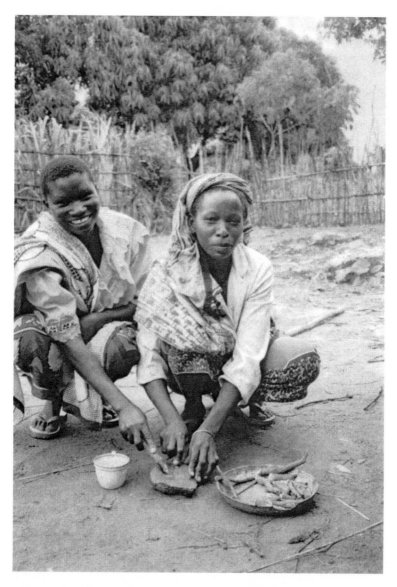

Figure 7.4. A mother (with a friend) at Binti Dadi's compound grinding up root medicine for her child with *degedege*. *Photo by author, 1999.*

Dadi bathed Jamia in medicinal water,[8] fed her medicine made from a combination of roots, and gave her medicine to wear on her ankle, wrist, and waist. After approximately a month of using this medicine of the *shetani,* Jamia began to be able to turn herself over in bed and pull herself up onto her feet again. Later, she began to feed herself.

The Story of Musa

On April 2, 1999, Maua, a 22-year-old mother, brought her one-and-a-half-year-old boy, Musa Kijina, to see Binti Dadi so that he could be washed with medicine (*kumwogesha mtoto dawa*) for *degedege.* A year earlier Musa's body had grown hot and he had started to convulse. At first, Maua explained, her son had a straight-forward case of malaria. Then, however, he changed, and with this change her evaluation of her son's "malaria" changed as well. "It climbed up to his head," she argued (*amebadilishana na malaria; ilimpanda mpaka kuchwani*). When Musa began to convulse, Maua took him to see Binti Dadi. If you go to the hospital, she told me, they say that the fever has gone into the head. Here at the traditional healer's, she continued, they say it is *degedege.* After Musa received treatments for both malaria and *degedege,* "life returned to him" (*hai kumrudia*). "But now," Maua said, "this year, during the period when the corn has started to blossom, the fever has begun with him again. . . . Therefore, in this period it is necessary to bathe [him] with medicine." This medicine protects (*kukinga*) her son, Maua told me. Musa only needed to be washed once, because these treatments were to "fill in" (*kuziba*). Mariamu chimed in, saying that too often mothers can "forget themselves." After the child has been healed, they hope that they do not need to have their child treated again. But children, Mariamu says, will give a mild jerk or start, demonstrating their continued vulnerability, and "show their mother that it is necessary to be sent [to the healer] again."

The individual accounts of Juma, Jamia, and Musa are versions of stories told to me over and over again. Although healers who treat *degedege* and doctors who treat malaria do not work cooperatively, in the patients' narratives the diagnosis and treatment of *degedege* and malaria are inextricably woven together. Mama Juma feared that the hospital medicine would bring on *degedege,* and indeed she attributed the convulsions Juma had after being treated for malaria in the hospital to *degedege.* She did not take him back to the hospital to be treated for malaria again until he had completed a series of treatments for *degedege.* When he finally received a second round of treatments for malaria and anemia, he did not convulse. Mama Juma saw this as evidence of the efficacy of the *degedege* treatments. The very possibility that Juma's malaria could be treated came to depend on his treatment for *degedege.* In Jamia's case, her parents as well as Binti Dadi and Mariamu read her chronic disabilities as an example of the consequences of

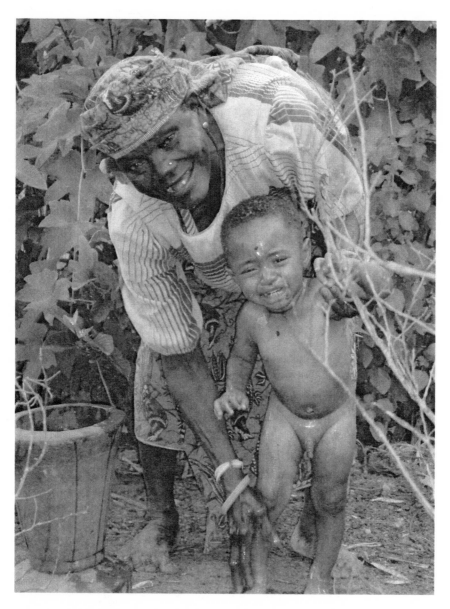

Figure 7.5. Binti Dadi giving a child a medicinal bath for *degedege*.
Photo by author, 2008.

focusing treatment on malaria and not attending to treatment for *degedege*. Treatments for *degedege* illustrate the therapeutic limitations of hospital medicine by marking the impractical specificity of a "cure" that leaves a child unable to walk or to feed herself. Maua reiterated these claims, adding that while the hospital explains *degedege* as a stage of malaria (one in which it "goes to the head"), healers insist on making a distinction between *degedege* and malaria.

Neither accounts of the movement of patients from one kind of healer to another or of the movement of medicine from one kind of space to another fully capture the dynamic and productive tensions in these efforts to find effective treatment. The similarities, connections, distinctions, and conflicts described in these case studies evoke the definitional contours of *degedege* and malaria (in all their fluidity) because they begin to account for the processes through which therapies enact their objects of intervention.

In the following sections, I describe the ontological politics at stake in the multiple and multifaceted events that shape *degedege* and malaria. Propositions central to the lives of Juma, Jamia, and Musa include the following: *mashetani* play with children, *mashetani* climb on the head of healers and tell them medicine, and Christian priests and Muslim imams evoke the *shetani* as the Devil. None of these descriptions involve essentializing *mashetani*. Rather, they begin to elicit the multivalent existence of the *mashetani* through their relationship with other entities and objects on the plateau. In this chapter, not only *mashetani* but also parasites, *degedege*, malaria, the blood room (*chumba cha damu*), the laboratory, Binti Dadi's home, and the bodies of the afflicted come to matter through encounters with each other. Each of these entities appears as a relational event. They stabilize as a trajectory of events. Analyzing and comparing the events that sustain *degedege* and malaria offers a way to describe *mashetani* and parasites without having to relegate one to the realm of belief or culture and the other to the realm of reality or nature. This approach de-essentializes entities that have become objects of therapeutic intervention (such as bodies and parasites) *and* statements of truth about them while still remaining committed to the positionality of these entities and the analytical connectedness of the statements.[9] Instead of struggling to make statements correspond to the world out there, the following sections describe how *degedege* and malaria are brought into relationship with each other in ways that are deemed effective, resilient, or desirable and then examine what is at stake in this (pro)positioning.

Degedege Practice

Children receive *degedege* therapies before they are actually sick, while they are sick, and/or after they have been healed. Although therapies vary from healer to healer and from patient to patient, treatments tend to consist of a series of medicinal baths, repeated doses of a thick drink of ground roots, and one or more types of medicine that the child wears. Healers sometimes use additional medicine to protect an otherwise healthy child from *mashetani*, and they give more specialized treatments in severe cases where the child has lost consciousness. While each of a healer's medicines is crafted with a specific purpose, specialists refer to the range of medicines used to address *degedege* as "medicines of the devil" (*dawa za shetani*).[10] Healers such as Binti Dadi use these remedies to negotiate and manage encounters between *mashetani* and the children with whom they attempt "to play."

Mashetani do not have immediately visible existences. As I was told, one cannot see such devils with one's eye. Only some people, primarily healers, can see them "inside their head." *Mashetani* are not constituted of human matter. They do not have skin, and Tanzanians have found no reason to believe that human skin would act as a natural barrier to them. In fact, no barrier between the person and these powerful nonhuman forces is self-evident. No a priori unit of space constrains interaction with a *shetani*, and therefore *mashetani* are not necessarily guilty of a violation of space. In order to protect children from *mashetani*, boundaries, edges, or barriers must be made. In each of the case studies above, Binti Dadi began treatment by marking off and claiming a bodily, material space by giving the child a medicinal bath. She covered every inch of the child with medicinal fluid, even the bottoms of the feet. This medicine renders the exterior surface of the child substantial and recognizable to the *mashetani* as an obstacle. The boundary is not visible; it is made of medicinal power.

Medicine for *degedege* is commonly said to provide relief and calm by "closing" (*kufunga*) a child. As Mariamu explained: "If a child has *degedege*, s/he will do this [she imitates the stiffening and jerking of a convulsing child] for a long time. However, after closing a child, s/he can be calmed—her/his collapsing stilled."[11] Closing a child involves building a boundary around her or him. To close a child with medicine gives that child a distinct defendable material integrity. Some medicine in southern Tanzania, then, works by (en)closing a person. The efficacy of the techniques healers use lies in their creation of a boundary that distinguishes the child from the *mashetani*.

At the same time that this medicinal boundary asserts a line that is not to be crossed, it also establishes the possibility of transgression. Bodily boundaries tend to be established after transgressions have occurred; put more precisely, the possibility of concretizing the contours of a body emerges through an encounter or event. The first step in managing such encounters is to declare that a transgression has occurred through asserting an enclosed and protected bodily space. The bath is the healer's first attempt to mark off a space, to create a frontier that can then be negotiated. The particular boundedness or exteriority of such a body is new, and it is unstable and fragile. The child continues to receive treatments to reestablish and strengthen the discrete boundedness of the body twice a day, morning and night. The medicinal baths further delineate the body's exteriority as they come to be articulated in relation to ingested medicine that constitutes the body's interiority. These processes of objectification enact a particular, situated kind of materiality.[12] They make the substance of the child—his or her very physicality—sustainable.

Furthermore, healers use protective or preventive medicine to re-close a child. When a child unexpectedly and involuntarily jerks, this sudden movement may be read as a sign of his or her vulnerability. Children are not considered ill at this point, but the jerking of their body indicates their need for medicine. Maua used the word *kuziba*, meaning to "stop up" or "fill in," when she referred to the use of Binti Dadi's medicines to protect her son from the affliction he had struggled with the previous year. When used prophylactically, Binti Dadi's *degedege* medicine "filled in" something. What it "filled in" were any places where the body's previously formed boundary may have broken down, where the definition of Musa's exteriority had weakened over time.

Degedege, then, is a struggle. It refers to a moment when there is an opportunity for either the *shetani* or the person to evolve. Healing acts are those that transform the event from one in which the *shetani* acts, therefore defining itself and demonstrating its existence, to an event in which the very substance of the person is enacted. A young child is most vulnerable to *degedege* because his or her bodily surface has not yet been medicinally solidified; no boundary between the child and the devils has yet been fixed.

The substances that have come to be referred to as *dawa za degedege* are substances that make the child's body more substantial, more material, more defined, and therefore stronger by denying *mashetani* these same qualities. Before treatment, *mashetani* could simply climb on the child and "play with" him or her. No aspect of the child reacted to or offered resistance to these devilish nonhuman agents. *Degedege* treatments render the exteriority of the child a recognizable barrier to *mashetani*. Healers strive to create a body from which devils turn away. On one hand, the hot coal placed in the medicinal bath and the shadow placed in the amulet scare devils away from the child. On the other hand, many of the fragrant leaves used to protect and declare the material space of a person are offered as gift to appease the *mashetani*. Treatments seek to materialize bodily frontiers that alternately induce fear or satiate the *mashetani* in an effort to prevent them from manifesting themselves. Medicine, I was told, is the food of the *mashetani*. When satisfied, these devils will leave. They will not feel compelled to act, to manifest themselves, to play—in essence, to enact an existence. Healers thus treat *degedege* by managing encounters in ways that discourage the emergence and evolution of *mashetani* and facilitate the definition and distinction of a human body.

Malaria Practice

This section describes malaria treatment and invites comparison with the account of *degedege* treatment above. Yet I refuse any easy conclusion that the children I describe with *degedege* actually have malaria and that healers are best described as misinterpreting malaria symptoms as encounters with *mashetani*. In this vein, I do not assess whether *degedege* medications "work" to reduce the symptoms of malaria or malaria parasites in the blood. Both of these approaches would leave nature and materiality behind the protective walls of "real" science and medicine while relegating much of the substance and many of the practices described above to the emotional, symbolic, or cultural—that is, to the powerful but limited working of "society." I make a different move as I compare the processes above with biomedical processes that address malaria in the Newala District Hospital, which is a short walk from Binti Dadi's compound.

While I seek a particular kind of symmetry in this comparison, all dimensions of the phenomena being compared cannot be held symmetrical at the same time. Symmetry is made through decisions about which things are to be held in the same "register" and, therefore, which things can be compared. In this chapter, I raise for analysis and comparison the processes through which therapeutic practices enact their objects of practice. The major difference that emerges between the treatment of *degedege* described above and the treatment of malaria described below is located precisely in the observation that these two sets of practices articulate very different objects of therapeutic intervention. I juxtapose the practices that elaborate a particular kind of body and bodily boundaries evident in *degedege* treatments with the practices that elaborate malaria parasites. This juxtaposition reveals the radical difference in space, authority, and systematic procedures between various kinds of treatment. For instance, individual healers are central to healing and treatment in *degedege* therapies. During *degedege* treatments, the healer, her ancestral shades and other disembodied guides, the medicine she uses, the patient, the environmental surroundings, and numerous other actors come together in a way that compels a particular intervention. Healing practices articulate an epistemological sensitivity to these contingencies. A healer may treat the same symptoms in two patients differently, just as two healers will likely treat the same patient differently. In contrast, a combination of institutional procedures, certain forms of equipment, and the flow of patients compelled by the hospital architecture emerge as particularly important to common malaria therapies in southern Tanzania. This contrast is all the more stark when considering the routine outpatient treatment of an endemic illness such as malaria in a rural district hospital that is understaffed. The emphasis in the latter context is on procedure and moving large numbers of patients through the clinic quickly and efficiently. Few words are exchanged between nurses and patients in the routine care of malaria. Doctors' and nurses' often deep concern for the health of people in the district and for the quality of their work does not manifest itself in an emphasis on doctor-patient relationships.[13]

I illustrate these differences both stylistically and substantively in my accounts of *degedege* and malaria treatments. This section on malaria practice reads differently from the previous section on *degedege* practice. The differences in narrative style capture the ways that objects of treatment, such as bodies and disease agents, are shaped in relation to the detailed processes through which these two maladies are treated. This difference is an effect of how healers, patients, doctors, and nurses in Tanzania (pro)position *degedege* and malaria. The individuality of healers and patients and the specificity of the medicine in my description of healers' treatments for *degedege* is as critical to this type of therapeutic intervention as the elaborate coordination of staff, use of technology, and clinical architecture is to doctors' and nurses' treatments for malaria. As a result, in the account that follows detailed descriptions of individuals are less visible and instead you will find more elaborate descriptions of categories of experts, kinds of equipment, and layers of procedure.

The hospital's procedure for malaria is initiated when a patient walks into (or is carried into) the hospital. Children under five years old receive free treatment throughout Tanzania in government clinics, but the nurses in maternal and child health clinics must see a child first before that child can be referred to a doctor. In the clinic, the nurses register the child's name and check his or her card to see if he or she has been weighed each month and is up to date on all immunizations. The nurse then sends the child and her or his caretaker to see a doctor, who jots down in the patient's notebook the child's various symptoms or complaints such as "headache," "general body weakness or malaise," "throwing up or vomiting," "cough," and "fever." The notebook is a record of the patient's intake dates, observations, requests for tests, test results, diagnoses, and prescriptions.

The list of symptoms propels decisions about whether to initiate a series of laboratory tests. In a case where the initial observations are similar to those listed above, the doctor directs the mother or caretaker to carry the child and the child's notebook to the blood room (*chumba cha damu*), where the child's blood will be drawn. She places the notebook in a cardboard box outside the doorway. After several notebooks have accumulated there, a laboratory assistant carries them into the blood room. Sitting behind a large table in the corner of the room, this laboratory assistant calls out the names written on the front of each notebook one by one. The parent or caretaking kin enters the room with the child when they hear their child's name called. A long low bench runs along the wall from the doorway to the table where the laboratory assistant sits. As parent and child sit on the edge of the bench near the table, the laboratory assistant gestures for the child's arm or foot to be extended across the table. She unwraps a razor blade and pricks the child's middle finger or big toe to draw blood. She puts the first drop on a glass slide, which is called the "observation slide." She then picks up a second glass slide and uses the edge of it to spread out the drop of blood on the observation slide. She numbers the observation slide with the blood smear and props it up against a box of clean slides or a pile of notebooks to dry.

While the blood smear is drying, the laboratory assistant squeezes a second drop of blood from the child's finger and dabs it onto a corner of a white sheet of paper. (Depending on the time of day this paper may be covered with other dabs of blood.) He or she compares the resulting dot to a color card that is designed to measure the levels of hemoglobin in an individual's blood. The card consists of ten bars of color that move from yellow through orange and light red to a deep, dark red. In the center of each bar is a hole. (The card and the white blotting paper are visible on the table in Figure 7.6.) The dot of blood on the paper is placed behind this card so that it shows through the hole, and the nurse matches the color of the blood to the color on the card. Each color on the card corresponds to a percentage of hemoglobin in the blood. The lightest yellow, for instance, indicates that there is no hemoglobin in the blood, while the darkest red indicates 100 percent hemoglobin. The nurse writes the corresponding percentage in the patient's notebook.[14] This percentage of hemoglobin in the blood defines whether or not the individual has anemia, which in this context is taken to be a sign of chronic malaria.

By the time this second test is completed, the blood smear is dry. The laboratory assistant dips the observation slide in a 99.8 percent methanol solution to fix the smear. She calls in another patient and repeats the procedure. Afterward, the laboratory assistant puts the patients' slides with their respective notebooks and carries the pile from the blood room to the laboratory, where there is a microscope. She puts a drop of acridine orange solution on the blood smear and puts a thin transparent cover over this solution. The Newala laboratory adopted this method of diagnosis in January 2000. In 1998, a Japanese organization donated the microscope currently used in the Newala laboratory, but it sat in a closet for two years because the laboratory staff had not been able to obtain the correct staining solution. During this time they used a different staining procedure and a much older microscope, the lens of which was covered with fungus, making it difficult to see parasites at all (Fabricius 1999). It is important to remember that the context of international funding and a long history of unequal relationships between the "First" and the "Third" worlds is critical to the broader story of science and the production of medical facts in southern Tanzania.

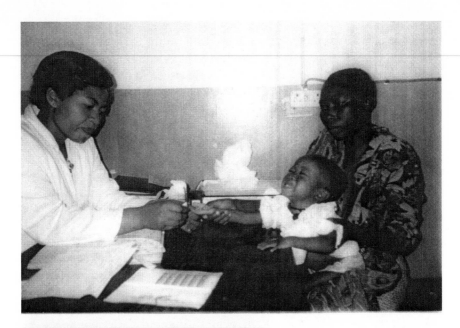

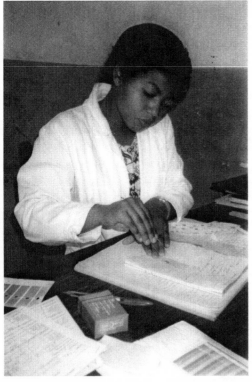

Above. Figure 7.6. A nursing student serving for the day as a laboratory assistant pricks a child's finger to draw blood for malaria and anemia diagnostic tests. *Photo by author, 1999.*

Left. Figure 7.7. A nursing student making an observation slide before screening blood for malaria in the laboratory in the Newala District Hospital. *Photo by author, 1999.*

Facing page. Figure 7.8. Blotting blood for a hemoglobin test. *Photo by author, 1999.*

The laboratory assistant slips the prepared slide into the two thin arms under the lenses of the microscope and selects the magnification. A magnification of twenty times what the naked eye can see is used to find the field—that is, the blood smear. Then the magnification is increased to a factor of forty or sixty times what the naked eye can see. The nuclei of the parasites appear as yellow dots with a small red dot visible at the bottom of each cytoplasm. This is how malaria parasites can be distinguished from red and white blood cells and from other possible parasites in the patient's blood. Malaria, then, becomes visible as a yellow dot with a smaller red dot clinging to it. The laboratory assistant counts the malaria parasites in the field of observation and records the number in the patient's notebook as the number of parasites seen over 200, which is considered the "average" white blood cell count for a field (these are not actually counted). The lab technician then carries the marked notebooks back to the blood room. Sitting behind the desk again, she calls out the name on each notebook. The caretakers pick up the appropriate notebooks and take them to one of the doctors' offices in the hospital so that he[15] can read the results of the test and prescribe the necessary medication.

The doctor is likely to prescribe Panadol, a brand name for a general pain reliever that also reduces fevers, along with chloroquine. If the child is well enough to be sent home, he or she is likely to receive chloroquine in the form of syrup and Panadol in pills that can be dissolved in a spoonful of water. If the child is

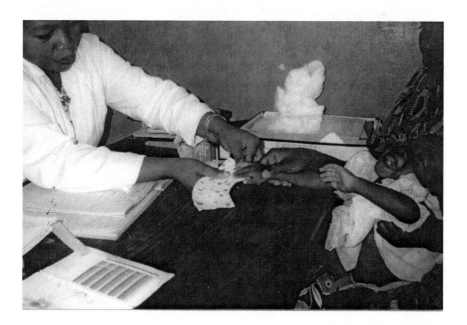

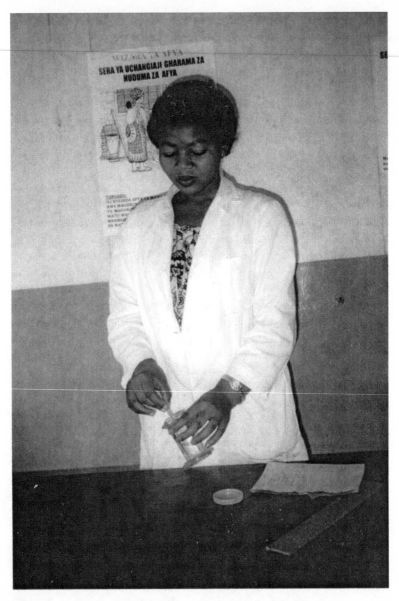

Figure 7.9. Dipping the observation slide in a 99.8 percent methanol solution to "fix" the smear. *Photo by author, 1999.*

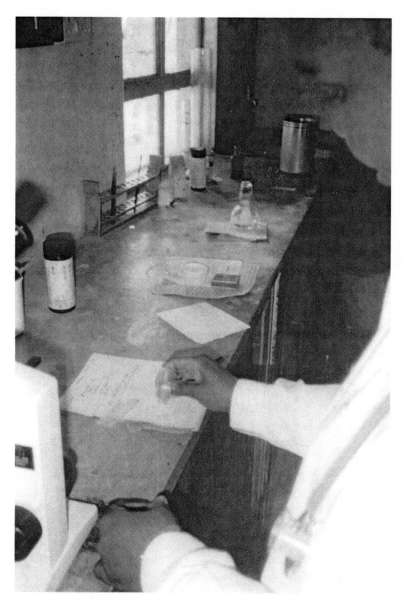

Figure 7.10. Staining the blood smear with acridine orange solution
for observation under microscope. *Photo by author, 1999.*

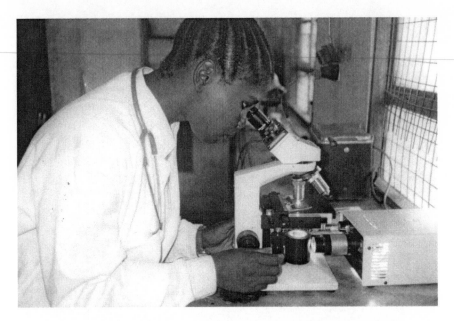

Figure 7.11. Looking at a stained blood smear to check for malaria parasites.
Photo by author, 1999.

severely anemic, he or she might be admitted to Ward 5 and given a blood transfusion. Children who are admitted will likely be given chloroquine by injection.
If a child is unconscious, a quinine drip is typically used to treat the child. If
the particular strain of malaria a child is carrying proves to be resistant to these
drugs, then he or she will likely be given Fansadar [R] or one of the increasingly
popular artemisinin remedies. Malaria medicine is understood to "work" by
penetrating the body—an already-bounded unit with an inside full of biological
material including hemoglobin, red and white blood cells, and parasites. In the
case of malaria in Tanzania, medical scientists and epidemiologists claim that the
invading element is most likely to be distinguished as the parasite *Plasmodium
falciparum*.[16] Malaria medicine of whichever variety works by entering the child
and attacking the problematic foreign element of the interior.

Propositions, Articulation, and Causality

The propositions in the description above articulate the biomedical disease entity
malaria in a web of relationships with medical instruments, experts, institutions, notebooks, razor blades, acridine orange solution, a Japanese development
organization, white blood cells, and many other actors that are too numerous

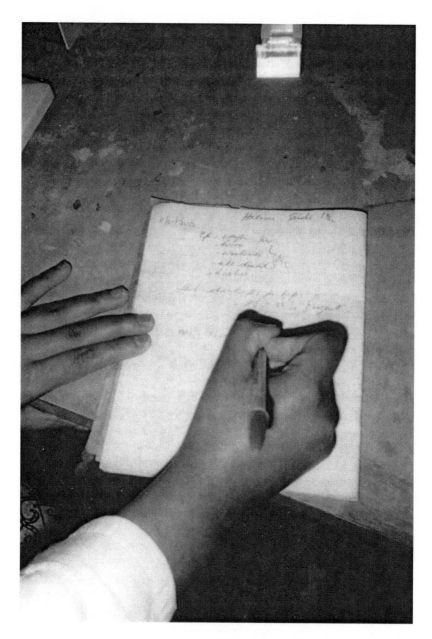

Figure 7.12. Noting the parasite count in the patient's notebook.
Photo by author, 1999.

to name here. In the process of diagnosing malaria, medical staff first come to understand the state of a body as a set of symptoms. Then through a series of laboratory procedures they further translate these complicated states—the fever, the malaise, the general aches and pains, the frequent crying of a child, the lack of energy, and the lack of appetite—using a blood smear into a small magnified field of stained dots and finally to a biomedical diagnosis and a chemical treatment. Parasites are continually reconstituted through these processes of parasitology as they are practiced in a rural hospital in southern Tanzania. Through the use of staining solution and a properly functioning microscope, small entities come into view, emerging as the object of therapeutic practice. Once they are visible, biomedical practitioners herald them as the cause of the child's discomforts and disabilities.

Theories of causation within biomedicine vary greatly. Typically, however, biomedical descriptions of infectious diseases center on identifying specific entities, such as parasites, amoebas, bacteria, and viruses. Diseases become knowable as these entities are isolated as causes. Ideally, it is possible to identify such entities for all complaints. In biomedical practice, isolating causal entities forms the basis for determining cures. Because parasites have come to be seen as causing malaria, identifying them and eliminating them delimits the cure. As one American doctor said to me, "I could take them [patients] into the laboratory and show them what is making them sick!" Such conviction in laboratory demonstrations highlights the importance for biomedical practitioners of articulating a disease entity through each diagnosis. Remember for example, Jamia, whose disabilities had become chronic although she had been "cured" of malaria. For the many clinical practitioners Jamia visited, the object or focus of therapeutic practice was a causal entity.

In contrast, a healer's convictions do not reside in a demonstration of the existence of *mashetani*. While medical laboratory technicians extract blood and introduce dyes and solutions that make malaria parasites react, healers seek to deny *mashetani* the opportunity to act and make themselves visible. Therefore, even while a description of a relationship between a child's convulsions and the play of a *shetani* may be seen as a kind of etiological explanation for affliction, *mashetani* do not emerge as the central point of intervention or as the target of the therapeutic practice. This distinction may appear at first glance to be an asymmetry in that my description of *degedege* practices focuses on the use of medicines whereas my description of malaria practices gives a detailed account of diagnostic procedures. This sense of unevenness, however, is the result of holding on to a notion that therapies must be divided into diagnostic and therapeutic procedures. The division between diagnosis and treatment is neither inevitable nor universal; it is one that is made through a culturally specific series of steps that insists on identifying a cause—an entity that is separate from the person and that contaminates or violates an individual's body, affecting it in an undesirable way.

Feierman (2000) suggests that in Sub-Saharan Africa, the process of moving from one healer to the next is a process of diagnosis by addition. Rather than searching for an underlying mechanism, healers and patients "explored the social and moral circumstances of an illness in ever-widening circles" (329). This argument convincingly opens up the category of diagnostic inquiry beyond reductionist procedures designed to identify single disease mechanisms through processes of elimination. Feierman expands the notion of causality by suggesting that African healing practices allow for the possibility of social and political causes as well as "natural" ones, but he stops short of insisting that causality is a historically specific condition evoked through particular kinds of knowledge and action. As a result, others have interpreted his work as advocating that biomedical and nonbiomedical therapies are "complementary strategies aimed at dealing with different *aspects* of illness causation" (Green 2000, emphasis mine). Such readings cast diagnosis broadly as a series of searches—sometimes widening, sometime narrowing—that seek to identify, isolate, and give shape to a cause, whether it be natural, supernatural, social, moral, or political. Yet diagnosis remains an inevitable and discrete part of therapeutic practice.

I would like to suggest that all forms of healing do not distinguish between diagnosis and treatment. To the extent that diagnosis is the act of identifying a causal agent, *degedege* healing practices do not fall into categories of diagnosis and treatment. The search for a cause does not propel the actions of healers. Curative treatments for *degedege* do not elaborate a causal agent. In light of this example, the concepts of cause and causality deserve the same careful treatment and analysis that anthropologists have given risk (Browner and Press 1996; Crawford 1984; Kaufert 1998; Lock 1998) and efficacy (Feierman 2000; Waldram 2000).

Barthes' "Semiology and Medicine" (1988) begins to lay out the operations that constitute biomedical diagnoses and sustain scientific notions of causality. He defines diagnosis as "the act of reading a configuration of signs" (209). Central to this definition is a distinction between symptoms and signs. Symptoms for Barthes are substantive and experiential. To describe symptoms, he suggests:

> Let us call it *phenomenal*; but a phenomenal which in fact has as yet nothing semiological, nothing semantic about it. The symptom would be the morbid phenomenon in its objectivity and in its discontinuity. . . . The word "symptom" had not immediately involved the idea of signification . . . We believe that the symptom is something to be deciphered whereas in fact it seems that medically the idea of a symptom does not immediately involve the idea of deciphering, of a legible system, of a discoverable signified; it is actually no more than the crude fact available to a deciphering labor, before the labor has begun. (204, italics in the original)

In contrast, signs emerge as the physician's organizing consciousness adds to or supplements the symptoms. Symptoms exist as "substance" but must be made legible, intelligible, and meaningful through signification. Physicians, Barthes argues, transform symptoms into signs through language because such signs are structural and semiotic. Deciphering "crude facts" converts them into signs (the signifiers) of a malady (the signified). In these accounts, biomedical intelligibility emerges as a product of the movement from symptom to sign.

While I question the ontological status Barthes gives to symptoms, the specificity of his description of the "*culture* of the notion of signs" offers the possibility of seeing the relationship between symptom and sign and the form of diagnosis it supports as "belonging to a certain history of the sign, to a certain ideology of the sign" (212). No less is at stake in this question than the historical specificity of diagnosis and the form of biomedical causality it elaborates. The medical cause of discomfort or disability emerges within the distinction between the symptom and the sign, the phenomenal and the semiotic, that Barthes outlines. Whereas symptoms are said to stand in their own right, signs are said to signify something. The "something" becomes the cause of disease and the object of therapeutic practice.

Expanding etiological arguments beyond biomedical notions of causality requires opening up ethnographic analyses to different articulations of the relationship of symptom and sign, substance and form. Substance itself cannot remain immune to semiological critique. Drawing on science studies, this book is committed to rethinking materiality within semiotic-material practice. When tracing the temporal-spatial trajectories through which "things" come into being, science studies scholars have noted that the articulation of cause is the final declaration of the work of scientific investigations. In situated studies of scientific practice, the attribution of cause is where investigations end, not where they begin. This insight requires us to rethink Barthes' view of medical practice, which he defined as "the intrusion of the operational which is a venture outside of meaning" (210). Considering the emergence of alternative materialities and the politics of their encounters requires us to examine the meaningmaking, the significations, and the relations of "the operational." Decentering scientific causality opens up a space for an even more radical reconsideration of etiology.

In this third part of the book, my accounts of therapeutic practice in Newala demonstrate the ways that objects of therapies—substances, symptoms, signifiers, and signified—are emerging within practice. The afflicted and the kin who are helping to manage the pain and debility of the afflicted as well as nurses, doctors, healers, other patients, and numerous nonhuman actors enact the matters of maladies through interactions—questioning, traveling, responding to changes in temperature, eating foods, sleeping, or ingesting medicines. When we consider materiality as emergent, the distinction between symptom and sign is not self-evident. Barthes' account, then, does not reveal the nature of physical substance and medical form as much as it begins to explain when, how, and to what effect biomedicine separates the phenomenal from the semiotic. Situating his analysis in this way suggests a modified definition of diagnosis. Rather than "the act of reading the configuration of signs," biomedical diagnosis might be better described as the acts of establishing signified and signifier, purifying substance and form, separating matter and language, and differentiating cause and experience.

An insistence on dividing all therapeutic practice into categories of diagnosis and treatment smuggles in a narrow conception of etiology and the forms of substance and materiality that make it intelligible. The god-trick that transforms this situated culture of the notion of signs into a universal aspect of therapeutic practice has reduced *degedege* to a symptom, a crude fact to be transformed by a physician's organizing consciousness. It eliminates the possibility of therapies that do not address a "signified" and instead interact with other kinds of objects of practice. It denies the existence of therapeutic objects that cannot be described as "a kind of two-faced unit, of which one hidden face . . . is by and large the disease and one exteriorized face, materialized, eventually fragmented into several signified, is to be constructed, interpreted, given syntax" (Barthes 1988, 205). Malaria practices facilitate the articulation of this "two-faced unit" while *degedege* practice refuse this articulation.

Biomedical processes that address malaria define, visualize, and isolate parasites in a drop of blood, while therapies that address *degedege* entreat the *mashetani* to turn away. In the process of rendering bodies with well-defined interiors and exteriors, *degedege* medicines deny the *mashetani* the opportunity to act and to make themselves visible. This is not to say that biomedical practices do not enact a body or that healers in Tanzania are uninterested in practices that aim to locate a cause. But modern and traditional practitioners enact bodies and bodily threats through particular practices and therefore these bodies and bodily threats are embedded in specific historical, political, social, and technological relationships. Read together, the previous chapter and this chapter illustrate that relationships between protective/preventative and curative practices in clinical and traditional healing are inverse. In the hospital, preventive practices create the future patient or population that will need treatment, while curative practices define the agent of affliction. At the healers' home, protective practices delineate the agent of affliction (such as the *mashetani* or jealousies), while curative practices create a bounded and defensible body.

This chapter focused on how scientific and nonscientific therapeutic practitioners bring into being the very objects of therapeutic care that are then used to justify interventions to treat *degedege* and malaria. Significantly, the body is not the focus of curative malarial treatments and *mashetani* are not the focus of *degedege* treatments. The biomedical body is taken for granted in malarial diagnosis and treatment. The "black-boxing" of certain forms of the biomedical body is evidenced in such small actions as using a standardized estimate of the white blood cell count under a more precise and individual parasite count.[17] *Degedege* healing practices take *mashetani* for granted. Healers do not attempt to eliminate *mashetani*; instead, they use medicine to persuade these devils to "play" elsewhere. Although such *degedege* treatments do not elaborate this etiological agent, they do clearly delineate bodily boundaries, rendering the body substantial in encounters with *mashetani*. Unlike narratives about malaria therapies, narratives about *degedege* therapies do not rely upon an a priori body that then becomes contaminated. Rather, healers propose that the very problem is that there is not enough of a body. In such a circumstance, the child cannot remain distinct or distinguishable in an encounter with *mashetani*. Thus, *degedege* treatments establish an independent material reality for the child.

These ontic and epistemic distinctions inform perceptions about the dangers *degedege* and malaria pose and the forms of intervention that are desirable. On the one hand, undiagnosed malaria leaves a child vulnerable. The processes of isolating, visualizing, and identifying malaria parasites in the blood of an individual make action to counter the threat possible. On the other hand, *mashetani* make themselves visual and demonstrate their distinctive characteristics by climbing on a person. They manifest themselves as a threat by distinguishing themselves (in the process of choosing a body to climb on) and by making themselves perceptible (through the child's convulsions). As Binti Dadi and Mariamu argued above, *degedege* medicines "close" the child; they manage the threat of the *mashetani* by disallowing their identification through a child. Each of these articulations of danger and threat evoke connections between collectives or assemblages of actors and entities. Briefly, from one position, devils called *mashetani*, healers guided by ancestral shades and other disembodied actors, medicine that renders bodies substantial in encounters with *mashetani*, and numerous roots and leaves are joined by a host of other actors that are too numerous to name here but are crucial to the compatibility of all these actors. From another position, parasites and germs, microscopes and the chemical solutions used with them, laboratory assistants, biomedical doctors and nurses, drugs produced in India and Europe, needles, and pills exist and thrive together, again with a host of other actants. *Degedege* and malaria are knowable through the encounters of these multiple entities, and conceivable interventions are shaped by the propositions that have brought them into being.

Furthermore, the ontologies of these two maladies shape the dynamics of their coexistence. Ontological claims structure the myriad translations through which healers, nurses, doctors and patients attempt to intervene. *Degedege* is malaria because malaria parasites cause convulsions. The needles of malaria treatments startle a child without a strongly defined body, provoking *degedege*. *Degedege* is a "traditional malady" that describes the dangerous encounter between *mashetani* and children. These translations of *degedege* and malaria, which seem so important for the making of both moral and epistemological judgments, are part of a process of renegotiating differentiations between the assemblage of actors and entities in which the maladies exists. Such negotiations are social, economic, and technological as well as material, and therefore the ontologies of *degedege* and malaria are not without political meaning.

Politics and Translation

Degedege and malaria matter in the context of treatments, and therefore debates about their relationship are most contentious among those who treat these maladies. In southern Tanzania, *degedege* and malaria have come to be compared and translated because hospital staff and healers disagree about where "startled" and convulsing bodies should go first. This disagreement is at the heart of both public health education programs and the forces that shape contemporary traditional medicine. The two sides, however, are not equal. Biomedical practitioners have the ear of the state. Public health narratives crafted and disseminated by the national health care service can be incorporated into health education classes at the maternal and child health clinic. Nurses currently tell women waiting to have their children weighed and immunized at clinics that *degedege* is malaria. Yet despite the institutionalization of this translation, it does not travel uninterrupted. Outside the hospital, discourses on malaria have not absorbed those on *degedege*. As the case studies above illustrate, the collectives that are drawn together and coordinated through *degedege* treatments remain central to the ways that the afflicted and their families articulate and manage threats to well-being.

The connections and separations that link and define *degedege* and malaria are forged within the context of an impoverished national health care structure, skewed international economics, changing environmental conditions, particular disease ecologies, long histories of expertise in "seeing" disembodied actors, and elaborate knowledge of plant, animal, and mineral substances. These economic, ecological, political, and historical factors position public health nurses and healers differently and consequently evoke different articulations of *degedege* and malaria from them. Public health nurses seek to draw an equivalence between *degedege* and malaria, while healers strive to hold these two maladies separate. Biomedical narratives assert that both maladies have a single cause, while healers' narratives distinguish between the two illnesses by referring to different objects of therapeutic practice than doctors and nurses do.

These arguments over whether *degedege* and malaria are the same thing or whether they are different illustrate long-standing contests about ontologies.

By focusing my analytical lens on how the objects of therapeutic interventions are brought into being, I have sought to sketch the processes through which similarities and differences between *degedege* and malaria are constituted. In so doing, I have not taken up declarations of belief or the many expressions of doubt, skepticism, and uncertainty that patients, caretakers, nurses, and healers make. An individual's or a family's decision to use a therapy does not necessarily indicate faith in that therapy or in the person administering it.[18] Patterns of treatment, however, and the diverse forms of objectification to which people subject themselves and their loved ones in the process of addressing an affliction do enact the ontic differences that are central to therapeutic negotiations in Tanzania. Tracing how therapeutic objects in *degedege* and malaria treatments are created illustrates the coordination of multiple events that articulate bodies and threats to those bodies. In practice, *degedege* and malaria and bodily surfaces and deadly parasites are intelligible as assemblages of relationships or propositions. The struggle between the absolutist politics of public health narratives (*degedege* is malaria) and the hierarchical politics of healers (children must receive *degedege* treatments before going to the hospital) is a struggle to maintain particular relationships and ensure the stability of particular propositions.

Ironically, the friction between these two positions opens bodies and disease entities to further translation. As the absolutist assertions of nurses interfere with the hierarchical claims of healers (and vice versa), they come to shape each other. Narratives about startled bodies and fierce needles describe a contingent and evolving pluralism. Experts and therapy management groups (Janzen 1978) act by reconfiguring the propositions that delineate *degedege* and malaria. Binti Dadi claimed that the treatments given to Juma for malaria startled him (*kumshtuka,* the same word use to describe the effect of the *shetani* playing with the child) and thereby brought on *degedege.* Mama Juma evaluated the efficacy of Binti Dadi's *degedege* treatments by her son's ability to submit to a second set of treatments for malaria without convulsing. Jamia's body was revealed as ravaged by *degedege* because her mental and physical disabilities continued after her malaria was cured. Nurses told Musa's mother that *degedege* is malaria that has gone to the head. In practice, the materiality of these bodies and of the threats to these bodies were composed through partial connections.

In these junctures, complicated and interdependent therapeutic ecologies begin to be visible. The coordination of doctors' assessments of symptoms, tests for malaria parasites, and evaluations of anemia, and healers' assertions about mischievous *mashetani,* medicinal baths, and herbal concoctions enact the subjects and objects of this southern Tanzanian ecology. Partial and strategic relationships constitute these hybrid bodies and disease entities. Attention to such situated connections not only contextualizes absolutist claims but also opens up a space in which to imagine less hierarchical, possibly more democratic, translations.

8

Shifting Existences, or
Being and Not-Being

The struggle of therapeutic practitioners—both biomedical and traditional—to articulate objects of knowledge that will travel between the hospital and the healer's home has, to this point, drawn our attention to moments of interference and encounter. Translation, however, requires some combination of political will, social desire, technological need, and ethical demand. What of times when there is no will to translate? Or when there is an active refusal to entertain the possibility of translation? This chapter is about maladies and objects of therapeutic care that remain inaccessible to biomedical practitioners and unintelligible to scientific medicine. It is about the spaces where there is absence, denial, and silence, at least from the perspective of medical science. To the healer, the unseemly growths, dirty breast milk, and oversized heads discussed below are telling clues about which actors are catalyzing the maladies in question, but to the doctor, these symptoms are insignificant and lifeless. For Binti Dadi each of these symptoms provides a glimpse into the unfolding of a person, body, devil, ancestor, and world. In the Newala District Hospital, however, they are neither cause nor symptom but rather non-events, even impossibilities. While at times healers resist the absences and silences forged by biomedicine, at other times they protect them, claiming them as their own, even reveling in them. For the spaces where scientific translation falters turn out to be exactly where the matters of maladies refuse to be subdued or domesticated.

The cartoon by Balozi that I described in chapter 1 captures the disruption of the inexpressible when knowledges, materialities, and healing truths in southern Tanzania encounter each other (see Figure 1.1). When my cartoon counterpart questions the healer, she asks, "Is true?" The subject of her inquiry is awkwardly absent. This space where speech stumbles and where substances are unrepresentable is what Judith Butler has called the "outside." For her the "outside" of any given normative regime holds the revolutionary potential of the uncontrollable, the unmanageable, the indivisible. It is that which escapes or exceeds the binaries that are central to modernist goals and scientific hierarchies (Butler 1993, 53). In this final chapter, I am called into the absence held open by my cartoonist friend's rough English. I explore the unspeakable, the spaces and things that are hindered by the biomedical gaze. What types of violence are visible from this analytical place? What threats and possibilities lurk in the unrepresentable and the unintelligible "outside"?

The Ethics of Absences

Mothers living in the district of Newala, like mothers in many parts of Tanzania, carry their babies long distances each month to take them to the hospital to be weighed. At times their children also receive immunizations, and if they are sick they might receive curative care. More often, however, women walk to the clinic just to sit through a health education lecture, stand in a long line to have their child weighed, and have this weight written on the child's "under-five card." I marveled at what the biomedical community calls the "compliance" of these women with such obligations even in the middle of critical agricultural seasons. What compelled these women who walked, cooked, and farmed with their children on their backs to look to the rising line on a growth chart for assurance of their child's health? Surely they did not need a scale to tell them that the child had gained or lost weight. Why were they willing to spend the good part of a day taking their children to the clinic each month?

At first, most people simply laughed at my probing questions and changed the subject. One day, however, Mariamu suggested that monthly visits to the clinic were not a choice. Early childhood preventative care was not as uncontroversial as it first seemed to me.

> **Mariamu:** Many people see the nurses who assess the health of the child because they like to know if the health of the child has increased or decreased [over the course of] each month.
>
> **SL:** But I would think that a mother knows. Like you, you hold Yanini every day. You know her weight.
>
> **Mariamu:** Eeh.
>
> **SL:** But you think it is good to [get her] measured?
>
> **Mariamu:** It is good because it has become a thing that is necessary, not a choice for people. It is required. Now we go to the hospital. If you do not go to have the child assessed, if s/he is sick you cannot get medicine.
>
> **SL:** Truthfully?
>
> **Mariamu:** Eeh.

SL: The nurses?

Mariamu: They refuse you and say, "Because you have not weighed the child, we are not giving you medicine." Truthfully, they take the child's card. If you don't have [an up-to-date card to give them], well [that's it]. It is necessary, not a choice, in all of Tanzania. Each section [of the country], even in the villages they weigh children. . . . If she sees on the card that you have not weighed your child, well, you will get problems. They will refuse you. They can cause you to return [home] without giving you medicine. Indeed, this is the reason people go to the hospital to weigh their children. But if it would be a choice, without being obligatory, many people they would not take their children to the hospital.

We were sitting with a group of young mothers when we had this conversation. They all voiced their agreement that fear of being turned away during a time of crisis motivated them to attend the maternal and child health clinic to have their children's cards filled out each month. Encouraged, Mariamu continued. She contended that not just the weighing of children but also the process of immunizing them was contested terrain.

[Once] they have measured the weight, they ask you, "The child has which problems?" If she is not ill, she may need to be stuck with the needle of protection [immunized]. You take her to get the shot. If the [early childhood preventative] assessments were not obligatory, well then many people we would not immunize the children here because it gives them a fierce fever for three days. Many people they would not go.

Over the weeks that followed, other women confirmed that these fears marked the contours of their "choice."

The Ministry of Health does not officially base access to curative care on regular attendance at under-five checkups. Furthermore, I could never confirm the rumors that nurses in the district hospital denied sick children medicine because parents had been delinquent in bringing their children to the weighing station. One doctor caught me off guard, however, when he admitted that although he was not aware of services being denied for this reason, he thought that such tactics were probably warranted. He exclaimed: "How else will you get people to come?" For him, such threats were insignificant in the face of the benefits children obtained from regular biomedical surveillance and immunization. He did not find the fears of these mothers disconcerting. The reason women sought out early childhood care for their children—whether from a sense of public health as a good or as the result of (rumored) threats by health care providers—seemed immaterial to him. He focused his concern strictly on whether or not people complied with the state's guidelines for early childhood preventive care.

This doctor's complacence implicitly poses the question of whether such threats matter. If they do matter, in what ways do they matter? What kind of violence do they perpetrate? After all, the women clearly experienced some pleasure in monthly clinic visits. They dressed their children in their best clothes. They sat and talked with friends and neighbors. They took a day off from their work in the fields. Many swelled with pride over the growth of their child and the compliments of the nurses. Was the cost of the under-five clinical surveillance routine simply a little time out of each mother's farming schedule? From this perspective, holding medicine hostage and releasing it only to well-disciplined bodies appears less detrimental than neglecting to take one's child to be weighed each month and immunized on schedule. I argue below that this moral evaluation by biomedical practitioners is a result of their refusal to acknowledge the objects of therapeutic care and forms of materiality central to healers and traditional healing practices.

The perspective of clinical practitioners is a product of the displacements, substitutions, and associations integral to the enactments of children's bodies through early childhood preventative care. The routine work of under-five visits compiles and cultivates a comprehensible body as part of a standardized population, as we saw in chapter 6. The practices of weighing, charting, and immunizing articulate children's bodies as a series of (relatively coordinated) trajectories. The physical body emerges through practices making it compatible with medical instruments (scales, needles, medicines, etc.) and a variety of clinical actors. These multiple compatibilities (partially) constitute biomedical corporeality. Through them, the body physical becomes a clinically intelligible matter. Bodies that are brought into being through other practices and technologies—that incorporate other compatibilities and that matter in other ways— are displaced by biomedical versions. They are also typically marginalized or seen as unintelligible in debates about health and development. Yet the prevalence and popularity of traditional therapies speak to the resilience of the bodies and threats they enact. Any serious effort to focus on the development of more democratic translations of traditional and modern medicine, as discussed at the end of the previous chapter, requires a sensitivity to ways that therapeutic practices formulate both intelligibility and unintelligibility.

Assessing Pendo's Fever

On March 31, 1999, Seif and Sabina carried the hot feverish body of their two-month-old son, Pendo, to Binti Dadi's home for treatment. They came from their home in Legeza, several kilometers east of Newala. When I greeted this family as they arrived at Binti Dadi's compound, Seif immediately described his son's condition. He explained that two days earlier, Pendo had been "startled by *degedege* . . . and his body was hot. [He] cried and cried, and was spitting up." Seif added: "We took him to the hospital, but the medicine of the hospital and this fever refused each other."

Mistakenly bringing a kind of causal interpretation to Seif's description, I jumped to the conclusion that Pendo had been feverish before his parents arrived at the hospital. Furthermore, I assumed that such symptoms would have compelled the hospital staff to assert that Pendo's symptoms, what might have been deemed his *degedege*, was a result of malaria. The degree to which my assumptions were incorrect was revealed in the following conversation.

SL: He was treated for malaria? Which medicines was he given?

Seif: He was given pills and liquid medicine.

SL: Is that so?

Seif: Eeh, the needle he has not gotten yet. He was given a preventative shot [immunized] the other day. It was Monday. This is the way the fever was seen.

SL: The doctor assessed him?

Seif: No, he was not assessed.

SL: Really?

Seif: Eeh, he was not assessed. They only stuck him with a needle. They said that it was preventative after being weighed at the clinic.

Seif claimed that before his son was immunized, he had appeared healthy and strong. "Indeed, [this is] his first malady. Eeh, this fever of his is the first. After being pierced with the needle, the fever came suddenly and it climbed until [he was] very hot and spitting up in his mouth." Despite the fact that Pendo's body grew hot and he started vomiting immediately after he was immunized, Seif did not suggest that the immunization caused his son's fever. Rather, he said that the vaccine and the fever "refused" one another. This refusal made Pendo's malady visible. "This was the way that the fever was seen."

Although when Pendo's fever presented itself he had not yet left the clinic, this fever did not receive any clinical attention. Pendo was not referred to a doctor at this time nor was any lab work recommended. The nurses only offered Pendo medicine to reduce pain and relieve fever.

SL: What did the doctors say? Why did they think that his body was very hot?

Seif: Eeh, they said the body was hot. That's all.

SL: For no reason?

Seif: For no reason.

SL: Eeh, then you came here.

Seif: Indeed, today [we] arrive to our place (*kufika kwetu*).

The nurses in the hospital most likely interpreted Pendo's fever as a reaction to the vaccine he received and therefore did not take it to be a sign of a significant malady. For them, the fever did not warrant inquiry or intervention. The fact that the reason their son's body was so hot was opaque to Seif and Sabina—"for no reason"—is what drove them to Binti Dadi.

Sabina had heard about Binti Dadi and her therapies from several other people, including her sister-in-law, who escorted the family to Binti Dadi's compound for their first visit. Although neither Seif nor Sabina had been to Binti Dadi's compound previously, Seif referred to it as "our place." Seif and Sabina also referred to Binti Dadi as *mama yetu,* our mother. These possessives implicitly contrast "our" medicine practiced by "our" people with hospital medicine. Through this assertion of a kind of kinship, Seif positioned the family's relationship with Binti Dadi as more fundamental than its relationship with the hospital. He assigned hospital medicine a more tenuous hold on his son's body than Binti Dadi's medicine. Even more important for my discussion here, by discerning that the difference between the hospital and the healer's home was that the healer's compound was a place of kinship where they already belonged, Pendo's parents carved out a place from which they could evaluate the clinic's refusal to ascribe meaning to their son's fever.

Although this place of kinship is outside the normative structures of scientific medicine, it is not free of history, technologies, types of expertise, moral codes, and processes of materialization. When I first asked Pendo's parents why they thought he was not well, his mother said that she did not understand her son's malady. His father, however, ventured a diagnosis.

> **Seif:** I know. It could be that it is a deficiency of food . . . of food that is fed to the child or food that he eats from his mother. He does not have strength in his body. Now this malady can have been brought to the child. He has been infected by this fever, which comes from the stomach.

> **SL:** Because the mother's milk is not strong enough?

> **Seif:** Eeh, he has no strength. Now, for what reason? Being fed nothing.

Complicating any easy association of a possible deficiency of food with straightforward nutritional requirements, he went on to explain that maladies of *mashetani* typically manifest themselves as problems with a women's breast milk. As I turned to Binti Dadi, however, she immediately reinterpreted Pendo's condition as the result of *makanje,* growths that "sprout" in the mother's vagina or in either parent's nose. She announced that Pendo's mother "must break up the *makanje* (*kuvunja makanje*). He has become ill . . . and now we will break the *makanje* and we will give him *degedege* medicines."

Upon hearing Binti Dadi's interpretation, Pendo's father accepted Binti Dadi's expertise and withdrew his earlier explanation.

> **Seif:** The meaning of *makanje* is small creatures that sprout in the nose. Others they can sprout tiny creatures. Just then, if the tiny creatures sprout, they have grown. They can cause danger [for] the child. That is, if they grow inside of the nose [of the mother] they can result in fever and pains for the child. His health is very hot and this puts the health of the child in danger. Then [Pendo's affliction] is not caused by insufficient food. The food is good, eeh.

While some enactments of physical bodies and bodily threats elude biomedicine, these bodies and threats are not outside of all regulatory regimes. As we learn with Seif, the bodies and bodily threats of traditional healing are not outside the norms that are imposed through Binti Dadi's therapeutic expertise. When Binti Dadi rejected Seif's interpretation of Pendo's condition, Seif willingly accepted her expert opinion. Pendo's fever became intelligible as the focus shifted from the child's hot body to the small pimple-like growths called *makanje.*

When fevers afflict a child repeatedly, healers in southern Tanzania look for *makanje.* According to Binti Dadi, *makanje* "sprout" within the body of the mother and/or father. Growths around the mother's vagina or anus and in either parent's nose make visible the habitation of the *mashetani.* Often, *makanje* present as very small pimple-like growths that do not protrude very far; however, I was told that they could grow to be as long as an adult's smallest finger. Every time Pendo looked at his mother or father, the sight of the mischievous devils frightened him, Binti Dadi said. She claimed that the repeated shock of seeing these devils brought on Pendo's fevers.

> Eeh, the child is startled (*anashtuka*) by his mother. If he looks at his mother, if he looks into the face of his mother, the child gives a start. There is a creature inside who scares the child.

Makanje are one way that *mashetani* startle children. The shock of devils calls for *degedege* medicine, which interrupts the dynamic that is developing between devils, parents, and child.

In Binti Dadi's diagnosis, the vaccine that made Pendo's fever visible fades to the background. As she draws connections between the startled child, the fever, and the various growths on the bodies of the parents, the vaccine plays a minor role in the cast of characters that shaped the trajectory of Pendo's affliction. The ability to move outside one discourse rests on the partiality of any dominant normative regime and on conditions that compel the development of alternative associations and translations. This is not an argument for things outside language. Throughout this book, I am advocating for ethnographic work that rethinks materiality in ways that do not isolate substance from semiotics. The dialogue in this section reveals how entities as diverse as Pendo's fever, his mother's growths, Binti Dadi's medicine, and *mashetani* become intelligible as a set of propositions that describe the specific substances of each through their encounters with the others.

Tradition as Matter Out of Place

Binti Dadi attributes *makanje* to rape by a *shetani*. The penetration of the needle used to immunize Pendo made visible this other penetration. *Mashetani*, she told me, visit women in the middle of the night. Throwing the husband onto the floor, they fornicate freely with the unsuspecting wife. *Makanje* emerge as glimpses of these devilish actors and are the embodiment of their acts of violation. To describe the meaning of *makanje* to me, Binti Dadi offered the following hypothetical example:

> The *shetani* comes to commit adultery with this mother (*kumzini mama*) while she sleeps. In the morning, her child gets a fever. This is the business of the *shetani*. The mother herself does not know [what happened while] she was sleeping. . . . Eeh, like you. So I told you first about the business of the *shetani*. It is like this if you live here. Jafari [her name for my partner Jeff] is there in the bed and the two of you are sleeping together. . . . Now it comes and removes Jafari and puts him on the floor. Therefore, you will say that you were sleeping with Jafari, but lo and behold Jafari was removed. Eeh, it slept—this *shetani*. You did not know [and] Jafari did not know the business of the *shetani*. Well then, in the morning your milk does not come. The child is hurting. You come to pierce your *makanje*.

The offending growths, which take up residence in the vagina, the anus, and the nasal cavity, manifest the raucous devil that rudely threw a husband to the floor and daringly raped his wife in his presence.

Mothers and fathers generally cannot feel these *makanje* (at least the smaller variety). The parents themselves are not considered ill.

SL: Eeh, but the mother does not feel sick?

Binti Dadi: No, she does all her work. She farms. She goes to the water. She pounds [grain with a mortar and pestle to remove the husks]. She cooks *ugali*. She eats. She is not hurting.

SL: She thinks she is well.

Binti Dadi: She is well.

Although the *makanje* reside in the parents, this malady does not disrupt their ability to perform their daily tasks. The parents continue their work without debilitating discomfort or pain. The mother is actually said to feel pain by or through the child (*mama anasikia maumivu na mtoto*). Mariamu accounts for these dynamics though "heat."

> The child was startled by the heat of the mother. Even the heat of the father can contribute to the heat of the child because he takes care [of his son], and he contributes.

Makanje within the mother affect the health of the child.

Many mothers seek treatment for this malady at least once during the first years of a child's life. Some mothers return multiple times to ensure the health of an individual child. Women often go with their child to a healer before their husbands are checked for *makanje*. Binti Dadi, like other healers in the area, removes such growths by cutting or piercing the surface of them (*kukunja*).[1] First, Binti Dadi leads the mother to a private place such as the latrine. Lying the mother down on her back and spreading her legs in the air, Binti Dadi examines the mother's genitals, her anus, and the area in between. She lances the surface of any growths with a sharp tool. Second, she examines the woman's nose. The mother kneels on the ground in the courtyard and the healer tips her head back, pushes her nose up and looks deep within her nostrils. If Binti Dadi identifies an *mdudu*, a small creature, in the mother's nose, then she pierces it with a sharpened stick. She describes the process as follows:

> Women come to make a cut in the[ir] noses. Blood comes out. Then the child gets happiness. . . . Eeh, small creatures have been sitting inside (*viko vidudu vimekaa*) like this, and they sit in the other nostril [as well], these small creatures in the nose. Then, well, you lance (*unakunja*). . . . I have killed those small creatures that brought trouble for the child by being in the nose of his mother. . . . When you pierce them, the child plays.

While little blood results from cutting *makanje* around the genitals, piercing the nose releases a stream of blood. Immediately after the *makanje* in her nostrils are pierced, the woman bends at the waist, allowing the blood from her nose to make a red pool on the ground. After the *shetani* has been removed in this way, Binti Dadi marks the child with the physical evidence of the devil's death. She dabs the blood that has fallen to the ground on the center of the child's forehead near his hairline and on the bottom of his left foot. When the blood stops flowing from the mother's nose, Binti Dadi pours water into the mother's hands and she washes her face. Then, without drying her face, the mother runs her hand from her forehead to her chin to scrape off the excess water and flicks it into her child's face. This water startles the child, countering the many times he was startled by the frightening sight of *mashetani* in his mother.

Next, Binti Dadi prepares medicine. She pulverizes several different leaves together in a mortar. She adds water as well as one hot coal from the fire. Binti Dadi scoops some of this water into her mouth and spits it on the rear end and

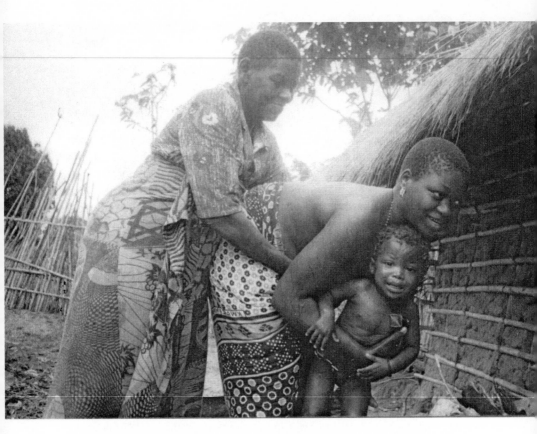

Figure 8.1. Binti Dadi bathing a mother and child during treatment for *makanje*. *Photo by author, 2000.*

the head of the child. The medicinal water, mixed with the saliva in her own mouth, further counters the malady by startling the child with the medicine and the strength of the healer. Binti Dadi then bathes the child by scooping the water out of the mortar with her hands and rubbing it over his body. After Binti Dadi bathes the child alone, the mother strips from the waist up. Standing next to the mortar, she bends ninety degrees at the waist, making her back parallel to the ground. She holds her child under her breasts. Binti Dadi uses the medicinal water to wash the mother's back and breasts. As the water pours off the mother, it falls onto the child. This second part of the treatment showers the child with medicinal water that is mixed with the "strength of the mother." Finally, Binti Dadi dumps the medicine water from the mortar onto the part of the thatched roof that hangs over the door to her kitchen. As the medicine drizzles down, the

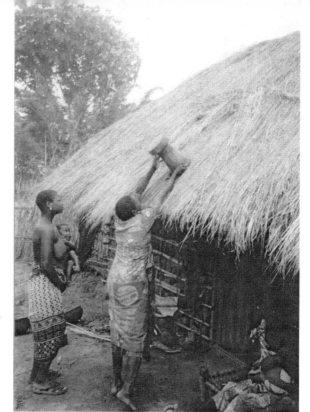

Figure 8.2. Binti Dadi pouring herbal water from a *makanje* bath on the thatch eaves of her kitchen. The mother and her child will walk under the dipping water. *Photo by author, 2000.*

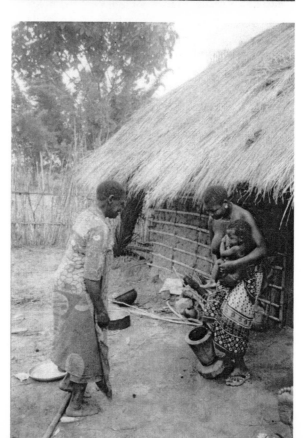

Figure 8.3. As the mother and her child return from walking under the shower of herbal water from the eaves, the mother knocks over the *kinu*, in which the herbal bath has been prepared, with her knee. *Photo by author, 2000.*

mother, still holding her child, walks under the spray toward the door and then turns around and walks back under the spray walking away from the door. Binti Dadi places the now empty mortar in her path. As she is returning, she hits the mortar with her knee, knocking it over.

If the father is to come to have *makanje* removed as well, he will usually come a few days after Binti Dadi lances the devilish creatures in the mother. She pierces the father's nose and uses his blood to mark his child. She washes the child again, although she does not bathe the father. The mother's bath under the eaves puts her in the path between the kitchen and the mortar, a path which is well trod with female steps. Her double pass through the dripping medicine references specifically gendered forms of power enacted through the intimate spaces of this part of the home and over the activities of nurture and feeding that happen there. This therapy gives space to her ability to sustain her child; it rejects the power of the *mashetani* that violated her. While the father "contributes" to the child, as Mariamu says, his contribution marks the boundaries of these gendered spaces of feeding and reproduction. In combination, treatments to remove *makanje* make the bodies of a mother, father, and child (more) compatible.

There are no clinical treatments in the Newala District Hospital to cure *makanje*. Clinical practitioners do not articulate these vaginal, anal, and nasal growths as signifiers of underlying disease or as entities that generate effects. As Mariamu asserts: "At the hospital, they do not know. It is traditional medicine." None of the women with whom I spoke ever went to the hospital with complaints of *makanje*. Often when I described *makanje* to doctors in the area, they looked at me quizzically, unable to imagine the problem. When I probed further, they claimed that the condition was "not harmful" or "not dangerous." Perhaps these *makanje* were "new growths" or "scar tissue," or "the sores of someone having a chronic sexually transmitted disease." Those in the nose might be "polyps," they hesitatingly offered, but they were "nothing to worry about," nothing that needed medical treatment.

Nurses tended to be more ambivalent. One of the deans of the nursing school attached to the Newala District Hospital confessed to me that she had once examined herself for *makanje*. While she quickly stated that she did not "believe" in *makanje,* she had submitted to her mother-in-law's pressure to check for *makanje* when her second child was battling a recurring fever. Using a small mirror, she examined her vaginal opening. In general, nurses tended to be familiar with *makanje*. Some had had *makanje* removed themselves. Binti Dadi spoke of such incidents when she asserted the reality of *makanje* and the credibility of her own therapies.

> Even the nurses [from the district hospital], they come to break the *makanje*. [They say,] "Binti Dadi I have come. I have given my child shots. I have been defeated. I see my child; she is afflicted. I have come to break the *makanje*.

Binti Dadi also claimed that the nurses at the hospital referred patients to her. Although doctors at the Newala District Hospital (who were all men, and none of them were Mmakonde) were unaware of *makanje* as objects that were relevant to the health of women and children in the area, nurses (who were mostly women and were often from families on the plateau) understood *makanje* as matters that needed to be dealt with outside the space of the clinic.

People on the plateau frequently glossed *makanje* and the treatments they require as "traditional" or "customary." Mariamu explained that these therapies "guard (*kudhibitia*) the child by our—the waMakonde—customs." Her reference to "our customs" echoes Seif's claims above to "our place" and "our mother." While such attributions assert a distinction between the hospital and the healer, this distinction is not easily reduced to a difference between the physical and the social, the modern and the primitive, the universal and the particular, or even the "Western" and the "African." Mariamu speaks of "custom" in order to name that which disrupts the hegemony of biomedical articulations of the social-material world.

> [Long ago,] there was no hospital. But people used the medicine of traditional healers and they were cured . . . they were completely cured. But now there is a great deal of medicine and many children they get maladies because mothers eat vitamin pills [in order to] increase their blood. Children, after they are born, after they arrive at a young age, three or four years, even one year, many children they are having no blood. Many children have the problem of having no blood. [Long ago] each child had good health, and if they were hurting a little, they went to remove *makanje,* then the child healed. But now there are problems because they break tradition. Because many doctors they break tradition by saying, "the medicine of traditional healers is not good." Because of this [many people] now go to the hospital. They do not have the opportunity to know many customs. Eeh, there is no knowledge of *makanje.* Some women can have *makanje* without being aware of it, and their children can have problems. Even if [the child] gets chloroquine, he will continue to have problems because he cannot go around custom. Many mothers go to the hospital and then they return to Binti Dadi. They say, "Wait! Let us go to Binti Dadi."

"Custom" here glosses the practices that lie outside the clinical setting, and are often deemed subversive. As Mariamu describes it, "custom" threatens the continuity of biomedical treatments and perhaps that of biomedicine. *Makanje* embody difference that cannot be controlled by biomedicine.

The hospital, Mariamu implies, has never succeeded in domesticating all signs of corporeal difference. It has never been the only site, even the primary site, in southern Tanzania for delineating the physical body and those things that threaten its existence. The supposed progress of biomedical expansion, however, has given new shape to the resilience and resistance of *makanje.* These growths now disrupt the expected trajectories of immunizations and malaria connecting them with devils, sex, healers, herbs, and a range of therapies. Binti Dadi's treatments may be seen as intersecting with the ills of a population that have been created through public health measures such as immunizations, but these intersections are not the explicit focus of her treatments. She, like other healers, cuts *makanje* to intervene in a child's affliction. Similarly, mothers and fathers submit to this pain and the startling sight of blood in an effort to stop the fevers that plague their child.

When Mariamu declared that "it is traditional medicine," she was referring simultaneously to the knowledge of and the physical manifestations of *makanje*. So-called traditional therapies articulate the substance of *makanje* in ways that do not contradict as much as they exceed biomedical explanation. *Makanje* remain outside the efforts of biomedicine to frame bodily experience, so their substance is vague and undefined in the clinic. However, in southern Tanzania, matter is not held hostage by medical science. Binti Dadi, her medicines, her *majini,* her *mahoka,* Mariamu, the mothers, the fathers, the mothers-in-law, and the sisters-in-law described above all actively attributed material qualities to inscrutable events.

The matter of these devils establishes a space from which to view the violence of biomedicine's effort to frame bodily practices. This violence is not inherent in preventative or curative medical practices; it is a result of a confluence of political, economic, and ethical regimes that support the hegemony of modern medicine. The doctor I mentioned above who tacitly supported subtle threats that motivate women to take their children to maternal and child health clinics for monthly checkups participates in this violence. In addition, ethnographies that depict traditional therapies only as a social commentary on modern medicine, bodies, development, and postmodern conditions extend the denials that erase the historical and contingent nature of biomedicine's claim on bodies and the things that threaten those bodies. Faithful description of the ecologies within which physical life unfolds in southern Tanzania requires accounts that are open to the possibility that matter comes into being in multiple ways.

Substantive Non-Events

Makanje are not alone in their capacity to elude the attempt of biomedicine to circumscribe what bodies are. Seif's initial (mis)interpretation of his son's fever as a weakness from insufficient food draws attention to the existence of other entities that biomedical practitioners refuse to perceive. The shout by Mariamu's composite patient above ("Wait! Let us go to Binti Dadi!") threatens the continuities that constitute biomedicine as a normative regime. In this section, I describe two other maladies—dirty breast milk and *nyokoli*—that are treated with traditional medicine in southern Tanzania. In the months and years that I worked with Binti Dadi, these maladies were some of the most common reasons that patients sought her help and medicines. Binti Dadi kept medicine for these maladies on hand and even moved some of the medicinal plants she uses closer to her compound because she treats these complaints so regularly.

Dirty Breast Milk

Any problems a mother has with breastfeeding can evoke a multitude of indictments against the *mashetani*. Most prominent is the assertion that one of these devils has come in the night and fornicated with her. This violation can materialize in the mother's breast milk. The first indication of the *shetani*'s habitation is the swelling of the nursing mother's breasts (*maziwa yanajaa*). As the *shetani*'s presence contaminates her breast milk, she begins excreting "only water" (*maji tu*). The milk becomes the poison of the devils (*maziwa yana sumu ya shetani*). When the breastfeeding child receives this poisoned water, she or he may throw up or have diarrhea. To treat this malady, the outside bark of the roots of two trees (*mala* and *mngulu,* sometimes referred to as *mungunu*) are gathered and pounded into a fine powder. This powder is then cooked like porridge. The resulting medicine is fed to the mother and child and then the remainder is smeared on the mother's breast and over the child's entire body.

Biomedical practitioners do not believe that a mother's milk can "turn to water" or "become dirty." Nurses and doctors tell mothers that pain in their breasts is likely to go away in a day or two if the baby breastfeeds frequently and the mother rests and drinks a lot of fluids. In clinical terms, breasts usually become too full or "engorged," because the child has stopped feeding as much or as frequently for some reason. If a duct becomes plugged, biomedical advice asserts that massage, frequent breastfeeding, and hot compresses are the best remedies. If the blockage leads to an infection or abscess, doctors will sometimes prescribe an antibiotic. Breast milk itself, however, does not become an object of therapeutic attention in clinical settings, and biomedicine is not mobilized to transform it.

Large Heads

Not all unruly substances emerge from interactions with the *shetani*. A common growth that healers in southern Tanzania consider malevolent, and therefore remove, is the *nyokoli*—a small, whitish pimple-like formation found in the throat of infants. This is not a malady of *mashetani* or the effect of jealous others; it is "just a malady" (*ugonjwa tu*). Most people in Newala were content to simply refer to it as a mundane or ordinary malady (*ugonjwa kawaida*). While it is not considered life threatening, the presence of the *nyokoli* is widely thought to influence the size of the child's head. If the growth is not removed, the child's head will grow too big.

Often Binti Dadi administered treatment for *nyokoli* preventatively. One afternoon, however, Mariamu described the arrival of a negligent mother who had allowed her child's head to grow unusually large by failing to have the *nyokoli* in his throat removed soon after it appeared.

> Yesterday, one child came in the morning. Her/his mother stays in Mtama. She came here to Newala for a problem. She is burying her uncle. But after the mourning [rituals], she brought the child [to Binti Dadi]. S/he had *nyokoli* [Kimakonde]—which is *kimeo* [Kiswahili]—a thing that sprouts here. [She points to the back of her throat.] The *kimeo* in the throat. Indeed after this [sprouted], someone in their [family] had neglected [to take the child to a healer and] to have it removed. Well, this child had grown large because they failed to remove it early. The child had a large head. Because they neglected early treatment, the child developed this problem.

To remove *nyokoli,* Binti Dadi looks deep into the throat of the infant. Identifying the small white dot, she wets her index finger with a little oil. (If she has prepared *nyonyo* oil for other reasons, that is what she uses. If that is not available, she uses vegetable oil.) Then she dips her finger in a black medicinal powder, *chanjele,* which adheres to the oil. Inserting this finger into the mouth of the child, she digs out the *nyokoli* with her fingernail. After the *nyokoli* has been removed, Binti Dadi smears more of the *chanjele* on the wound in the back of the child's throat. Finally, she streaks some of the *chanjele* in two lines that span the length and width of the child's head: the first along the top of the child's head starting on the forehead and going back toward the nape of the neck and the second going from one ear to the other. She binds the head together with this cross of medicine.

Salima, the waMakonde wife of a German doctor who worked at the Newala District Hospital in the late 1990s, recounted her experience of taking their daughter to a local healer to have a *nyokoli* removed when the child was two months old. Her husband, who walked in unexpectedly on our conversation, was shocked to learn almost a year after the fact that his daughter had undergone this treatment, and he was puzzled about what was removed. When Salima described the growth and explained that if it had not been removed their daughter would have had a large head like one of their neighbor's children, he scoffed. When he demanded to know why she had not told him of the treatment, Salima responded only by saying that the *nyokoli* was not about the medicine of white people (*dawa za wazungu*) but was rather about custom (*desturi*). Echoing Mariamu, she evokes custom to refer to a space outside the evaluation and logic of "white medicine." In the process of dismissing her husband's concern, Salima juxtaposed the collective of entities active in biomedicine and their genealogy through colonial and development practices with the collective of entities engaged through traditional medicine.

In the hospital nursing school, I was shown pictures in medical school textbooks of entities that these nurses and instructors interpreted as *nyokoli*. They assured me that they were harmless and insisted that they had no connection to the size of a child's head. In 1973, the Department of Child Health at the University of Dar es Salaam published a pamphlet entitled *Care of the Newborn Baby in Tanzania* in which the authors described "small white cysts on the hard palate." These "cysts," the pamphlet claimed, "are normal" and "will disappear in a few months without treatment" (Hamza and Segall 1973, 4).[2] *Nyokoli* are lost in this clinical translation. They are represented as inert and lifeless and not as productive sites for the generation of events.

When I told Binti Dadi and Mariamu that I had gone to the hospital and seen pictures of *nyokoli*, Mariamu responded simply, "*Hakuna*. There are none." She incredulously denied the possibility that pictures of this phenomenon were available at the hospital. How could doctors and nurses know about these lumps if they did not have the ability to remove them, affect them, or act on them? She asserted: "This is the medicine of Binti Dadi. She was put at ease by God for saving children to remove this. You break a pimple (*kuvunja chunusi*). Then, in that place, you smear medicine." Healing in southern Tanzania is what Farquhar (1994a) has described elsewhere as a "knowing practice." Mariamu rejected my report that clinical practitioners who do not treat small pimples in the back of infants' throats as clinical matters have pictures of them. She insisted that *nyokoli* are unintelligible within biomedical discourse. In so doing, she claimed that the power to represent *nyokoli* and to intervene to treat them lies in the purview of other experts in other spaces. For people on the plateau, knowledge of the body and its threats are imagined as intimately connected to therapeutic intervention. Correspondingly, representations emerge as a part of therapies.

Both traditional and modern practitioners create absences and silences. The same separations and connections required to formulate objects of therapeutic attention also lead to obfuscations. The privileged position of scientific knowledge allows biomedical practitioners to deny the existence of objects of therapeutic practice that are unknown or unknowable in the clinic: the clinic circumscribes ontological possibilities. In contrast, the more vulnerable political and economic position of traditional healers compels them to more explicitly locate the existence of objects of (both biomedical and traditional) therapeutic practice in forms of expertise, institutional structures, technologies, and temporal trajectories. Healers then situate and pluralize ontological possibilities. Mariamu seized on the ability (and willingness) of Binti Dadi and other practitioners of traditional medicine to identify and articulate objects of therapy as outside the languages of science and medicine in order to demonstrate the limits of biomedical knowledge. She denied the possibility that these small white growths might be translated into a biomedical context, for the incommensurability of *nyokoli* with biomedicine holds open a space for alternative matters. This incommensurability neither describes particularity nor is it complementarity. Rather, it illustrates the limit of a normative regime's ability to domesticate all it encounters.

Corporeal Emergences and Correspondences

Not all bodies in southern Tanzania are bound by skin. Attempts to translate treatments for *makanje* and other traditional maladies into current medical scientific practices are complicated by assumptions about corporeality. Biomedicine starts with the assumption that after birth the body of the parents and that of the child are discrete entities. This is the starting place from which doctors and scientists articulate connections or relationships between the parents and the child. For instance, in biomedicine, although genetics may speak of the kinship of bodies, disorders in a child cannot be addressed through the body of the mother or father. Traditional healers, however, take connections and relationships as a starting place from which to understand corporeality. Traditional healers say that treatments for *degedege, makanje,* dirty breast milk, and *nyokoli* "close" the afflicted person. Medicinal baths, lines and crosses of blood or medicine drawn on the skin, amulets, and "ropes" of medicine worn around the waist, ankle, wrist, and neck of a patient all bind and tie together the very substance of that person. Bodies are not essentially discrete objects; their separateness, solidity, and stability are created through the interventions of healers. In other words, bodily boundaries in southern Tanzania are created and maintained through medicine.

Therapies attribute corporeal qualities to inscrutable events. Each treatment, however, enacts the body in a particular way; we might say that each treatment enacts a particular version of the body. The correspondences and resonances between different ways of "getting" and "closing" a body establish a habitus in which corporeal matter becomes intelligible. To evoke these correspondences in a way that keeps them as productive and flexible as they are for healers, I turn my attention to additional ways that healers stabilize bodies and their relationships in the world.

The Dangers of Sex

In some parts of the continent, including some areas of Tanzania, people describe sexual fluids as contributing not only to conception, but also to the growth of a child in the womb. Sexual fluids that are inappropriately distributed can harm a fetus or a newborn. Ethnographies and histories of African health and healing have detailed therapeutic practices that address prolonged or difficult labor as evidence of adultery. Therapeutic diagnoses that attributed problems in childbirth to the adulterous relations of one of the parents-to-be caused great distress to medical missionaries, both for the gatherings they would bring to the hospital ward and for the forms of corporeality they enacted in the hospital (Hunt 1999). These therapies demanded that the man or woman who had strayed outside of marriage publicly confess their actions. In southeastern Tanzania today, such confessional therapies still provoke the concern of doctors and nurses. The project coordinator at Médecins Sans Frontières in Mtwara argued that some women chose to give birth at home rather than in the hospital in order to have the option of using such therapies to ensure their health and that of their child. Other scholars have suggested that since government hospitals prohibited the presence of family members in the maternity wards, some women have delayed their departure for the hospital during a complicated labor in order to receive such therapies.[3]

In Newala, if a pregnant woman or her husband engages in sexual relations outside marriage, the child in the womb is thought to "climb up" (*anapanda juu*). These adulterous acts prompt the child to move from a position low inside the woman's belly toward her heart. This position is linked with a long and dangerous labor. Therefore, some elders and *mkunga* demand that both the mother and her husband confess the names of anyone other than their spouse with whom they have had sexual relations during the pregnancy of the child about to be born. The safe delivery of the child is then attributed to these confessions. The act of confession by the mother not only affects her own body, it also affects the body of the child within her who is "climbing" in response to her parents' illicit behavior. The father's confession does not affect his own body at all, but it does affect the bodies of his wife and of the child still in the womb. These displacements and associations establish the body of the child in events that involve the mother, the father, and the womb.

In the hands of some midwives, however, the confessions of adultery have become less central. Binti Dadi, for instance, now uses a medicine that coaxes a fetus down into position so that a woman may give birth easily without explicitly confessing any of her extramarital affairs or demanding such a confession from her husband. While the use of this medicine implies that one or both parents have committed adultery during the time of the pregnancy, thereby acknowledging the effect of the parent's sexual relations on the state of the womb, this medicine works directly on the child in the womb. Binti Dadi rubs the medicine on the mother's stomach in downward strokes starting at the chest and ending just above the genitals.

After children are born, their physical states remain vulnerable to their parents' sexual relations. The parents' sexual activity with each other threatens to destabilize the body of the child. Tanzanians link the resumption of sexual relations too soon after the birth of a child to the deterioration of the physical state of this infant. Elders declare that in the past, parents had to wait for approximately two years after the birth of a child to resume intercourse. After this time, medicine facilitated the resumption of sexual activities and ensured the continued health of toddlers by protecting them from the harmful effects of their parents' intercourse. Sex between a husband and wife before this time was referred to as adultery (or crass fornication, *tendo la zinaa*) rather than as an act of marriage (*tendo la ndoa*).

As expectations about sex and fidelity change, when and how medicines are used to intervene in these events also change. Binti Dadi claims that these days, men and woman who want to have sex after the birth of a child often demand such medicine early. The availability of modern contraceptive methods seems to have contributed to this demand. Women who are still breastfeeding an infant can now prevent the birth of another child while also preventing their husbands from seeking out the company of other women, a practice that might lead to the husbands having children out of wedlock or taking another wife. In response, Binti Dadi has modified her traditional medicines. New parents who want to resume their sexual activities before the recommended two-year timeframe or while the child is still breastfeeding regularly have options. Binti Dadi now makes medicine that protects the child from the harmful effects of this folly. The infant's body continues to materialize as part of the relationship between mother, father, and child, yet under contemporary conditions new traditional medicine is needed to ensure its health.

Healer as Mother

A new mother named Sabini sat in Binti Dadi's compound with Mariamu and me one the afternoon recounting her experience of conceiving and delivering her son.

SL: Did you use medicine from the hospital? Before getting pregnant?

Sabini: I got pills.

SL: Pills?

Sabini: To increase [my] blood by vitamins.

SL: And did you use the pills?

Mariamu: I got vitamin pills as well.

SL: Did you eat [the pills]?

Sabini: I left those other ones. [Taking them would have been a sign of] ignorance, because if you continue [taking the vitamins] for a long time, they are a problem. The nurse in the clinic did not give me much medicine; she told me, "You have to eat vegetables and many leaves." Now me, I delayed [taking the hospital medicine]. I continued drinking *kombe* and medicinal leaves for the purpose of defending the health of the child who would be born. Because I saw one mother, she was a nurse in the clinic. . . .

SL: A midwife here in Newala?

Rather than allowing Sabini to clarify this question for me and continue her story, Mariamu interrupted. She wanted to correct Sabini's vague assertion that implied that she had continued to drink *kombe* throughout her pregnancy. Indeed, this was the problem, according to Mariamu. Sabini had used *kombe* to get pregnant but had not continued to use it once she had conceived.

Mariamu: Eeh, now I gave her medicine. After getting medicine, she got pregnant. [During] this pregnancy she did not drink medicine again until it reached six months. She only drank the medicine of the hospital, but she did not want to use traditional [medicine], not even *kombe* and herbs. The child was born after nine months but he had only one and a half kilos. A very small one. He was covered with oil [a reference to *lugano*].

SL: Is he alive now?

Mariamu: Eeh, he is here. Because she broke tradition, the child was not born healthy. The *kombe* helped to give her [the mother] health in the face of the *mashetani*. These devils were banished [by the medicine]. If a person has had devils, if a person has gotten a malady [*ugonjwa wa mashetani*] . . .

Mariamu turned to Sabini accusingly and reminded her that: "You have had *kombe*. You came to see Binti Dadi." Sabini slightly sheepishly agreed: "Yes, I came to see her."

Mariamu claims that Sabini had difficulty conceiving because she was plagued by *mashetani*. Sabini came to Binti Dadi's compound for help and received medicine that banished these devils, enabling her to conceive. After she became pregnant, she did not continue to use this medicine frequently (as, for instance, Mariamu herself had continued to do during her pregnancy with Yanini). Mariamu argues that the *shetani* returned and bothered the fetus. As a result, the child weighed only one and a half kilos when he was born (less than three and a half pounds).

As central actors in the conception and gestation of Sabini's child, Binti Dadi and her medicine continue to be critical to his continued health and well-being.

The child's physical vulnerabilities are imagined (at least partially) as disruptions of the relations that made his conception possible. Because his existence, his corporeality, owes itself to Binti Dadi's medicine, Sabini's failure to medicinally reinforce and fortify this child's body opens up the possibility of malady. Binti Dadi and this child maintain lifelong obligations to one another. She and her medicine cannot be easily abandoned, nor can she easily turn away from the needs of this child. To mark this relationship, Binti Dadi refers to Sabini's child as "my child." He will grow up referring to Binti Dadi as "my mother," like many of the grown children whose conception Binti Dadi facilitated. These possessive claims do not undermine Sabini's rights to motherhood. But they do acknowledge the work of Binti Dadi's medicine in the conception. The physical body of the child emerged as a relationship that involved the mother, the father, and the healer. The attribution of corporeal qualities to the events that followed from these relationships shaped and continue to shape this child's body.

Exchanging Fluids

Mariamu used her saliva and her breast milk to cultivate the growth of Yanini's body. She spit into her hands and massaged the back of Yanini's head, shaping it, coaxing it into a narrower cone. She squeezed out drops of breast milk in order to straighten Yanini, particularly her joints. "We arrange her like this," Mariamu told me.

> We set her right [tunamtengeneza]. You use the water of the child. You do this to her in order to return the head so that it sits well . . . the head of the child. For [when] doing this frequently, the head sits well. If the child has a big back of the head [ana kisogo kikubwa] well then it will return. . . . I spit saliva to do this . . . to lick her in the custom of long ago, in [the custom of] the elders, indeed they were doing this. For to do this is to smooth [kulainisha]. The child gets the mother's saliva each day to smooth her. Indeed, like when you rub the breast milk, you straighten [kunyoosha] the child for milk. . . . In the morning, early, you straighten her, then you bathe her with water [and] you dress her as usual. Helping her in this way she can get a body quickly [kumpata mwili haraka]. That is to say, you cannot cause pain [by doing this]. Each day you straighten her; then her body, it will come. It will pull itself [kujivuta] well. She will be well. If you neglect to straighten her for the day, she can cry a great deal.

Techniques of caring for a newborn involve massaging the child with breast milk so that s/he will "get a body" and with saliva so that the child's head will "sit well." The fluids of the mother inform the shape and nature of the body as it "pulls itself" into being.

The strengthening, smoothing, and straightening that are critical to the child's initial acquisition of a body resonate with both protective and curative therapies.

The strengths of the healer and of the mother repeatedly emerge as central to the administration of medicine. Medicine is stronger when a healer administers it herself. The power of her hands influences the potency of the medicine. In both *degedege* and *makanje* treatments, as the healer begins to bathe a child, she first scoops water into her mouth and then spits it onto the child's head or buttocks. The healer's saliva becomes part of the medicine. Above, in describing the treatment for *makanje,* I recounted how the child was held under the mother as he was being bathed so that the water flowed over the mother, bringing her strength to her child. Everyday encounters with the saliva, breast milk, and the strength of one's "mothers" (both the biological mother and the healer) tend to the well-being and life of children and cultivate bodies that will be compatible with curative remedies when they are needed in the future.

Medicine in southern Tanzania conceives, engages, and transforms the matter of the body. The mass that is pushed out of the womb is considered to be relatively vague, undifferentiated. Adult bodies have evolved through years of effort.[4] The corporeal qualities of adult bodies have stabilized in a series of therapeutic events that draw together the configurations of actors that are necessary for the relations that sustain the substance of their life. In this way, their physicality is more established than that of a child. Adults do not need to "get a body" as much as they need to maintain and fortify the physical discreteness and stability that they have fostered through years of addressing maladies of God, of Mashetani, and of Person. As a physical body grows more defined and more discrete through encounter, suffering, and therapy over time, its character unfolds and its nature comes to be known. The matter of the person becomes intelligible in the sense that correspondences, resonances, and compatibilities have been established that sustain life and facilitate curative care when it is necessary. Maladies, debilities, and misfortunes become events against which healers can take effective action.

Seeing the Limits of Existence

Selinger (2003) observed that "how people look at 'materiality' depends in part on what people are willing and unwilling to see" (11). In some cases, staunch refusals "to see" reveal the ways that the social and political are implicated in the real (and vice versa). This chapter discusses matters that medical science and clinical practitioners are unwilling to see. Doctors in southern Tanzania deny the very existence of the maladies healers strive to transform. They declare *makanje,* dirty breast milk, and *nyokoli* inconsequential and immaterial. Mariamu and Binti Dadi asserted the salience of their expertise by refusing the possibility of translation between their practices and those of the clinic. They argued that their clinical colleagues could not describe, know, or intervene in (some of) the threats that commanded their attention. They attributed the inability of biomedical practitioners to understand *makanje,* dirty breast milk, and *nyokoli* to the limits of their knowledge system rather than to the limits of the existence of such matters.

Medical science attempts to fix power relations in part by establishing what is visible, palpable, and representable. Healers argue that the things biomedical practitioners find unintelligible are substances that are out of place. What is unintelligible to doctors and nurse exists in a space of struggle, a space of defiant multiplicity.

In southern Tanzania, the enactments of some bodies and some threats have become morally obligatory. I first illustrated this connection in relation to the requirement that traditional birth attendants learn about hygienic birth practices (chapter 5). I showed another example of this in chapter 7 in my discussion of parents who treated their children's *degedege* before treating their malaria. These parents ran the risk of being considered ignorant and immoral. Similarly, international health development organizations and the state suggest that the requirement that mothers submit their children to regular biomedical surveillance from birth to five years of age is based on an ethical imperative. Mothers "should" take their children to the clinic. The doctor in the opening section of this chapter relied on such normative reasoning when he accepted the possibility that hospital medicine was being reserved for children who had consistently attended their monthly early childhood checkups. Medicine, he implied, should be reserved for those who have proven themselves worthy. Whether or not this notion is just depends on who or what can be blamed for sickness and death. Healers also appeal to ethical regimes; for instance, when they point to the consequences of abandoning "custom."

Refusing to conflate the limits of biomedical discourse and the limits of corporeal existence gives grip to the work of healers. By maintaining the incommensurability of their therapeutic system with biomedicine, they resist being figured only as the Other of biomedicine or as the solution to postcolonial ills. In each of the examples described in this chapter, the discreteness and solidity of the body emerges in the context of interactions between mothers, fathers, healers, saliva, breast milk, sweat, and medicine. The body as an object of knowledge and therapeutic practice becomes visible as a loosely connected series of events and the relations they establish.

The challenges *makanje,* dirty breast milk, and *nyokoli* pose do not reside in the existence of some scientifically more effective traditional medicine lurking within diverse indigenous healing practices. Nor is the social commentary traditional healing might offer on clinical practice and modern life the most profound threat it poses. The prevalence of traditional healing practices does not (necessarily) attest to the failure of biomedical therapies to be holistic enough or to engage "the patient" sufficiently. In practice, healing exceeds its role as foil for clinical practice and resource for medical science. The ontic denials described in this chapter disrupt the very processes of othering that aim to produce traditional medicine as a complementary category of practice, and instead strive to enliven and preserve the uncontrollable, unmanageable, and irreducible.

Conclusion

Postcolonial Ontological Politics

> If post-colonialism is the time after colonialism, and colonialism is
> defined in terms of the binary division between the colonizers and the
> colonized, why is post-colonial time also a time of "difference"? What
> sort of "difference" is this and what are its implications for the forms
> of politics and for subject formation in this late-modern moment?
>
> —Stuart Hall, *When Was the Postcolonial?*

Traditional medicine is a highly politicized and deeply intimate battle over
who and what has the right to exist. As a modern category of knowledge and
practice—forged through encounters between traditional healers, scientists (from
Tanzania, Britain, China and elsewhere), biomedical practitioners, government
bureaucrats, and international development organizations among others—it
embodies the frictions central to postcoloniality. It grounds arguments for a
history that is not bound by colonial categories of knowledge, in the intimate
care of loved ones and the bodies of kin. Close attention to struggles for control
over the right to determine what objects are central to life and the relations that
sustain them reveals a new story of colonization, post-independence socialism,
and its collapse in the face of economic liberalization. Postcolonial healing tells
this history as a series of struggles over rights to existence and over the particular
forms of materiality that support different claims to existence. In other words,
postcolonial healing reveals contemporary struggles not only over material and
conceptual resources but also over who gets to determine what is material and
what is immaterial, or "merely" conceptual.

By bringing arguments about the nature of knowledge to bear on African
therapeutics, this book strives to take alternative materialities seriously. It investigates how the entities and objects critical to therapeutic practices in southern
Tanzania are brought into being. Healers and their medicine live in a world where
national governments intervene in the lives of their citizenry through biomedicine, where scientific knowledge formulates the boundaries of care, and where
pharmaceutical drugs constitute paths of transnational power. While biomedicine
has reconfigured the landscape of therapeutic practice in Africa, Tanzanians have

never found it a sufficient resource for addressing all the forms of affliction they encounter. They strive to find ways to position themselves in relation to the world as it has been transformed by medical science, a world that offers both narrowed and expanded possibilities of "what is," or at least "what might be."

The power of precolonial healers and the efficacy of precolonial medicine derived (in part) from their influence over forms of social organization and patterns of political-economic engagement. Colonialism and postcolonial development unmoored healers and their medicine by undermining indigenous political and economic institutions, catalyzing the migration of populations, and forcing changes in settlement. Feierman (1985) suggests that the power of healers and the efficacy of traditional medicine cannot be evaluated outside of their meaningful incorporation into modern structures of governance. He concludes, however, that healers are unlikely to obtain a central role within the modern nation-state. The ways of knowing that are critical to African healing expertise have been systematically excluded from the forms of knowledge that are linked to statecraft. I agree that resting our intellectual or political hopes for more democratic forms of therapeutic knowledge on the official integration of traditional healers seems unsatisfactory if not futile. Traditional birth attendants are a case in point. Through training initiatives, policies on referring patients, and relations with clinical staff, they are now included in the government's health care system. Yet their official work has been so diluted and constrained that it hardly bears a resemblance to the social and therapeutic roles traditional midwives formerly played. This case illustrates how difficult it is for traditional practitioners to maintain an influential role in shaping the social and political determinants of health from inside the national health care service. Their "incorporation" into the national health service has meant (re)formulating "traditional" expertise and therapies in relation to biomedical disease entities and national health development goals. Therefore, while TBAs provide a detailed picture of the making of one form of commensurability, they offer a rather unimaginative example of how diverse therapeutic practices might be coordinated.

Although the professionalization of birth attendants and healers has been central to the ways that traditional medicine is institutionalized in Tanzania, the impact of this professionalization on healing practices has been rather limited. Many healers are wary of initiatives that see them as only one more type of clinical healer. They are painfully aware that efforts to incorporate them and their medicine into institutionalized medical care have (so far) reinforced hierarchies of knowledge instead of disrupting them. Traditional healers often bristle at the dismissive ways that doctors and scientists interact with them. Traditional healers, however, do not systematically reject biomedicine or medical science. They do not see their practices as wholly incommensurable with the clinic. Instead, healers on the Makonde Plateau are constantly reconfiguring the boundaries that mark the inside and outside of biomedicine as they strive to address the complaints, debilities, worries, and pain of those that come to them. Through their everyday encounters, healers suggest forms of integration, coordination, and engagement with biomedicine that disrupt the hierarchies of medical institutionalization, challenge the privileged position of science to articulate matter, and reject divisions between the physical and the social. While the asymmetries that shape the relations of healers with biomedicine and medical science are overdetermined, the encounters between healers (and their herbal remedies, *mashetani, majini* and other objects of healing practice) and biomedical practitioners (and their clinics, notebooks, drugs, parasites, viruses and other objects of clinical knowledge) are unpredictable. For this reason, I remain intrigued by the moments when biomedicine interpolates healers or healing and those when healers (mis)translate themselves into medical science. I submit, however, that the subtleties of these interpolations and (mis)translations can be more accurately accounted for through the emergence and maintenance of objects of healers' treatments than through healers' participation in and marginalization within governmental structures.

Thus, this book has trained attention on the processes through which objects of healing knowledge and therapeutic care are formulated in southeastern Tanzania. It locates these processes of objectification in historical, political, social, and technological relations. My focus on healers (and healing practices) highlights the dynamism and creativity of their efforts to articulate the objects their therapies address. By attending to the generative work of objectification, I propose a method for attending to the subtleties of the relationship between traditional and modern medicine in practice. The power of healers and the efficacy of their medicines are neither opposed to the power of clinical practitioners and the efficacy of pharmaceutical substances nor explained through medical science. I have explored the moments when biomedicine interferes with traditional healing (and vice versa), and I have traced the new or refigured objects of therapeutic care forged within this interference. Postcolonial healing, I argue, is about the complex ways that bodies and agents of affliction are transformed ontologically (as well as epistemologically).

From Pluralism to Ontological Politics

To address the range of therapeutic practices they encounter, anthropologists have often evoked the concept of "medical pluralism." This approach makes the broad landscape of healing and therapy its object of study. As they described the coexistence of biomedicine and other forms of healing, these anthropologists countered the notion that the expansion of biomedicine and the modernization of health care would lead to the erasure of local healing knowledge and practice. Instead they focused on the diversity of healing options, the complexity of therapeutic itineraries, and the efforts to professionalize healers. The analytic of pluralism has contributed to richer, subtler descriptions of the therapeutic worlds that exist in Africa. The best studies have demonstrated that traditional medicine—although it is a product of missionization, colonial violence, international development, and global economics—is not fully defined by the dictates of biomedical science, the needs of the nation, and the demands of capital. Some scholars have argued that biomedicine itself is an "ethnomedicine." In other words, these scholars do not see biomedicine as existing outside of or isolated from the historical, technological, social, and biological changes that took place in the nineteenth and twentieth centuries. This perspective has had radical implications for the ways we might account for relations between types of medicine. It holds open the door for studies of therapeutic systems that are more methodologically symmetrical than previous studies were.

Symmetry, however, keeps moving, keeps slipping out of sight as our ethnographic stories try to account for the continuities of imperial power. Inspired by debates in both anthropology and science studies, I argue that institutionalized types of pluralism maintain the forms of difference that were originally central to imperial power by continuing to privilege certain ontological possibilities. For example, as the Tanzanian state builds more laboratories to investigate traditional medicine with the help and support of the international development community, it articulates differences in healing by grounding therapeutic efficacy only in the particular forms of materiality that medical science recognizes. The violences through which colonialism made existence a political question are not only naturalized, but also reframed as liberating in the hands of the postcolonial state. Any attempt to analyze the hierarchies of knowledge that structure contemporary African therapeutics requires us to rethink the ontological ground of our studies of medical pluralism.

This book has taken its lead from healers. Healers neither repudiate nor maintain allegiance to the ontological boundaries of biomedicine or to scientifically defined and bureaucratically controlled forms of traditional medicine. While at times healers articulate a space outside of biomedicine, marking its limits, at other times they use bits and pieces of clinical medicine to formulate new techniques for discerning the matter of maladies, of bodies, and of the range of entities that sustain and threaten life. Healers link knowledge with practice and insist on the multiplicity of the body and its threats. Law and Urry (2002) have raised the issue of how to think through the multiple, the fleeting, and the politics of those things that are not, as distinctly twenty-first-century issues. These are certainly postcolonial issues. To be concerned with the complex, the elusive, and the inconsistent is to be concerned with the life of types of power that live in the interstices of the dominant political, economic, technological, and ethical regimes.

While this approach is sympathetic to medical pluralism, it destabilizes any assertion of a priori boundaries between discrete "types" of healing. Pluralism requires us to hold something steady; when we do this, other things can be seen to vary in comparison. This type of analysis creates categories for therapeutic practices: it identifies maladies, therapies and technologies, and their effects by type—traditional, modern, Islamic, Christian, spiritual, herbal, and so forth. The iconic image of medical pluralism in anthropology texts is the shops of healers that are located just outside hospital gates. I find this type of analysis inadequate. In this book, I have suggested instead a focus on interferences, on the times and places where disruption, (mis)translation, and interpolation have generated multiplicities. This analysis does not seek to describe a plurality of healing practices (that is, many types of healing) but instead looks at the times and ways that healers, clinical practitioners, government bureaucrats, medical scientists, and patients implicate the modern in the traditional, the clinic in the home of the healer, science in the nonbiomedical, and vice versa. Postcolonial healing incorporates the traditional and the modern in flexible ways at a range of levels. Binti Dadi tests new medicines on rats. Kalimaga distances himself from forms of historical knowing based on immediate relations with *mashetani* and *mahoka* and structures his investigations as amateur clinical trials. Most healers address some biomedical disease entities and rearticulate traditional maladies through new propositions that articulate relationships with these biomedical disease entities such as the statement that *degedege* is malaria that has gone to the head. Postcolonial healing challenges ethnographers to find ways to describe healing in all its diversity without fixing difference in a priori assumptions about what is material or physical and what is immaterial or conceptual.

To consider variations in what counts as matter, I approach therapeutic objects and entities—needles, parasites, under-five cards, *mahoka, majini, mashetani*, saffron ink on white plates, and jealousies—as propositions that achieve solidity through their encounters with others. The *mashetani* of the late twentieth and early twenty-first centuries, for example, have materialized as discrete actors in relation to hot and convulsing bodies, healers' gestures and movements, the *udi* on the wrist of young children, pharmaceutical drugs, and so forth. *Mashetani* come to be known as a series of events. This focus on interferences makes it possible for the subject and the object, the semiotic and the material, the social and the natural, and the epistemological and the ontological to emerge together within my account.

This approach does not deny differences in the time of the postcolonial. It does not even deny the power of the differences that are central to scientific practice and statecraft, such as nature and culture, the modern and the traditional. It does, however, allow us to see how healers establish alternative frames for interaction in efforts to establish positions from which to negotiate. As healers reformulate the objects of their therapeutic attention, they disrupt modernist hierarchies of knowledge. By creating new relations between herbal medicines and scientific technologies, between ancestors and laboratories, cures for witchcraft and the efficacy of pharmaceuticals, they offer alternatives to the dominant order of things. Their efforts to assemble, refigure, translate, elaborate, visualize, and defend objects of African therapeutic knowledge and practice suggest the possibility of more radically democratic forms of politics than do struggles to control already defined elements of the world.

Discerning Difference, Compelling Politics

This analytical turn to practices of objectification in the time of the postcolonial has raised a number of theoretical and methodological issues. Considering this turn in the context of Stuart Hall's incisive questioning in the epigraph, however, pushes us still further.[1] If colonialism made existence political and if postcolonialism is about the continuities and discontinuities of imperial power, then what forms of politics are possible when we raise the question of the ontological? When taking into account practices of objectification (including the political, economic, and social determinants of ontological commitments and the ways that matter comes to be defined through specific efforts to see, act, and intervene), what sorts of choices might be available and to whom?

A long history exists of situating politics in choice. It assumes that people have a place from which negotiate. It assumes that choices are limited only for those with less power, for those who can't move. It assumes that options exist and that a playing field exists on which choices are being made. Most fundamentally, however, it assumes that if there are multiple discrete options, then politics exists to some extent in our choices—choices about interpretations, beliefs, where to go, whether to use medicines or not, and so forth. Similarly, as scholars, our politics might be seen to lie in our choice of which position we view the world from. We can cultivate particular sensitivities that enable us to see the world from different perspectives. In this way we can choose a standpoint that is in solidarity with particular groups of people: women, the poor, Africans. From this perspective, if we don't cultivate these sensitivities then we are colluding with those in more dominant positions. The notion of ontological politics opens up new possibilities for scholarly engagement. It does not limit choice to options defined by differences black-boxed in therapeutic objects and entities.

My approach builds on the large body of work that has elaborated the complexity around notions of choice for patients' seeking therapy. By acknowledging the role of kin and other community members in the management of individual illnesses—what Janzen (1978) originally called "therapy management groups"—ethnographies of African healing have discredited analytical frameworks that assume that it is single individuals who make choices about treatment and that such choices, when they are made, are "rational." Therapeutic itineraries are a product of negotiation and compromise. When this insight is brought to bear on processes of objectification central to therapeutic care in Tanzania, then objects of healing emerge as the effects of multiple decisions about medicine, books, technologies, measurements, and narratives made through the collaborative work of healers, patients, and kin as well as ancestors, devils, parasites, and viruses. There is not one belief or one choice; instead, there are many arguments, compromises, and trails. Power lies in the cumulative effects of negotiations. One of the most profound of these effects is in the formulation of objects of therapeutic intervention and care. Politics, then, seems to lie less in choices between types of medicine or kinds of healers and more in the generation or innovation of objects of knowledge and practice that compel new desires, pleasures, and senses of well-being.

The development of contemporary traditional medicine has been driven by a range of compulsions we might call politics. The state has been "compelled" to deal with traditional medicine. Its interest has emerged in response to the demands of postcolonial governance and the need to gain legitimacy in the eyes of its citizenry as well as in relation to the goals of international health development and the inequalities of global resources. As the World Trade Organization strives to shape intellectual property law, as China shows interest in Tanzanian plant material, and as healers organize nationally and regionally, the objects of governmental concern have shifted. Efforts to control global resources, trade agreements, national budgets, patients, disease entities, and regional security have evoked myriad responses in the name of traditional medicine. The hospital, in turn, has been compelled to confront the challenge of traditional medicine when patients arrive full of medicine, stash it under their hospital bed, or demand discharges so that they can go to see healers. Nurses and doctors have chosen to respond to the presence of traditional medicine in the clinic in different ways, depending on the specifics of each case, the types of medicines that are at issue, and their own experiences. Clinical staff may turn a blind eye as patients slip out between doctors' rounds to see a healer or as kin smuggle medicine and even healers into the clinic for their loved ones. At times, when nurses see little hope for the patient with available treatment, they may implicitly or explicitly refer patients to healers for help. References to traditional medicine gives some nurses a way to act and to care at moments when diagnostic procedures reveal a disease for which there is no available cure, when pharmaceutical drugs fail to stimulate the desired effects, and when the hospital pharmacy stores are empty. At the limits of biomedical potency, traditional medicine has gained purchase. Neither bureaucrats, doctors, nurses nor "traditional" practitioners in Tanzania can avoid mediating diverse forms of therapy. They must find ways to order the world, to create assemblages that facilitate intervention, and to define a trajectory for transformation.

In this book, I have been primarily concerned with the choices and compulsions that have driven healers. Healers have had to respond to biomedicine, to the state's version of traditional medicine, and to the growing interest in commercially produced herbal preparations. Their responses have created unpredictable distinctions and solidarities between traditional and modern medicine, between nonscience and science. As healers deny medical science the role of sole arbiter of the forms of materiality and senses of physicality that are actionable, they open up a space to talk about the relationship between practices of objectification and the choices they make possible. The corporeal truths of bodies and threats that are generated by healers under conditions that are not of their own choosing may be evaluated in light of the kinds of survival they make possible, for whom, and at what cost. The matters of African maladies—biomedical and otherwise—may be evaluated in light of the forms of justice they imagine. After all, struggles about the right to define existence are also struggles about the right to define what it means to be human, to live, to prosper, and to die.

Epilogue

Binti Dadi has hundreds of children. She is well known for helping women "get pregnant quickly" (*kupata mimba haraka haraka*). Each child that her roots and leaves and *kombe* have helped to bring into the world she calls "my child" (*mwanagu*).

Over the past decade, I have watched her prepare countless concoctions to help women and men who want to have a child. In the process, I have dutifully noted down the plants and trees used to make medicine; the conversations between Binti Dadi, Mariamu, and the women seeking children; the details of the therapies; the therapeutic itineraries of women who have sometimes sought care in a variety of settings before coming to Binti Dadi; and the births of children. During the first few years that I shadowed Binti Dadi, an old Sony Walkman sat in a corner recording the sounds and voices of these women's visits. I had them all transcribed into the red school notebooks I bought in the Newala market. The notebooks into which the complaints, fears, and prayers of these hot days found their way now sit in the closet in my study, the familiar curly round handwriting used by so many educated women in Tanzania starting to fade. In the beginning, when my immediate goal was still a dissertation and this book part of a vague, as-yet-unformed future, I read through them all and marked pages with little Post-it notes. Each note was designed to draw my attention to patterns among therapies or particularly interesting exchanges or dramatic events. On later trips, I used digital files and videotapes. A few of these stories have found a home in the pages of this book.

All anthropologists, I suspect, feel that the lives of their friends, adopted kin, interlocutors, and interviewees are never fully captured in their tellings. Not all the fragments of the stories held on old cassette tapes or in field notes can come together in the *sadaka*, the thank you, that we offer through our writing. Yet the dust gathering on the stories I collected seems particularly poignant as I look back at my more recent field notes and notice a glaring absence of writing on the day that Binti prepared medicine for my partner, Jeff, and me.

We had arrived in Newala for a visit shortly after the rains had finished in 2008. I was spending six months in Dar es Salaam beginning a new research project.

Eager to see our friends, Jeff and I made the *safari* to Newala as soon as we could. We noted the changed roads along the coast. The long-awaited paving had begun between Dar es Salaam and Mtwara, the provincial capital and the town where one turns west to head to Newala. All but sixty kilometers was smooth blacktop, raising our hopes for other changes that might bring greater ease to our friends' lives in the south. (On the way home those sixty kilometers managed to eat up three days when our car broke down in the middle of what the long-distance truck drivers familiar with the route called "bandit country.")

When we peeked our heads through the slits in Binti Dadi's fence there was much elation. Binti Dadi, though now perhaps in her mid-nineties, danced delightedly. We spent two glorious days lounging in her courtyard; catching up; laughing; wondering at her granddaughter Yanini, now nine and a half years old; delighting in her daughter Sofia's new house; and savoring the company of Binti Dadi and Mariamu. Word spread quickly that we were back in town. The infamous neighbors who had cut down Binti Dadi's tree so long ago merely shouted their greeting from next door. All other visitors poured into the compound.

In the midst of so much excitement, Binti Dadi chose a relatively quiet moment—when the teenagers had Jeff's attention and Mariamu and Yanini were helping an elderly blind friend, whose leg I had once watched Binti Dadi heal, find a comfortable spot on the grass mat—to ask me the familiar question. This time she asked in almost a whisper, "So, when are you going to have children?" Over the years she had asked this question in many ways. She had also taken it upon herself to publicly defend my childlessness many times, asserting to others that "Stacey must finish school."

Binti Dadi is a strong, independent-minded woman, and as a healer she bent many of the expected gender norms. One day in 1999 when I arrived at her house and asked after her husband, I learned that she had unceremoniously kicked him out the night before. "If he is sleeping at another woman's house he can eat there too," she said, abruptly ending any conversation on the topic. Over the past decade he has occasionally come by to visit his grandchildren, but she has never invited him or allowed him to stay. As long as I have known Binti Dadi she has been amused by the possibilities that the different expectations of gender in America might offer Tanzanian lives. One day in a tea shop, she caught Mariamu and me by surprise and left us shaking with suppressed laughter. She had fallen, and we had taken her to the hospital for an X-ray of her arm. Unfortunately, the electricity in the hospital was on the blink, so we three decided to go to a small shop just outside the hospital gate for a milky, sweet cup of tea and a *chapati* while we waited for the power to return. Such *mkahawa* (coffee and tea shops) are male spaces. As we entered, the animated voices we heard inside turned to whispers. The tension in the air clearly invigorated Binti Dadi. She seemed to forget her arm, which we later learned was broken. She watched the men survey us in the doorway and her eyes twinkled as she saw that some of them decided to leave. In response, she gladly took their seats, gesturing to Mariamu and me to sit down. Two sips into the tea and one bite into the *chapati* she turned to me and said in an unusually loud voice, "Stacey, is it true that all men in America help their wives carry water?" She had been to the small home Jeff and I had down the road, and she delighted in the fact that Jeff would collect the water and bring it to her for washing her hands before the meal. The whispering around us stopped. I raised my eyebrows. This comment really got to the heart of gender relations and the ways they have changed on the plateau.

Historically people had to go off the plateau to collect water. When Binti Dadi was still a girl, men and women shared this task, carrying heavy jars of water up the 1,000-foot escarpment on alternate days. The complicated demands of colonialism, national citizenship, migrant labor, Christianity, and Islam as well as the growth of social services have transformed life and the gendered roles that sustain it on the plateau. In addition, since the 1950s, there have been various schemes to pipe water up the plateau. By the turn of the millennium, communal pumps were bringing water up the plateau most days, shrinking the distances that people had to walk with a twenty-liter plastic bucket on their heads and reducing the elevations they had to climb. Across the plateau, women dominated the long lines at these communal pumps. Only occasionally were they joined by a few young men who were working as servants.

Binti Dadi continued to project her voice across the teashop, "Do all men clean the dishes after the meal in America?" Binti Dadi clearly enjoyed her meals at our house, but she had never spoken to Jeff or me directly about our relationship or home life. Mariamu tried to concentrate on her *chapati* and gulped her tea to help suppress the laughter rising up from her belly. I found my voice and provided Binti Dadi with the conversation partner she was requesting.

Binti Dadi was not committed to what others in Newala might view as proper gender relations. Yet as she turned to me on that afternoon of our return visit in 2008 there was a new seriousness in her voice. Despite the fact that she had never gone to school, she clearly supported my extended studies. Now, however, I had finished my doctorate and I was teaching at a university. I could no longer use the familiar excuse that "I don't want to get pregnant yet; I am still in school." The question delicately phrased with a "when" was really an effort to know whether we *would* have children. I confided in her that we had been trying for the past two years. I left out the details of the various lab tests to which Jeff had submitted and the poking, prodding and radioactive dye to which I had submitted, only to be told that biologically we should be able to conceive unassisted. I simply echoed what I had heard so many times in her compound. "The doctors say that there is nothing wrong," I said, adding that "their tests indicate that there is no reason that we should not be able to get pregnant."

For a decade, Binti Dadi and other healers had given me protective medicine during my work on the plateau. Like them, I was exposed to *mashetani* and other potentially mischievous nonhumans each day as I helped administer medicine, and this heightened exposure warranted caution. I have always been very healthy during my time in Newala. Therefore, I had never been a patient; I had never sought curative care. Binti Dadi's bluing cataract-covered eyes examined me in an unfamiliar way for just a moment, and before a new set of visitors moved into hearing range, she said, "Don't go back to Dar es Salaam yet. Come again tomorrow."

As Mariamu, Sofia, Jeff, and I ran errands together the next morning, Binti Dadi was working. When we arrived at her compound in the afternoon the air was quiet. There were no visitors. A few children came in as we told about our morning, but they were soon all settled onto a grass mat in the corner of the compound. Binti Dadi had prepared medicine for us as a gift. She sat under the eaves of her kitchen on an old rope cot. After handing Mariamu and Sofia a bundle of leaves tied together with grass, she began to slowly take out her saffron ink, her battered white plate, and a liter bottle of water. As always when she is writing *kombe,* her body stilled and the brightness and animation that usually defined her faded. Her eyes grew blank. She was far from us as she began drawing the iconic star and moon. The white enamel of the plate disappeared as her red ink writing slowly filled the space. Long millipede-shaped *mashetani* emerged as well as patterns and manifestations known only to her.

As she wrote, Sofia brought out the small *kinu* that Binti Dadi uses to pound medicine. Mariamu selected some of each of the three kinds of leaves tied up in Binti Dadi's bundle and crushed them together in the mortar, making a rough moist green pulp of the freshly picked leaves. When Binti Dadi stopped writing, she looked intently at the plate. She turned it methodically to examine each mark. When she looked up, her familiar sparkle had returned. She poured water into the plate and swirled it around until a uniformly pink solution remained. With a single steady hand she poured all but one swallow of this solution into the water bottle, without spilling a drop. She drank the last swallow herself before handing the plate to Sofia. Sofia placed the green mass of pounded leaves in the plate and then added fresh water from another bottle. She stirred the moist broken leaves, turning the water bright green. After several minutes she took out a tea strainer and strained the leaves from the water. She repeated this several times with fresh leaves Mariamu had pounded and filled a second water bottle with the green solution.

When the *kinu* had been moved to the side and the white plate had been rinsed, Binti Dadi called Jeff and me over. She instructed us to sit on either side of the threshold of the mud-and-wattle building that included her kitchen and a storage room where she keeps dried food and medicine. I sat just inside the threshold of this building and Jeff just outside the threshold. Binti Dadi first poured a little of the *kombe* into the original white plate. She called over the granddaughter who had laid claim to me so long ago. Together Binti Dadi and Yanini both held the plate while tipping some of the pink solution into my mouth, while Binti Dadi muttered. I could make out only a few words, a few references to Mungu (God). Binti Dadi and Yanini then repeated this action, tipping the remaining solution into Jeff's mouth. When the *kombe* was finished, Mariamu handed Binti Dadi the bottle of herbal medicine that she and Sofia had prepared. Binti Dadi poured some of this into the white plate. She and Yanini brought the plate up to Jeff's mouth. Eager to show his appreciation, Jeff drank until Binti Dadi smiled and gently told him not to take too much. Mariamu and Sofia's laughter still hung in the air as Binti Dadi and Yanini brought the plate of sweet herbal medicine to my mouth and she again whispered her prayers, her words to God and to the devilish *mashetani*. After this last drink, we rose from our respective sides of the threshold.

It was not until we were driving back that I thought about that step I took over the threshold back into the courtyard where Jeff as well as Binti Dadi, Yanini, Mariamu, and Sofia stood. I stepped from the deeply gendered space of the kitchen, the hearth, and the storeroom for food and medicine. I stepped from the space for fire, for women, for cooking, for births.

Two weeks after leaving Binti Dadi, we conceived. Nine months, two weeks and three days after leaving, we three—Jeff, Binti Dadi, and I—were gifted with a baby girl. Our families are now bound together even more strongly. Over the years, many people throughout Tanzania have come to know me as Binti Dadi *mdogo*. Binti Dadi half-joked in private and in public that her *mashetani* would likely one day climb on me. Long before the afternoon of this medicine, I had grown to call Binti Dadi my mother and Mariamu and Sofia my sisters. Now we are no longer fictive kin. We share a child. Because healers that contribute to conception are implicated in the new life, Binti Dadi has gained a daughter and my child Tsadia will grow up calling Binti Dadi her mother.

Each time I see my daughter, I am reminded that what counts as the substance of life is an intimate question. Ontologies are not removed from sign, from symbol, from prayer, from friendship, from love, or from action. They are political; they are about power. They are about the obligations and responsibilities that come with the emergence of things that matter.

Glossary

binti	Daughter (of)
dawa (za mitishamba, za kitabu)	Medicine (of the bush, of the forest)
degedege	Traditional malady described by a sudden stiffing, convulsions, a hot body, and foaming at the mouth
kanga	Cloth worn by many women in Africa
kombe	Form of medicinal therapy in which the *mashetani* communicate with a healer through writing that is then read as the diagnosis and added to water to make the treatment
ndoto	Dream or vision
jini/majini	Nonhuman actors who climb on a healer's head and who sometimes have medicinal knowledge they share with their host
kinu	Mortar used to pound grains and medicines
kivuli	Shadow
mahoka (Kimakonde)	Ancestral shade
makanje	Traditional malady in which *mashetani* manifest as pimple-like growths in a mother's nose, anus, or vagina and/or father's nose
mashetani	See *shetani*.
mdudu/wadudu	Bug or small creature/bugs or small creatures
mganga/waganga/uganga	Healer/healers/healing
mMakonde/waMakonde	A person who identifies as a Makonde person/people who identify as Makonde
mzee/wazee	Elder/elders
njozi	Visions
nyama/wanyama	Animal (or meat)/animals
shehe	Qur'anic teacher
shetani/mashetani	Devil or demon/devils or demons
uchawi	The use of medicines for harmful purposes
uganga	The use of medicine for beneficial purposes
wivu	Jealousy

Notes

Prologue

1. *Binti* means "daughter of." For a girl child, it is used after a given name and before the father's name—for instance, Fatma *binti* Dadi.

2. Binti Dadi and Binti Mayaula were related through their maternal grandmother, who was also remembered as a great healer and who visited Binti Dadi in her dreams.

3. Throughout the book, I translate *mahoka* (Kimakonde) as "ancestral shades." Each person is said to leave a *mahoka* on the earth when they die even as their *roho* (soul) is said to leave their body. These *mahoka* visit living relatives in sleeping and waking "dreams" and are central to the transmission of healing knowledge. For a more detailed description, see chapter 4.

4. A respectful title for an older man in Kiswahili.

5. *Safi* literally means "clean," but here it connotes "impressive" or "striking."

6. All conversations unless otherwise noted occurred in Kiswahili.

7. Kalimaga's first language is Kiyao. An mYao is someone who identifies as part of the Yao, one of the prominent groups found in southern Tanzania.

8. The AIDS counselor in the Newala District Hospital translated this malady as herpes zoster, or shingles (personal conversation, June 5, 2003).

1. Orientations

1. Dr. Mhame (2000), who has headed the traditional medicine units in both the National Institute of Medical Research and the Ministry of Health in Tanzania, estimates in a paper for the United Nations Conference on Trade and Development that traditional healers serve as the first point of contact for 60 percent of Tanzanians seeking health services and that a majority of the population "depends on traditional medicine for primary health care" (1).

2. My thinking about these issues has been influenced by the conversation in science and technology studies about boundary objects. See especially Star and Griesemer (1989).

3. For particularly influential examples see Comaroff (1985), Comaroff and Comaroff (1997), Hunt (1999), Livingston (2005), Stoller (1995), Weiss (1992, 1998), White (2000), and West (2005).

4. This phrase is borrowed from Tiffany (2000).

5. Idhe and Selinger's edited volume *Chasing Technoscience: Matrix for Materiality* (2003) evokes the contours of this literature in interesting ways through interviews with and essays by Donna Haraway, Don Ihde, Bruno Latour, and Andrew Pickering as well as analytical essays comparing the work of these four individuals.

6. Concern with the ontology of scientific objects has been central to much work in science studies, from Bruno Latour and Steve Woolgar's early study of thyrotropin releasing actor (TRF) (1979) to Annemarie Mol's work on atherosclerosis (2002). The collection of essays edited by Lorraine Daston in *Biographies of Scientific Objects* (2000) is a good introduction to key positions in the field. Another key reference point is Andrew Pickering's *The Mangle of Practice* (1995). Marc Berg and Annemarie Mol's edited volume *Differences in Medicine* (1998) brings together studies of diverse objects of medical care enacted through different medical specialties and disciplinary practices. Panels at the 2004 joint meeting of the Society for the Social Studies of Science and the European Association for the Study of Science and Technology addressed some of the emerging issues related to the ontology of scientific objects ("Onto Ontics and Ontology: Working, Testing, and Appreciating Nature-Cultures" organized by John Law, Annemarie Mol, and Helen Verran, and "The Ontology of Scientific Objects," organized by Jenene Wiedemer). Another session at the conference on Annemarie Mol's *The Body Multiple: Ontology in Medical Practice* (2002) discussed Mol's contribution to this literature in an "Author Meets Critics" roundtable. The ontological debates in science studies circles have been productively engaged by medical anthropologists exploring the history of particular diseases (e.g., Young's [1995] study of posttraumatic stress disorder), the diversity of biological experience (e.g., Lock's work on menopause [1993b, 1993c] and brain death [2002]), and the ways that disease categories travel (e.g., Cohen's [1998] examination of Alzheimer's and aging in India).

7. Classic science studies literature that sets the stage for these debates include Barad (1999), Galison (1999), Latour (1988), Rheinberger (1997), and Shapin and Schaffer (1985). For an overview of the anthropology of new medical technologies, see the edited volumes by Gary Lee Downey and Joseph Dumit (1998) and by Margaret Lock, Allan Young, and Alberto Cambrosio (2000). Important advances in this conversation have also been made by Joseph Dumit in his work on PET scanning (2003) and new medical objects.

8. This point was elaborated in Gabrielle Hecht's (2006) paper on uranium in Africa and the broad discussion it provoked among the audience at the Society for the Social Studies of Science meeting in Vancouver.

9. The phrase "ontological politics" is borrowed from Annemarie Mol's work (2002). It has also been further developed by John Law (2004) and Helen Verran (2001).

10. For a history of "African medicine" in South Africa, see Flint (2008).

11. The scientific development and bureaucratic modernization of traditional medicine is part of a longer history of empiricism. Many have argued that such forms of knowledge took shape as technologies of control intertwined with techniques of governance designed to dominate territories and manage colonial populations (Arnold 1993; Latour 1993; Mitchell 1988; Prakash 1999).

12. *Shorter Oxford English Dictionary on Historical Principles*, 5th ed., vol. 1 (Oxford: Oxford University Press, 2002).

13. Klaits (2002) has written more extensively on Christian rejections of the existence of demons and the power of witchcraft in Botswana as a moral strategy.

14. See especially Prakash's critique of Latour (1999, 12–13). Redfield (2002) also convincingly argues that it is necessary to bring science studies together with postcolonial studies. Although his focus on space exploration keeps him tightly focused on technoscience "proper" and he does not consider the sticky politics of "other" nonscientific or "traditional"

knowledges, his argument that provincializing Europe calls for the provincialization of science is germane here.

15. See introductions to postcolonial technoscience by Anderson (2002) and McNeil (2005). In addition see the work of Castaneda (2002), Haraway (1989, 1991), Harding (1994, 2006), Hayden (2003), Latour (1993), and Verran (2001). During the 2006 Society for the Social Studies of Science annual meeting Joan Fujimura and Amit Prasad organized a panel entitled "Intersections and Dialogues across Postcolonial, Feminist, and Laboratory Studies of Science," which advocated for a rigorous engagement of science studies with postcolonial theory. Also, Dumit and Rajan (2007) are beginning important work that links the alienation of "first world subjects" with the exploitation of "third world subjects" by drawing together their individual research on pharmaceutical marketing in the United States and clinical trials in India, respectively.

16. This term is borrowed from Timothy Mitchell (1988); it is also used by Jean Langford (2002).

17. Comaroff (1993) suggests "that the development of British colonialism in Africa as a cultural enterprise was inseparable from the rise of biomedicine as a science" (306). The intimate processes of colonizing African bodies and making African colonial subjects have been examined through the medicalization of birth (Hunt 1999), the popularization of hygienic practices through public health campaigns (Anderson 2001, 2006; Bashford 2003; Burke 1996), and the operationalization of medical knowledge through urban planning (Curtin 1992; Mitchell 1988). See also Vaughan (1991) and Arnold (1993) on medicine and colonialism.

18. Appadurai (1996).

19. For an ethnographic discussion of this theoretical argument, see Feierman's (2000) article on Ghaambo medicine in northeastern Tanzania and Adams's (2002) article on the scientific investigation of Tibetan medicine.

20. Michael M. Phillips, "Persuading Africans to Take Their Herbs with Some Antivirals: U.S.-Backed Program Pushes Doctors, Healers to Treat AIDS Patients Together," *Wall Street Journal,* May 5, 2006, A1. Phillips captures a debate between healers and researchers about whether to legally recognize certain therapeutic actors in South Africa. Similar debates are occurring within the context of research projects at the Institute of Traditional Medicine (Edmund Kayombo, personal conversations, 2004 and 2008).

21. Throughout this book, I use the concept of articulation to account for the constitution of postcolonial bodies and bodily threats. The anthropological literature on medicine, particularly by scholars working on Ayurveda and Chinese medicine, offers a range of resolutions to the problem of accounting for the ways bodies are constituted and cared for as assemblages. Jean Langford (2002) refers to "fluent bodies" that emerge within the context of postcoloniality and its ambivalences. Judith Farquhar (2002) unsettles the string of dichotomies attached to distinctions between traditional and modern medicine by writing of "historical bodies." Volker Scheid (2002) approaches his description of contemporary Chinese medicine through a notion of "synthesis," which is particularly compelling if one mulls over Hegel's version of synthesis as a new idea that resolves conflict between the initial proposition (for the nurses in my account, biomedicine) and the antithesis (for the nurses, traditional medicine). Ayurveda and Chinese medicine, however, have been entangled with nationalist projects and propelled by state investment in ways that contrast sharply

with the situation in Africa. For this reason, I describe bodies in southeastern Tanzania as being more or less clearly articulated (Langwick 2008a). This description draws on the dual meaning of the notion of articulation—to make intelligible and to join. Joining—as an elbow might join different parts of the arm—captures both the distinction using a spatial metaphor (there must be something on either side of the joint) and the sense that something whole is at stake. See also Latour (2004).

22. Micropolitics is a term that has developed in relation to Foucault's (1978) argument that contemporary power must be examined in the aspects of everyday life that shape modern subjects and subjectivities. The micropolitical perspective locates power in the emergence of gestures, desires, pleasures, appetites, skills, aesthetics, and objects of knowledge rather than in antagonistic oppositions between people and (economic or governmental) institutions. Here I illustrate how healers in concert with patients contest the diffuse and decentered forms of contemporary power that manifest in changing forms of affliction, options for care, ethics of bodily practice, and techniques of developing therapeutic expertise.

23. For further discussion of the role of nurses in mediating the use of traditional maladies in Tanzanian hospitals, see Langwick (2008a).

24. See responses to Harding (1994) by Farquhar, Kuriyama, and Cohen (all in Harding 1994).

25. A growing social science literature on the professionalization of traditional medicine in many parts of the world has begun to reveal epistemological if not ontological struggles over which practices, technologies, and knowledges will be institutionalized. Much of this discussion has appeared in the journal *Social Science and Medicine*. See for example Baer (2006), Baer et al. (1998), Cocks and Dold (2000), Cho (2000b) Janes (1999), and Pigg (1995).

26. For other work that examines *mashetani* in surrounding areas, see Erdtsieck (1997) and Giles (1987). Focusing on southwestern Tanzania and the Swahili coast respectively, the work of these scholars suggests that the life of the *mashetani* varies by region.

27. The *mashetani* of George Lilanga, who some refer to as Tanzania's best-known artist, are easily recognizable. Lilanga was born of Makonde parents from Mozambique was raised in the district of Masasi located west of Newala in southeastern Tanzania. His vision reflects the life of the border area around the Ruvuma River. As a young man he decided to try his luck in the capital city of Dar es Salaam, so he left southeastern Tanzania and began an artist journey that would bring the distinctive life of the devilish spirits who populated his dreams to a broader audience. For more on Lilanga, see Goscinny (2001).

28. There is no English word that conveys the history, fear, and hope that *mashetani* does. At times, when it is awkward to use the Kiswahili, I translate *mashetani,* with some trepidation, as (small "d") devils. Others have chosen to translate *mashetani* as "spirits." In Newala, however, I find "devils" to be more faithful to the jarring, suspicious, and playful connotations that speakers on the plateau—healers, patients, church leaders, and Muslim *shehe*—invoke when they refer to *mashetani*. Devils, I hope, also suggests the ways that these actors share a kindred spirit with the mischievous and promising monsters, cyborgs, and vampires of much science studies literature (e.g., Haraway 1997). Like these similar narrative figures, *mashetani* have specific category crossing work to do (Haraway 1997, 79). The crossings they make between the human and the nonhuman, the embodied and

the disembodied, the visible and the invisible, the material and the immaterial and the medical and the religious draw on the use of *shetani* in Kiswahili translations of Christian and Islamic texts. The term "devils" gestures to (some of) the contemporary politics of this category-crossing work.

29. This struggle to create an analytical language in which nature and culture are not thought separate is also seen in Lock's "local biologies" (1993b) and Rabinow's "biosociality" (1992; and "Artificiality and Enlightenment: From Sociobiology to Biosociality," in Rubinow 1996).

30. For this approach I am indebted to Judith Farquhar's (2002) richly evocative ethnography of historical bodies and their appetites in China, Volker Scheid's (2002) study of experts and objects of contemporary Chinese medicine, and Margaret Lock's (1993b) work on "local biologies." The latter has opened a new space in medical anthropology from which to ask questions about the emergence and historicity of the physical body in cross-cultural perspective. Questioning the universal application of medical and epidemiological truth claims, she argues that the order and disorder of bodies as well as sickness and healing are the products of specific social, cultural, material, and historical contexts. In *Encounters with Aging: Mythologies of Menopause in Japan and North America* (1993b), for example, Lock has shown that Japanese women report symptoms as their bodies stop menstruating that are significantly different from symptoms that are generally taken to be universal in biomedical discourse. Lock suggests that this finding, in conjunction with established differences between Japan and North America in the epidemiologies of heart disease, osteoporosis, and breast cancer, supports the notion of "local biologies." By illustrating the cultural specificity of human biological experiences, Lock's work has the potential to raise questions about the variableness of bodily materialities. The focus of her studies on menopause and brain death, however, do not allow her to discuss nonbiomedical actors and entities.

31. For relevant studies elsewhere in Africa, see also Hunt (1999), Livingston (2005), and Thomas (2003).

32. For a beautiful example of this linkage, see Rachel Prentice's forthcoming ethnography of surgical training and practice.

33. Many in northern Mozambique also identify as Makonde. Tanzanian Makonde and Mozambican Makonde lay claim to different origin stories (Liebenow 1971).

34. As Iliffe (1969) has noted, the Germans neglected the southeast during their period of colonial rule (1888–1918). He describes the area as follows:

> Open savannah country of low fertility, it was colonized during the nineteenth century by Ngindo, Mwera, and Makonde groups, probably moving north from Mozambique. Raided sporadically by the Ngoni, and crossed by the slave caravans from Kilwa to Lake Malawi, the area was politically fragmented. The Germans met much uncoordinated resistance from groups in the immediate hinterland of the coast. On the Makonde Plateau a Yao warlord, Machemba, defied several expeditions until forced back into Mozambique in 1899. Taxation was always difficult to collect in this area. Whenever possible, the Germans left it alone, for it had little apparent attraction. Between the district offices on the coast and the garrison in Songea, three hundred miles away, there were only a handful of askari [guards] and a non-commissioned officer in a grass-roofed stockade in Liwale. (17–18)

35. Rather than emphasizing the virtues of flexibility or egalitarianism, these descriptions of "statelessness" are most often used to imply a lack of the sophistication and cultural richness associated with more centralized and hierarchical (and patriarchal) forms of social organization found in the north.

36. Most living on the plateau today see accusations of resistance to development in the southeast as an excuse to justify the post-independence government's continued neglect of this region. The road from Mtwara to Dar es Salaam has been in the process of being paved for decades. In the late 1990s, the bus trip from Mtwara to Dar es Salaam could take anywhere from twenty-four hours to six days if you were unlucky enough to get stuck in or behind a broken-down vehicle in the rainy season. Newala was another eight hours west by bus, on roads that were alternately sandy and bumpy. The difficulty of transportation made the markets of the larger cities inaccessible to many farmers and craftspeople.

37. Many people have farmland both on and below the plateau. Only a few are able to harvest enough to sell some of their vegetables to neighbors or in a small roadside stand. Many complain that they can no longer produce a large enough harvest for even their own family's consumption. Although the temperature is moderate, because of the sandy soils and pattern of rainfall on the plateau, there is only one growing season. This current situation contrasts sharply with notes in the Newala District Book that suggest that in the first half of the twentieth century Newala was known as "the 'granary' of the surrounding plains country." Author unknown, report inserted into the Newala District Book, early 1950s.

38. District books are continuous logs that were kept by colonial officers stationed in each district. The Newala District Book is a collection of observations, notes, and comments and occasionally essays (by British district officers or others) that caught a district officer's attention.

39. Memorandum by M. Sillman, Agricultural Officer, Newala District Books, ca. 1945–1949, Tanzanian National Archives, Dar es Salaam (hereafter TNA).

40. This is the same Dr. Leader Stirling noted in Kalimaga's story above.

41. For more on modernist purifications, see Latour (1993).

42. For other explorations of the limits of symmetry, see Strathern (1999a, 1999b, forthcoming).

43. I draw on the concepts of interference (Mol 2002), synthesis (Schied 2002), and complexity (Mol and Law 2002) to provide this alternative analysis, even while remaining sensitive to assertions of difference and their link with assertions of authority. Instead of starting with contemporary claims that distinguish science from society and then working to explain how this distinction comes to be made through processes of purification and mediation, these scholars focus on issues of complexity, starting with the incompleteness of such distinctions from the beginning.

2. Witchcraft, Oracles, and Native Medicines

1. "Madawa na Waganga-Kienyegi" (Medicines of Traditional Healers), M.10/14, 80–82, Newala District File, District Commissioner's Office, Newala District.

2. The 1928 ordinance was amended in 1935 and 1956. These colonial ordinances were consolidated into Act 12 of 1998 and then revised as Chapter 18, The Witchcraft Act, in the most recent edition of *The Laws of Tanzania* (Dar es Salaam: Government Printers of Tanzania, 2002).

3. Ciekawy (1998) locates the production and use of the English term "witchcraft" in colonial and postcolonial statecraft.

4. The public at issue here is not the same as that evoked through modern public health campaigns.

5. For more extensive exploration of healing in the German colonial period, see Feierman (1974, 1990).

6. Historians of the Maji Maji Rebellion have noted that it was not just a coordinated resistance to German colonialism but the Germans entered in as a much broader pattern of negotiation between different African groups over labor, territory, and other resources (Becker 2004; Monson 1998).

7. Evans-Pritchard discusses poison oracles in detail in *Witchcraft, Oracles, and Magic among the Azande* (1937/1976). Although his commonly cited distinction between witchcraft and sorcery does not find much resonance farther south on the Makonde Plateau, there are numerous similarities between his rich ethnography and the colonial record about poison oracles in Tanganyika. Evans-Pritchard himself suggests that the beliefs about witchcraft he describes are "found among many peoples in Central and West Africa" (1). His Sudanese informants lived at the "north-eastern limit" of the distribution of (at least some) of this knowledge about witchcraft.

8. In the 1960s, Gilbert Gwassa and John Iliffe at the University of Dar es Salaam worked with their students to collect oral histories of the Maji Maji Rebellion. The unpublished essays and transcripts of the interviews were bound as the "Maji Maji Research Project, 1968, Collected Papers" (Dar es Salaam, 1969), available at TNA.

9. Schaegelen in the Kilosa District Book in the Tanzanian National Archives, quoted in Iliffe (1979, 192).

10. Joseph Mtimavali in Maji Maji Research Project I/N/5/69/4, University of Dar es Salaam, quoted in Iliffe (1979, 188).

11. Eradication campaigns were not the only new strategies for dealing with witchcraft, however. After the Maji Maji Rebellion in the early 1900s many people in southern Tanganyika converted to Islam. Alpers (1968, 1972) has explained this as a way of coping with macroeconomic and wider social issues that Yao people faced, arguing that they found their own ways of appealing to localized and ancestral spirits inadequate. Whatever the reason, after refusing both Islam and Christianity for years, many people in the southeast, including the Makonde who dominated the area of the plateau, accepted Islam at this time. These conversions created new networks, and books from Cairo, Mecca, and Jakarta began to circulate through the area. Experiences with *majini* (spirits) increased. An important aspect of the work of Muslim teachers was the use of Qur'anic verses to heal, protect, and animate their own bodies and the bodies of others with the word of Allah. These new experts provided people with different ways to deal with witchcraft. Illife (1979) writes: "Faced by the government's ban on killing witches, coastal Muslims employed a quasi-Islamic rite, *halubadili,* wherein the angels who had won the Battle of Badr for Muhammad's followers

were invoked to make all participants in the rite immune to witchcraft and to kill those who practiced it" (215). Such practices drew on older practices concerning the oracle, institutionalized religious forms such as Islamic practices of protecting the body through ritual and prayer, and perhaps also Christian communion.

12. Terence O. Ranger, "Witchcraft Eradication Movements in Central and Southern Tanzania and Their Connection with the Maji Maji Rising." Seminar paper, University College, Dar es Salaam, 1966. Available in the East Africana Collection, University of Dar es Salaam Library.

13. Liebenow (1971) notes that "toward the end of the colonial period the witch-finders were utilized by the administration to go through various districts collecting witchcraft paraphernalia and were actually paid for their services. I encountered a witch-finder, Nguvu Mali, in Lindi and Kilwa districts in 1955, and I even assisted the district commissioner of Kilwa in burning artifacts that Nguvu Mali has collected and stored at the boma" (62).

14. I would suggest that over time this distinction has grown less clear. Due to the interest of Islamic and Christian leaders in fighting *uchawi*, religious idioms have also come to be mobilized in some practices that combat it.

15. For similar arguments about other parts of British Africa, see Ciekawy (1998; about Kenya) and Livingston (2005; about Botswana).

16. Enacting colonial legislation that defined practices to prevent or eliminate witchcraft as "occult" was not unique to Tanganyika. All Anglophone colonies implemented similar legislation. In addition, similar methods of marginalizing indigenous practices addressing life and well-being that were considered strange, dangerous, threatening, or false by colonists can be traced outside of Africa. See, for example, Wiener (2003), who writes about magic in colonial Indonesia as a European category "mired in relations of power" (130).

17. Montague, British Secretariat, DSM, to Kitching, May 17, 1934, Document 274, Box 5, Folder 7, 1933–1948, Witchcraft, vol. 2, Accession no. 16, TNA. The comments from officers trickled in over the following three years. It appears that the lack of urgency was due in part to the fact that some officers were on leave.

18. [Initials illegible], reply to Montague, the Secretariat, DSM, July 7, 1937, Box 5, Folder 7, 1933–1948, Witchcraft, vol. 2, page 280, Accession no. 16, TNA.

19. A. E. Kitching to Montague, July 22, 1937, Box 5, Folder 7, 1933–1948, Witchcraft, vol. 2, page 284, TNA.

20. Ibid., page 285.

21. *Oxford English Dictionary* (Oxford: Clarendon Press, 1989).

22. The 1928 Witchcraft Ordinance described the offense as causing or trying to cause "fear, annoyance or injury in mind, person, or property to any other person by means of *pretended* witchcraft" (my italics), or taking advantage of others by seeking some sort of gain or reward from such pretenses. Witchcraft Ordinance, No. 33 of 1928, *Tanganyika Territory Ordinances Enacted in the Year 1928* (Dar es Salaam: Government Printer, 1928).

23. I have borrowed this phrase from Wiener's (2003) chapter entitled "Hidden Forces: Colonialism and the Politics of Magic in the Netherlands Indies," in Pels and Meyers's edited volume *Magic and Modernity*.

24. A comparison with "witchcraft" in Francophone African countries, where colonization did not bring a variant of the Witchcraft Ordinance (which can found in all former British colonies in Africa), might be useful here. Geschiere (1995/1997) writes that in Cameroon

post-independence African elites actually saw the previous colonial regime as being soft on witchcraft because the French colonial courts required material proof of disturbances caused by witchcraft. After independence, the new Cameroonian government initiated judicial action against witchcraft, and since 1980 there has been a growing precedent for courts to accept increasingly wide interpretations of evidence against witches.

25. The efficacy of these techniques against witchcraft was at least partly due to their administration in the public sphere (i.e., in the presence of the community). For a more detailed argument concerning efficacy, see Feierman's essay about the medical world of Ghaambo in Tanzania (2000), in which he argues that "efficacy . . . can be defined in terms of the way a therapeutic act leads the patient's personality to mesh with a medicine, or to mesh with the personality of a healer. Efficacy can also be defined in terms of the effect of an herbal remedy that changes the patient's position in a web of kinship relations" (340).

26. This same denial of the "real" has plagued scholars. For this reason, studies of witchcraft in African communities have previously taken psychological (Malinowski 1925/1982; Kluckholn 1944; Krige 1947/1982) and sociological (Middleton and Winter 1963; Marwick 1970) analytical stances. Most recently, scholars have focused on witchcraft as an idiom that talks about, comments on, or interprets new kinds of economic and political powers at play in postcolonial Africa (e.g., essays in Comaroff and Comaroff 1993 as well as Geschiere 1995/1997 and West 2001). While this is subtle and important work, witchcraft remains in the realm of representation. The historical effects of the construction of a category of practice in British colonial law and policy called "witchcraft," which carried connotations from the history of this term in Europe, are difficult to examine and are rarely discussed (even when European and African conceptions of witchcraft are compared, as for example in Austen 1993). Last and Chavunduka (1986) and Feierman (1985) have argued that certain healing practices were driven underground and that others were changed as a result of legislation against witchcraft in British colonies. They speak of how the violence of the colonial regime against "witchcraft" and against any healing practices that might have been thought to be linked to witchcraft was so devastating that healers transformed their practices in order to protect themselves and those who sought their services from harsh reprimands. While they do not explicitly approach the ontological shifts that such changes in African therapeutics inspired, they do set the stage for such analytical work.

27. See Good (1994) for a discussion of the "problem of belief," including distinctions between belief and knowledge as they have been applied in anthropological scholarship (chapter 1).

28. Newala District Officer to Provincial Commissioner, Mtwara, 1944, Box 5 Folder 7, 1933–1948, Witchcraft, vol. 2, pages 308–309, Accession no. 16, TNA.

29. For a broader discussion of the strategic use of "belief" and the political implications of mobilizing this concept, see Barbara Herrnstein Smith (1997).

30. A great deal of scholarship has addressed the complicated issue of visibility in so-called modern medicine (e.g., Jones 2000; Koch 1993) and in various fields of science (e.g., Galison 1997; Rasmussen 1997). From the camera to the production of microscopic slides and the much more recent computer simulation of DNA, discovery in scientific medicine has been closely tied to technologies that enable the visualization of biological actors.

31. This information is drawn from the annual reports of the East African Agricultural and Fisheries Research Station at Amani from 1928 to 1960. In 1948, the Amani research station became the East African Agriculture and Forestry Research Organization. During the early 1950s the research station expanded to include twenty-seven senior research officers in some fifteen divisions. During this period of growth, another botanist, Dr. B. Verdcourt, worked under Dr. Greenway. Because of the botanists' increased effort to name specimens and Dr. Verdcourt's specific interest in mollusks and snails, the research stations reports make little mention of medicinal plants during the mid-1940s to the late 1950s. These annual reports are available in the East Africana Collection at the University of Dar es Salaam library.

32. Chief Secretary, DSM, to Director of Medical and Sanitary Services, November 3, 1933, Native Affairs, Vol. 2, page 7, Accession no. 21845, TNA.

33. Ibid. Much later, beginning in the 1970s, this view faded away and the Tanzanian government made several attempts to register all healers. See chapter 3 for more information.

34. Geschiere's *The Modernity of Witchcraft* (1995/1997) and the flurry of research that describes witchcraft as a practice deeply embedded in (and often a commentary on) "modernity" aptly illustrates that assumptions that modernization or "civilizing missions" would eradicate witchcraft were wrong. Some even suggest that witchcraft is on the rise in postcolonial Africa (e.g., Bastian 1993; Colson 2000; Rowlands and Warnier 1988). Although it is difficult to quantify, "witchcraft" certainly remains a flexible sign and powerful category of practice in its present-day articulations. For investigations of ways that witchcraft has become a form of critique of changing patterns of accumulation in contemporary states and is thereby linked with development practices, see Abrahams (1994), Austen (1993), Bastian (1993), Comaroff and Comaroff (1993), Englund (1996), Green (2003), Meyer (1992), Masquelier (1993), Mesaki (1993), Sanders (2003), and West (2001, 2005).

35. File note from Chief Secretary, DSM, to Director of Medical Services, DSM, October 13, 1933, Native Affairs, vol. 2, pages 4–5, Accession no. 2184, TNA.

36. Extract from Proceedings of Conference of Directors of Medical Services, held in Nairobi, July 1939, Native Affairs, vol. 1, page 3, Accession no. 21845, TNA.

37. Extract from views on the matter raised on the agenda by Agricultural Director of Medical Services, Zanzibar, at the Conference of Directors of Medical Services, Nairobi, July 1939, Native Affairs, vol. 1, page 2, Accession no. 21845, TNA.

38. Wembah-Rashid was first educated in mission schools in Masasi. He eventually went on to receive a Ph.D. from a major university in the United States. Much of his writings reflect his background as a Christian, a socialist, and a Chama Cha Mapinduzi Party loyalist. He played an active role in the independence government of Tanzania and was a fervid socialist in the 1970s. At the end of the century he worked for a Finnish nongovernmental organization concerned with enhancing agricultural development and broadening political participation in southeastern Tanzania.

3. Making Tanzanian Traditional Medicine

1. A growing body of literature on "alternative modernities" (e.g. Gaonkar 2001; Ivy 1995; Rofel 1999), or what Bruce Knauft (2002) calls "vernacular modernities," argues for

the importance of paying attention not only to "non-Western" modernities in Africa, Asia, and Latin America but also to the ways that flows of people, ideas, goods aesthetic forms and cultural products between countries in the global South have shaped other notions of modernity. Brian Larkin (1997) first popularized the concept of alternative modernities in Africanist literature with an article that explored how Hindi films in Nigeria presented an alternative to Euro-American images of "the modern." Ferguson's (1999, 2002) has been particularly important in his insistence on politicizing the academic and colloquial references to "modernity" and "modernities" in Africa.

2. This image accompanied five different news stories in government papers over an eight-year period. The first time the image appeared was in *Sunday News* on September 12, 1976, with an article titled "Village Medicine Man." It was reprinted in the *Sunday News* on June 12, 1977, with "Traditional Medicine Proves Its Worth"; in the *Daily News* on July 12, 1978, with "New African Health Strategy"; and on August 16, 1978, with "African Herb-Based Drug Plants Soon." Six years later, on February 19, 1984, the image was resurrected one more time for "Traditional Healers and 'Health for All.'" In the pages of the *Sunday News,* the category of traditional medicine in Tanzania after independence is about clinics, herbs, jars with labels, research, international translators, and China. No matter what the story, it appears, there could not be a more appropriate image.

3. Iliffe (1998, 202, quoting from P. S. Mganga, "Visit to China," *Afya* 2, no. 2 [February 1968]: 4–7). This observation was made during the throes of the Cultural Revolution in China (1966–1976). While the question of whether to integrate "Western" and "Chinese" medicine began as a policy debate in 1912 in China (Croizier 1968), it emerged as central to the set of practices that Communist Party leaders began to refer to as Traditional Chinese Medicine (TCM) in the period 1945–1963 (Taylor 2005). The Cultural Revolution turned attention away from the more theoretical, disciplinary work of the 1940s and 1950s by closing down many academic and research institutions, professional journals, and other forums for study, research, and debate (Farquhar 1994a). Some argue that TCM became more clinically focused because of Communist Party policies that sent many teachers of Chinese medicine to rural areas to practice and initiatives to train "barefoot doctors" (Scheid 2002). Not until the 1980s did the drive to scientize and modernize TCM motivate ambitious new programs in theoretical and clinical research. Thus, the Tanzanian team went to China at a time when intellectual and theoretical pursuits were being repressed and the field of Chinese medicine was seen as a tool for socialist development (Iliffe 1998, 211). They witnessed a moment when a simplified form of Chinese medicine was being promoted in order to meet the state's rural development goals. In contrast, Zhan (2009) describes the dynamism of more contemporary Traditional Chinese Medicine as it evolves through specific translocal encounters.

4. The *People's Daily* (China) reported on October 11, 2000, that "over the past decades, China has dispatched 16 groups of medical experts, totaling some 858 people to Tanzanian [*sic*], to help uplift the level of medical service in the country." See "Tazara: Eyewitness of China-Tanzania Friendship," available at http://english1.people.com.cn/english/200010/11 /print20001011_52355.html.

5. In addition, since China's work to build the Tanzam Railway between Tanzania and Zambia in the 1970s, the number of Chinese people living in Tanzania has increased. Traditional Chinese Medicine clinics have been serving this community as well as their

Tanzanian neighbors for some time (Hsu 2002). It is interesting to note that the number of Traditional Chinese Medicine clinics in Dar es Salaam has grown substantially since 2000. Some of the doctors in these clinics and the herbal medicine sellers in local shops have only recently come to Tanzania to establish their businesses. Some do not speak English or Kiswahili, but they are able to find Tanzanians who speak Chinese to work as their translators and assistants. See also Langwick (2010).

6. *Sunday News,* April 28, 1985. Dr. Elimweka Mshiu, the first director of the Traditional Medicine Research Unit in the Faculty of Medicine at Muhimbili Hospital, marked the beginning of the Tanzanian government's interest in traditional medicine with this circular.

7. J. N. R. Kasembe, *Science, Technology and Development in Tanzania,* Country Report for ECA/UNESCO Regional Symposium on the Utilization of Science and Technology for the Development of Africa, Addis Ababa, 1970, S&T/CR/39.P.10. Available at the East Africana Collection of the University of Dar es Salaam library.

8. Interview with R. L. A. Mahunnah, director of Institute of Traditional Medicine, September 22, 1998.

9. Iliffe 1998, 211; Semali 1982; interview with Mahunnah, September 22, 1998.

10. "Local Cures Must Not Be Ignored," *Daily News,* August 31, 1976, 3.

11. "Chemist Defends Local Medicine," *Daily News,* September 27, 1975, 1.

12. "Traditional Medicine Is Good," *Daily News,* November 14, 1976, 7. This article is an interview of Peter A. Kitundu by James Mpinga.

13. "WHO Discussing African Health Methods," *Daily News,* February 11 1976, 2.

14. "WHO Hails Healers," *Daily News,* March 8, 1976, 2.

15. Both papers evolved from the *Tanganyikan Standard,* which was the most influential newspaper during the British administration. The *Daily News* began in 1972 as a result of Tanzania's early socialist policies. In 1970, Julius Nyerere nationalized *The Standard,* which had been privately owned by the London Rhodesia Mining and Land Company, a British multinational corporation. Shortly afterward, *The Standard* merged with the *Nationalist* to form the *Daily News* (Akhahenda 1984). Its sister paper *Sunday News* had begun earlier in 1954. The Tanzanian government currently owns the *Daily News* and *Sunday News,* both of which continue to be reliable archives of the government's viewpoint; they tend to report on government meetings, state resolutions, and development initiatives. They have typically reserved critique for people or entities that the government feels are standing in the way of its efforts to develop the country. Therefore, the ways that *Daily News* and the *Sunday News* have represented traditional medicine from 1974 to the 2004 chronicles the postcolonial state's use of this modern category of knowledge and practice to promote (and resolve) different ideological agendas over time. For a more detailed history of Tanzanian newspapers, see Sturmer 1999.

16. "Traditional Medicine Is Good," *Daily News,* November 14, 1976, 7.

17. "We Cannot Ignore Local Healers, Says Expert," *Daily News,* September 27, 1976, 5.

18. "WHO to Help Train Health Personnel," *Daily News,* December 12, 1977, 3.

19. "African Herb-Based Drug Plants Soon," *Daily News,* August 16, 1978, 4.

20. World Health Organization (1978b).

21. World Bank (1980).

22. "Herbalists Meet in Tanga," *Daily News,* November 15, 1979, 3.

23. The National Institute for Medical Research Act, 1979 (Act No. 23/79).

24. "Call to Probe Tanga Medicine Man," *Daily News,* June 11, 1980, 5.

25. "'Learn from Local Healers,'" *Daily News,* October 7, 1981, 1. Quote by Ndugu E. N. Mshiu, director of the Traditional Medicine Research Unit at the Muhimbili Medical Centre, from his speech to the Pan-African Congress of Dermatology.

26. "Herbalists to Get Society," *Daily News,* December 22, 1980, 3.

27. "'Control Herbs Dispensing,'" *Daily News,* July 18, 1981, 5.

28. "Ministry Cautions on Herb Use," *Daily News,* November 9, 1981, 3.

29. "Drugs from Local Herbs Ready Soon," *Daily News,* June 25, 1985, 1.

30. "Herbs Enter Conventional Medicine," *Sunday News,* July 28, 1985, 5.

31. Iliffe (1998) argues that "the major break with [colonial and early post-independence] health policy came at the TANU party conference of September 1971, which ruled that rural health services should have top priority in socio-economic development plans" (203).

32. Compliance with this task was marked by President Bush's visit in February 2008 and the accolades that Tanzania received for its work to create a business friendly environment.

33. In 1989, key policymakers at the World Bank and other international organizations sought to transform the economies of socialist countries by means of "structural adjustments." which required such thing as privatizing industry, floating currencies on the world market, and cutting social service programs such as education and health care. The consolidation of this vision came to be known as the "Washington Consensus" (Harvey 2005, Chachage and Mbilinyi 2003, Shivji 2008). For an early description of the Washington Consensus, see Williamson (1990).

34. "Cost sharing" is the term used for policies that required that patients contribute to the cost of their care in government-run hospitals, health clinics and dispensaries.

35. Iliffe (1998, 210–211).

36. For further analysis, see Sanders (2001).

37. "Tanzania Leader Condemns Witchdoctor Killings," *Reuters Africa,* April 3, 2008; Khadija Yusuf, "Deadly Harvest of Body Parts," *The Standard,* May 5, 2008; "Tanzania Albinos Targeted Again," *BBC News,* July 27, 2008.

38. See Green (2003), as well as the broader literature on development and witchcraft listed in note 32 of chapter 2.

39. Daniel Dickinson, "Tackling 'Witch' Murders in Tanzania," *BBC News,* October 29, 2002; "Tanzania Suffers Rise of Witchcraft Hysteria," *The Independent,* November 28, 2005. HelpAge International brought this issue to the attention of the UN Convention on the Elimination of All Forms of Discrimination Against Women. For more information, see "Help Age Urges Action on Older Women's Rights in Tanzania," available at http://www.helpage.org/News/Mediacentre/Pressreleases/m7BO.

40. Cost-sharing measures for health care services in Tanzania were introduced in 1993 (Lambert and Sahn 2002, Meena 2008).

41. One example of such research is I. Hedberg et al., "Inventory of Plants Used in Traditional Medicine in Tanzania. II. Plants of the Families Dilleniaceae—Opiliaceae," *Journal of Ethnopharmacology* 9, nos. 2–3 (1983): 237–260, which was the result of col-

laborative research between botanists and pharmacologists at the University of Uppsala in Sweden, the Tanzanian Government Laboratory, the University of Dar es Salaam, and the Institute of Traditional Medicine at the Muhimbili Medical Center.

42. "Malaria: Boil Leaves," *Daily News*, May 3, 1985, 4.

43. Throughout the 1990s, the need for a framework through which Tanzania could systematically review the ethics of health-related research being carried out within its national borders remained acute (Kitua, Mashalla, and Shija 2000). While the Commission for Science and Technology served academic researchers, no government office was tasked with monitoring non-academics who were collecting herbal medicines. Not until 2001 did the Tanzania National Health Research Forum publish the *Guidelines on Ethics for Health Research in Tanzania*, which had been developed by the National Health Research Ethics Committee. Recently, the National Institute for Medical Research established an ethical review board for all medical research involving human subjects. Mechanisms for enforcement remain unclear, however (Ikingura, Kruger, and Zeleke 2007). Because the Tanzanian government does not have adequate capacity to monitor research efforts that do not involve collaboration with Tanzanian academic or research institutions, botanical poaching in the name of independent scientific research poses a challenge.

44. "Nigerian Herbalists to Cure AIDS?" *Sunday News*, October 13, 1985, 1; "Local Herbs 'Usable in Hospitals,'" *Daily News*, March 21, 1987, 3; "Medicinemen in AIDS Research," *Daily News*, October 20, 1987, 5; "Give Funds to Our Herbalist," *Daily News*, November 3, 1987, 5; "'AIDS Victims Free to See Medicine Men,'" *Daily News*, May 12, 1988, 3; "Herbalist Allowed to Treat AIDS Patients," *Daily News*, October 14, 1988, 3; "Herbalist Asked to Treat AIDS Patients," *Daily News*, October 20, 1988, 3; "Hospitals Now to Dispense Herbs," *Daily News*, November 9, 2002, 1.

45. HIV/AIDS workshops for traditional healers, traditional birth attendants, and initiation specialists held in Chilangala on May 13, 2003, and in Newala on May 14, 2003. These workshops were conducted by nurse-trainers from the Newala District Hospital.

46. David Scheinman, "Traditional Medicine in Tanga Today: The Ancient and the Modern Worlds Meet," *Daily News*, December 5, 2002.

47. Interview with David Scheinman, March 1999. Shaman Pharmaceuticals has since closed and reopened under the name Shaman Botanicals (McMillen 2004).

48. "Hospital Now to Dispense Herbs," *Daily News*, November 9, 2002, 1.

49. Yet to the extent that scientists and government officials envision such medicine as an alternative to globally produced pharmaceutical drugs, they explore an enduring (albeit transformed) notion of self-sufficiency (Langwick 2008b).

50. Interview with Mahunnah, September 22, 1998.

51. Ibid.

52. In 1994, Mr. Chiliko, who had been trained as a pharmacist, was appointed in the Ministry of Health's Office of Traditional Medicine. He was many years Mnaliwa's senior, and he entered the office as her supervisor. He remained in the Office of Traditional Medicine until 1997, when he retired from the Ministry of Health. In 1995, E. S. Lugakingira was appointed to the Ministry of Health's Office of Traditional Medicine. For a brief time, the Office of Traditional Medicine had three full-time staff members. In 1996, however, Mnaliwa left to complete a one-year diploma in community health. When she returned, the Ministry of Health appointed her to the Office of the Registrar

of Medical Council. She did not return to the Office of Traditional Medicine until the beginning of 2000. In the meantime, another person, Dr. Paulo Mhame, joined the Office of Traditional Medicine to fill Chiliko's position after his retirement. Mhame headed the Office of Traditional Medicine from 1998 until 2001. In 2001, he was transferred to the National Institute for Medical Research and was assigned the task of building the Traditional Medicine Research Unit there. However, he returned to the Office of Traditional Medicine in 2006.

53. *Kilenge* is also a children's game played with four sticks. Another implication, then, is that traditional medicine may be interesting to play, but it is not substantive enough to ever move beyond being a game. I thank Masangu Matondo of the Department of Languages, Literatures, and Cultures at the University of Florida for this second interpretation.

54. *The Laws of Tanzania* (Dar es Salaam: Government Printers of Tanzania, 2002).

55. "Hospital Now to Dispense Herbs," *Daily News,* November 9, 2002, 1.

56. Alternative medical disciplines are officially defined in this law as "knowledge and practices established and accepted internationally such as homoeopathy, chiropractic, massage, aromatherapy, acupuncture, ayurvedic medicine and others." *The Traditional and Alternative Medicines Act No. 23* (Dar es Salaam: Government Printer, 2002), 6, available at http://www.lrct.or.tz/documents/23-2002_The%20Traditional%20and%20Alternative%20Medicines%20Act,%202002.pdf.

57. "Traditional medicine" is officially defined in this law as "a total combination of knowledge and practice, whether applicable or not, used in diagnosing, preventing or eliminating a physical, mental or social disease and which may rely exclusively on past experience and observation handled down from one generation to another orally or in writing." Ibid., 7.

58. Tanzania's status as China's largest aid recipient in Africa has recently changed with the substantial loan and aid packages that China has extended to central African countries that have large reserves of oil, timber, and gems. Joshua Eisenman, "China and the Developing World," paper presented at the Institute for African Development, Cornell University, Ithaca, New York, October 11, 2007. For more on China's increasing interest in Africa over the past decade, see Eisenman, Heginbotham, and Mitchell (2007).

59. "Tanzania Supports China's Reunification," *China Economic Net,* July 18, 2004, available at http://en1.ce.cn/National/Politics/200407/18/t20040718_1265051.shtml.

60. Interview with Sabina Mnaliwa, April 13, 2000.

61. This resonates with Hsu's (2002) study of Tanzanian patients in Traditional Chinese Medicine clinics in Dar es Salaam. As one patient told her, to be "modern" was "to be open, to advertise, and sell openly, and not to be secretive." Hsu commented that "this, [the patient] thought, was what the Chinese were doing" (307). While Hsu illustrates the flexibility of Tanzanian patients' claims that Chinese medicine is either modern or traditional, she also notes the salience of "the 'look' of the medicines, in pill or tablet form, aluminum foil or plastic packages, [which] made them [appear more] similar to biomedical drugs" (307).

62. There is some indication that this phenomenon is not limited to Tanzania or to other formerly non-aligned states. See "FG Seeks China's Cooperation on Herbal Medicines," *This Day* (Lagos), September 20, 2007. In addition, it is consistent with broader shifts in China's foreign policy toward Africa in the 1990s; see Taylor (1998) and Brautigam (2003).

63. Mnaliwa's reference to "everyone" raises the question of who these new traditional medicines appeal to. Who constitutes the public that has a "tendency to accept" (mass-produced) herbal medicine? She never explicitly described this public. If Lugakingira's medicines can be used as an example, however, it appears that this newly commoditized medicine circulates among a fairly restricted group. The prices of Lugakingira's vials and capsules (Tsh 40,000 per box) put them out of the reach of all but elite professionals, who are mostly urban and who mostly live around Dar es Salaam.

64. Interview with Mnaliwa, April 13, 2000.

65. Pudenciana Temba, "Sarungi Advises Herbalists to Form an Association," *Daily News*, August 2, 1991, 5.

66. Ibid.; Pudenciana Temba, "Local Herbs for Lab Analysis," *Sunday News*, August 4, 1991, 1; "Traditional Healers' Role Important," *Sunday News*, August 4, 1991, 4.

67. For other examples of healers in Tanzania who are innovatively shaping their practices to fit contemporary economic contexts and modern bureaucratic forms, see Gessler et al. (1995) and Green (2003).

68. "'Fake' Healers Flood Arusha," *Daily News*, January 12, 1993, 3.

69. F. wa Simbeye, "Call for Traditional Healers['] College amid Suspicions of Witch-craft," *Daily News*, July 5, 1999, 3.

70. Ibid.

71. "Herbalists to Start a Lab?" *Daily News*, April 26, 2003, 4.

4. Healers and Their Intimate Becomings

1. This representation turns the practices and lifeways of some into resources to be exploited by others who claim they have unique access to the dynamics of progress. Healing seems particularly susceptible to what Haraway (1989) has called "the cannibalistic Western logic that readily constructs other cultural possibilities as resources for Western needs and actions"(255). In a search for more productive ways to engage references to "tradition," some scholars have suggested analyzing "modernity" and "tradition" as circulating signs. Stacy Leigh Pigg (1996), for instance, has shown how in Nepal, claims to "the modern" or "the traditional" actively position a speaker within social constellations generated by the demands of development. Others have marked the ways that clear distinctions between the traditional and modern are disrupted when healers invoke the quintessential elements of modernity in their own practice. Vincanne Adams (2001) describes how Tibetan healers strategically align themselves and their therapies with science and against religion in the context of a repressive political landscape and questions assumptions that nonbiomedical healers are traditional or religious or holistic.

2. In Kimakonde, one of the major languages of the southeastern region, people do not distinguish between traditional and modern medicine. When people are compelled to articulate this division, they switch to Kiswahili.

3. Although anthropologists fear that the distinction between the traditional and the modern relegates the traditional to a stagnant baseline against which modern progress can be judged, this division is not easily conveyed in Kiswahili. Tanzanians do use the distinction between the traditional and the modern to articulate a distinction between the historical and ahistorical. The modern has no temporal depth in Kiswahili. Modern

medicine (*dawa za kisasa*) is literally the "medicine of now" (*kisasa*). Privileging the present, the "medicine of now" ignores the emergence of biomedicine and its change over time. Only the colloquial and now rather infrequent references to *dawa za kizungu,* medicine of the whites, refers to any sense of medical history in Africa. The history evoked in this racialized reference is that of the expansion of biomedicine through colonialization and missionization, not of its emergence through medical science.

4. While a relationship with time is a central feature of healing, it is not always the characteristic by which healers are identified. Tradition is not necessarily brought to the fore in the naming of healers. Locally, for instance, healers are often referred to as *fundi,* a word used broadly for all sorts of technicians and craftspeople. A *fundi* is a person with the skill to create something. Healers refer to themselves in a number of ways. Sometimes, particularly in urban areas, they take on "healing names" and assume titles such as "Doctor" or "Professor." In Newala, however, this is not common. Sometimes healers will carry forward a family name that identifies their lineage of healing. Generally, well-known healers are addressed as elders and as mothers and fathers.

5. In 1995, 135 traditional healers had been registered in the Newala District; "Madawa na Waganga-Kienyegi" (Medicines of Traditional Healers), M.10/14, Newala District Files, District Commissioner's Office. Many more remained unregistered.

6. Healers who derive their power from institutionalized religions such as Islam and Christianity—for example Muslim prophets and Christian faith healers—are also typically excluded from the category of traditional healers. Sometimes, however, specialists who work with the Qur'an (and are referred to as *waganga* [healers] but not as *waganga wa jadi* [traditional healers]) are indiscriminately swept into this awkwardly broad, everything-but-biomedicine category of traditional medicine in official state rhetoric. Similarly, I never heard practitioners of Traditional Chinese Medicine referred to as traditional healers, but as I suggested in the previous chapter, the state hopes to regulate Chinese practitioners under the Traditional and Alternative Medicines Act.

7. Swantz (1974) refers to this process in his description of divining by the Zaramo in Dar es Salaam. He writes: "The method of divining used by the largest group of traditional medicine men in Dar es Salaam is the Islamic form of geomancy. This method employs incantations from the Quran as well as making calculations and evaluations of each case from a book known as Satrikhabari by the local people. . . . It seems that all Islamic diviners in Dar es Salaam have studied the book called Satrikhabari, Sw., and use it in their practice" (193).

8. Ngubane (1981/1992) has noted a distinction in southern Africa between two kinds of indigenous healers—the *inyanga* (Zulu), who is usually male and uses African medicines without clairvoyant techniques, and the *isangoma,* or diviner, who is usually female and uses clairvoyant techniques. The *isangoma* has a relationship with spirits that is credited as a reason for her clairvoyance. A similar distinction does not appear to be made in southeastern Tanzania. A person with knowledge of medicinal substances is more likely to be known as a salesperson than as a healer. The notable exception to this in Newala is Maasai healers who sometimes travel from their northern homes to southeastern Tanzania to sell medicine in the market there. People in Newala evaluated Maasai expertise differently than they did the expertise of local healers. They called the Maasai healers and referred to them as *waganga wa jadi,* but they did not attribute the

knowledge of these Maasai to relationships with ancestors, familiars, or any other sort of disembodied actor. The Maasai themselves mobilized a variety of distinctions that are too complicated to address here.

9. In Arabic, a *shaykh* is a teacher or a guide to Sufism.

10. Awadhi gave several examples of the circumstances in which *faraki* medicine is typically used and has been used successfully. First, perhaps as a demonstration of the power of the *shehe* from whom he learned *faraki,* he told me about a time when one of the wives of this *shehe* wanted to go to Dar es Salaam. She left by foot to go to Dar (about 450 kilometers away), and she arrived, he said, in only ten hours. He also said that if you fall in love with someone but that person doesn't love you, medicine can be used to make the person fall in love with you. He claimed that with this medicine you can find yourself married within weeks. He also said that medicine might be used to make a bully leave a village.

11. These squares are found in many places throughout Africa and are said to reflect the highly esoteric science of Sufi mysticism.

12. Discussion during the workshop Healing Divides: Migrations, Transgressions, and Transformations of Healing Knowledge in Southeastern Africa at the University of Pennsylvania, Philadelphia, January 30–February 1, 2003.

13. Although Fatu Chenga, like many healers, had a difficult time remembering dates, she did say that she began treating patients in 1966, during her initiation. Therefore, it seems that she returned to this healer in the mid-1960s.

14. In an ethnographic study of Wasukuma in northern Tanzania, Marlene Reid (1982) also observed that afflictions attributed to *uchawi* "were usually those that had symptoms related to swellings and internal pain" (133).

15. There is no gender in Kiswahili; Binti Dadi made these statements using the third-person singular. However, because the *majini* or *mashetani* who come to teach Binti Dadi about various types of medicine typically appear as her grandmother, I have used the pronoun "she" here.

16. Sometimes also heard or seen as *mihoka.*

17. In a 1902 essay entitled "Some Animistic Beliefs among the Yaos of British Central Africa," Rev. Alexander Hetherwick of the Blantyre Mission discussed the "foundation of the Yao religion" as "the *lisoka,* the soul, shade, or spirit which every human being possesses, and which is the inspiring agent of his life." The plural of *lisoka* is *masoka* in Kiyao and appears to be similar in some respects to the Kimakonde *mahoka.* Just as the *mahoka* is critical in the dreams of healers, the *masoka* "is recognized [by the Yao] as the chief agency in dreams. . . . The *lisoka* is supposed to go out and visit the scenes and persons it dreams about, and in turn is visited by the *masoka* of others, dead and living. Pains in the body on rising from sleep in the morning are usually attributed to such nocturnal visits, while disease or pain of a severe type are ascribed to castigations by the whips of the *masoka* or more frequently of the witches who prowl around during the night watches" (90). While on the plateau *mahoka* were said to be one aspect of the dead, Rev. Hetherwick understood the *masoka* among the Yao in the late nineteenth century to be an aspect of each living person that persisted after death. He wrote: "In dreams or in fainting fits the *lisoka* leaves the body but only to return to it with the awakening consciousness. At death, however, it leaves its earthly abode never to return. It is now spoken of as having gone to *mulungu* or *mlungu*" (91).

18. This reference to the bush implicitly translates *nandenga* (Kimakonde)—a nonhuman said to live in large trees—as *majini* (also discussed in chapter 7).

19. Similar philosophies of therapeutic knowledge are found throughout the region. See, for example, Reynolds (1996, especially page 38).

20. The length of time that Mariamu spent with this healer in his compound implies that this treatment could have been (or could have led to) an initiation. While the *ngoma* is a discrete event, initiations for healers are less so. This ambiguity is an effect of the fact that it is only clear in retrospect if a person will be healed and if that healing will result in intimate relations with nonhumans who are knowledgeable about medicine. The emphasis Binti Dadi and Mariamu place on the fact that Binti Dadi "stole" her daughter marks the rupture in Mariamu's relationship with this healer. She does not claim that this period was an initiation, and she does not maintain any obligations or responsibilities to this person as a guide, teacher, and healer.

21. Therapies enact a series of spatial distinctions inside and outside the courtyard. In chapter 8, I describe the treatment for *makanje,* growths in the nose of fathers and in the nose or vagina of mothers that harbor *mashetani* who continually startle a young child each time he or she looks at a parent. This treatment divides up the space of the home into the buildings and the courtyard, reestablishing gendered dominions. Treatments for infertility do the same (see the epilogue).

22. According to both colonial (e.g., see Tanganyika Standard 1946), and contemporary Tanzanian accounts (Wembah-Rashid 1974), witches and sorcerers bolster their power by eating the dead. *Wachawi* go to the graves of those they have killed and ritually feast on their corpses. Healers' relationships with the dead through ancestral shades are sharply distinguished from *wachawi*'s relationships with the dead through corpses. Yet, when accusations of witchcraft are leveled at healers there is slippage between talking with the dead and eating the dead.

23. This medicine, then, provides the corollary to Bruno Latour's claim that "we have never been modern," for here we see that "they" have never been traditional! Latour's critique of modernization theory argues that claims to modernity have rested on the purification of culture and nature and humans and nonhumans. He argues that we have never been modern because despite our claims, our knowledge production practices mix up culture and nature all the time. Modernist efforts at purification result only in a need for translation. It appears here, however, that this so-called traditional society also invests a great deal in the purification of humans and nonhumans, and those who don't are dangerous. See Latour (1993).

5. Traditional Birth Attendants as Institutional Evocations

1. Whether or not training for TBAs is effective and how well TBAs contribute to the reduction of maternal and infant mortality and morbidity rates are currently topics of hot debate in public health circles (Bolam et al. 1999; Dehne et al. 1995; Matthew et al. 1995; Rosario 1995; Smith et al. 1997).

2. For an historical analysis of this representation, see Langwick (2006).

3. For evidence of the generation of the TBA as a global actor through the initiatives of the WHO and various UN agencies, see Langwick (forthcoming a).

4. Joyce Safe, "Traditional Birth Attendants in Maternal and Child Health Care, Tanzania." Tanzanian Ministry of Health, ca. 1992, p. 1. I acquired this source from the Ministry of Health in Dar es Salaam.

5. The Safe Motherhood Initiative (SMI) was launched in 1987 through the collaboration of three international organizations—the United Nations Population Fund, the World Bank, and the World Health Organization. The campaign aims to raise awareness about maternal mortality and advocate for interventions to reduce it.

6. Leader Stirling's (1947) memoirs of clinical work on the plateau point to this sort of exchange. More detailed evidence of clinical collaboration with "old women" in neighboring Congo, see Chapter 5, "Babies and Forceps," in Hunt (1999). Informal connections between traditional midwives and healers and biomedical practitioners continue today. For more on contemporary exchanges, see Langwick (2009).

7. Safe, "Traditional Birth Attendants in Maternal and Child Health Care, Tanzania," ca. 1992, 7.

8. District reports, 1996, Ministry of Health, Dar es Salaam.

9. P. Mmbuji and Joyce Safe, "Assessment of the Effect of Training Traditional Birth Attendants on Community Based Maternity Care and Pregnancy Outcome in Tanzania," 1997, p. 4. This was a research proposal for Maternal and Child Health/Family Planning (Safe Motherhood Initiative); I acquired it from the Ministry of Health in Dar es Salaam.

10. The WHO's Safe Motherhood Initiative covered a broad spectrum of issues related to pregnancy and birth, and it provided funding for most of the TBA training workshops and supply kits in Tanzania. See World Health Organization (1988).

11. Only in unusual circumstances might a woman be part of this village leadership structure. For example, in the Kitangari training workshop described above, only one of the seven village leaders who attended the first day of training was a woman.

12. District Maternal and Child Health Coordinator L. M. Kaluma, Maternal and Child Health Clinic, Newala District Hospital, to ward-level leaders, November 11, 1992, with the subject heading "Mafunzo ya Wakunga wa Jadi"(Traditional Birth Attendant Training).

13. Mmbuji and Safe, "Assessment of the Effect of Training Traditional Birth Attendants," 4.

14. The salience of these distinctions between the targets of training are reflected in the titles of these manuals—*Mwongozo wa Mkufunzi wa Mkunga wa Jadi* (Training for the Trainers of Traditional Birth Attendants), *Mwongozo wa Kufundisha Wakunga wa Jadi* (Instructions for Teaching Traditional Birth Attendants), and *Mwongozo wa Utekelezaji wa Huduma ya Wakunga wa Jadi Tanzania* (Instructions for the Executors of Care of Traditional Birth Attendants), usually referring to village leaders.

15. I have borrowed the phrase "ecology of expertise" from Awiha Ong (2005).

16. It is interesting to note how this change in posture has changed the mothers' experience of birth. When women demonstrated this position to me, they showed me how they would pull on their ankles during contractions. Pulling rather than pushing was encouraged. In addition, this change in position (as others have noted) illustrates the shift in the primacy of an authority figure. From a sitting position, women could "catch" their own babies and therefore did not need an expert present during a normal birth. Indeed, it seems that many women used to (and a fair number still do) give birth alone. This is more difficult from a lying position, which favors the actions of another person.

6. Alternative Materialities

1. As Last (1992), Whyte (1997, 2005) and Feierman (2000) have all described, there is a great deal of uncertainty among Africans as they mobilize various therapies to address their maladies or misfortunes. If so much uncertainty is found among people seeking treatments, then one might expect even more questioning, uncertainty, and multiple positionings with regard to the less urgent (even if not less significant) process of protecting one's child from future illnesses. Even as I explore these popular protective processes, I will try to also explore the controversy and doubt that is inevitably part of the process of seeking out protection.

2. Quoted from a paper given by Margaret Lock in the "Author Meets Critics" session for Annemarie Mol's book *The Body Multiple: Ontology in Medical Practice* at the 2004 joint meeting of the Society for the Social Studies of Science and the European Association for the Study of Science and Technology, Paris, August 27, 2004.

3. These resonate with but do not correspond directly to the differences in medicine I described in chapter 4.

4. One exception, however, is the work of Nicole Sindzingre and Andras Zempleni (1992) among the Senufo in the Ivory Coast, Burkina Faso, and Mali. They found that the idea of "sickness of God" among the Senufo was quite different than the idea of such illness Janzen found in Lower Zaire. "Sicknesses of God" in this more northern area is a "negative etiological category" that encompasses all things that "neither common understanding, nor divination, can assign a hypothetical cause" (317).

5. Feierman uses the word "illness" in his work; see, for example, Feierman (1981) and Feierman and Janzen (1992).

6. These findings are similar to those of Susan Reynolds Whyte (1997) in Uganda. She writes: "Diviners say frankly that if the line of treatment they are proposing does not help, the family should go and divine elsewhere" (23).

7. When an American missionary in Mtwara, the regional capital in southeastern Tanzania, soundly berated me for sending a gift of medicine to my sister's newborn child to protect her from devils, I discovered that church members do not uniformly dismiss the notion that some maladies are caused by *mashetani*. In the course of his argument, this missionary cited several instances when, to his mind, the use of medicine to address the *shetani* opened up a person to Satan (as it is understood in Christianity). The missionary claimed that the medicine in effect called Satan in for an engagement, and in this encounter the evil one could "win." In the stories of people he had seen and helped, this missionary claimed to have seen such medicine lead the people who used it to be possessed by Satan. As a result, he expressed his concern for the life and soul of my sister's innocent newborn in America.

8. Unlike the Kiswahili word *mashetani*, which in some contexts was used to refer to the older Kimakonde *mahoka* (which are always spoken of in the plural), *nandenga* (also Kimakonde) was often (but not consistently) spoken of in the singular as *shetani*.

9. *Nyoka* means snake in Kiswahili. Perhaps someday linguistic research will explore the history of the root of this word in Kimakonde.

10. Because this medicine is prepared and administered by healers whose knowledge and cures have different genealogies, practices vary not only by individual need and affliction, but also by healer. And yet there is an idiom of care (a set of narrative and practi-

cal technologies) that is mobilized throughout the area. Talk of illness and healing is so common that one rarely enters a public space, whether it be an office or a canteen, where the conversation does not turn at some point (or at many points) to stories of those who need treatment, those who fear they are dying, or those who have recently died. Sickness is particularly common during the rainy season. I attended many funerals, perhaps once a week, during this dangerous season. People who had more extensive networks than I did attended many more. The regular activities of caring for the sick and dying prompted Tanzanians to exchange their opinions often about a wide range of maladies. Although many women refrained from offering opinions about the sources of the problems that afflicted themselves or their children when they visited a healer, outside the sphere of experts most people drew on their extensive shared experiences to vividly describe the problem and to posit possible ways of dealing with the misfortune.

11. Writing *kombe,* as described in greater detail in chapter 4, is a process of communicating with guiding spirits and allowing the conversation to manifest as script on a white plate in red ink. The writing is then read and water is added to the plate to make a pink medicinal solution that may be drunk or used for washing.

12. This medicine was reminiscent of that used in the Maji Maji Rebellion (1905–1907). When I asked Chinduli about this rebellion, he implied that the medicine he used was the same medicine healers used to protect Africans who fought against the Germans. He also claimed that all the individuals who were protected in this fashion returned home alive.

13. These actions probably have an old genealogy. They have almost certainly been transformed as a result of changes in living conditions, villagization policies, and population density. For instance, another healer, Mama Libongo, told me that waMakonde used to bury the umbilical cord of a child in a cool, breezy open space far from people.

14. One of the items Binti Dadi and Mariamu use in making medicine to protect the wearer from *uchawi* is the throat or windpipe of a lion (*kikolomo kutoka simba*). The part of the lion's throat that produces the growl becomes a medicine that will strike fear in anyone with evil intentions.

15. Allan Young (2004) develops the concept of "fictive embodiment."

16. For anthropological studies of the historical emergence of and the political-cultural nature of the immune system, see Donna Haraway (1993), Emily Martin (1990, 1994), and David Napier (2003).

17. I thank Patricia Robinson of the College of Medicine at the University of Florida for sharing her understanding of immunology with me and for describing some of the changes in immunology since the proliferation of research on HIV/AIDS.

18. These agents and processes are described in contemporary standard explanations of immunization, such as the 1997 edition of *Roitt's Essential Immunology.* Here I have chosen to relate both the stories of the science of immunology and the stories of nurses in the Newala District Hospital because the range of agents at play in such institutional settings is shaped by the standard biomedical arguments as they are taken up in international health development efforts. Most directly, the World Health Organization uses these articulations of biomedical science in its guidelines for immunization, and in turn these guidelines structure national requirements. Therefore the agents of affliction at play, even in rural African hospitals, are best accounted for through both global and local discourses.

7. Interferences and Inclusions

1. See for example Frederick Johnson's *A Standard Swahili-English Dictionary* (1939).

2. Medecins San Frontieres, "Changing National Malaria Treatment Protocols in Africa," press dossier, Nairobi, Kenya, 13 February 2002. The practices and problems discussed in this chapter occur against a background of significant inequalities. For discussions of the political and material conditions of disease in Sub-Saharan African and particularly in Tanzania, see Anderson and Marks (1989), Packard (1989), Raikes (1989), and Turshen (1984, 1989, 1991).

3. Mariamu spoke the words "injection" and "chloroquine" in English.

4. See also Makemba et al. (1996).

5. One of the more sophisticated examples of such biomedical translations by an anthropologist is Peter Winch's (1999) evaluation of the Bagamoyo Bed Net Project. In his empirically rich study, he praises the project for promoting insecticide-treated bednets (mosquito nets) using rhetoric that Winch claimed did not judge local medical knowledge. This malaria prevention program in the more northern coastal town of Bagamoyo did "not state that local illnesses, such as those caused by spirits, do not exist, or that they are the same thing as *homa ya malaria* [Kiswahili, malaria fever]. Instead it was stated that *homa ya malaria* can cause *degedege* and other serious illnesses" (51). This framing asserts that malaria causes *degedege*. As will be discussed later in this chapter, scientific models of causality are in themselves powerful cultural translators. If malaria causes *degedege*, then *degedege* is no longer the primary or most effective object of treatment or action; malaria is. In the end, the effects of claims that "*degedege* is malaria" and claims that "malaria causes *degedege*" do not distinguish the two statements as significantly different. Malaria is asserted as the more fundamental affliction. Significantly, in the context of public health debates concerning *degedege*, this approach also rationalizes why malaria needs to be treated first.

6. For more examples of such help-seeking behavior in Tanzania, see Oberlander and Elverdan (2000).

7. In Kimakonde, such medicine is known as *mnchandamila, bwabalawa, mpungama-hoka, mpungamedi, mala, namamba, nahimana, nchinjimala,* and *munjulu.*

8. Binti Dadi prepared this medicinal bath by pounding the leaves of *mnchandamila, mnchingimala, mmamana, mnembelembe,* and *mmala* together in a large wooden mortar (*kinu*) and then adding water and one hot coal.

9. I draw on Latour (1999), who has argued that paying attention to the propositions scientists construct as they produce knowledge is one way of tracing the emergence of scientific entities. Propositions are actions, whether verbal or otherwise, that engender "*occasions* given to different entities to enter into contact" (141). They differentiate by inviting reactions, relations, and positions. Propositions enable the contours of a phenomenon to be identified, seen, named, and transformed. Latour focuses his work on propositions made by scientists; in this book I extend this analytical approach to doctors, nurses, and traditional healers.

10. The medicine with which Binti Dadi washed the child was intended "to reduce the heat of the body." However, it is important to remember that children who are well may

also be washed for protective reasons. The verb *kupona* (to heal) is derived from the verb that means "to cool." The roasted medicine that Binti Dadi rubbed into a cut on the end of Juma's nose is for removing the devils or *mashetani* who are bothering the child. The medicine that is taken orally is, according to Binti Dadi, "for the purpose of giving the child a drink so that she can defecate to remove the speed of the sickness." At the root of all these forms of healing is a notion of cooling.

11. "Collapsing" can also be translated as "drying." "Stilled" can also be translated as "calmed or settled."

12. For a nuanced discussion of how processes of objectification in the production of clinical knowledge shapes specific forms of agency, see Cussins (1998) and Thompson (2005).

13. Feierman (1985) has begun to trace the history of the sometimes extreme "depersonalization and decontextualization" that one is likely to find between biomedical practitioners and patients in African hospitals (110).

14. At least one of the doctors with whom I spoke did not rely on these percentages for a diagnosis. He claimed that in attempts to match the color of the blood to the color on the card there was too much room for human error. He had seen patients' notebooks that indicated that the levels of hemoglobin were so low that the patients should not have been able to walk around or have the energy to sit up. And yet often these patients would be sitting, talking, and able to walk. In such cases, he claimed, looking at the color of the palm of the child's hand or pulling back the lower eyelid and examining the color of the inside of the lower eyelid was a more reliable diagnostic technique.

15. From 1998 to 2003, all of the doctors at the Newala District Hospital were male. During this time, the vast majority of nurses in the hospital and all of the nurses in the maternal and child health clinic were female.

16. For examples of medical research on the effect of *Plasmodium falciparum* malaria on children in Tanzania, see Kitua et al. (1996, 1997) and Vounatsou et al. (2000).

17. Latour (1987) originally borrowed the term "black box" from cybernetics. Following Latour, many science studies scholars have now come to use this term to refer to scientific theories or technologies that have achieved such a consensus that their use in other experiments goes unquestioned. Black-boxed theories, formulas, or technologies can be mobilized uncritically in combination with other theories, formulas, or technologies to explore a range of new research questions.

18. Pigg (1996) traces how villagers position themselves within a complicated landscape of modernization and development through declarations of "belief" in shamans. For a broader discussion of belief in anthropological discourse, see Good (1994).

8. Shifting Existences, or Being and Not-Being

1. The verb *kukunja*, which was used to describe the process of removing *makanje*, is commonly used to mean "to fold, wrap up, crease, wrinkle, tumble, [and] make a mess of" (Johnson's *A Standard Swahili-English Dictionary*). I heard the verb used frequently to refer to both wrapping up food or medicine and folding clothes or cloth.

2. In the United States, such cysts on an infant's palate are referred to as "Epstein's pearls" and are said to disappear of their own accord without consequence. I am indebted to Dr. Marian Bouchard for this connection.

3. Interestingly, while no TBA denied that such confessions were demanded during certain births, they disagreed with the notion that such practices kept women from delivering in a clinic. TBAs told me that while such confessional therapies were not common, they were confident that in instances where it was necessary for the woman to confess, an arrangement could be worked out that would make it possible for her to do so in the clinic.

4. Others have focused on the bodily practices related to the care of children. Gottlieb (2004), for instance, explores how Beng parents in the Ivory Coast adorn their infants and carefully study their desires in an effort to read which ancestor has come back through their new body. The "culture of infancy" she describes is shaped by the notion that children come into the world through the afterlife. As a result, they arrive knowing everything, speaking all languages. For them, the process of growing into adulthood is a process of forgetting, of locating one's self, of specifying one's knowledge. Because my focus here is on therapeutic practice and questions of ontology, I account for Mariamu's care within the argument I have been developing about the body. Her care of Yanini could, however, be brought together with other stories of ways people on the plateau care for and engage with infants in order to explore questions about personhood and aging.

Conclusion

1. Mol (1994) and Mol and Mesman (1996) also ask which types of politics are made possible by analyses that describe objects of medical knowledge as effects of practice, that is as events that are significant only insofar as they enable intervention.

References

Archives and Manuscripts

District Commissioner's Office, Newala District

"Madawa na Waganga-Kienyegi" (Medicines of Traditional Healers), M.10/14, Newala District Files

East Africana Collection, University of Dar es Salaam Library

Annual reports of the East African Agricultural and Fisheries Research Station at Amani, 1928–1960.

J. N. R. Kasembe, *Science, Technology and Development in Tanzania,* Country Report for ECA/UNESCO Regional Symposium on the Utilization of Science and Technology for the Development of Africa, Addis Ababa, 1970, S&T/CR/39.P.10.

Terence O. Ranger, "Witchcraft Eradication Movements in Central and Southern Tanzania and Their Connection with the Maji Maji Rising." Seminar paper, University College, Dar es Salaam, 1966.

Ministry of Health, Dar es Salaam

District Reports, 1996.

Joyce Safe, *Strategy for Reproductive Health and Child Survival, 1997–2001.* Dar es Salaam: Ministry of Health, 1997.

Joyce Safe, "Traditional Birth Attendants in Maternal and Child Health Care, Tanzania." Tanzanian Ministry of Health, ca. 1992.

Joyce Safe, *Training of TBAs in Tanzania.* Dar es Salaam: Ministry of Health, 1997.

P. Mmbuji and Joyce Safe, "Assessment of the Effect of Training Traditional Birth Attendants on Community Based Maternity Care and Pregnancy Outcome in Tanzania." A research proposal for Maternal and Child Health/Family Planning (Safe Motherhood Initiative). 1997.

Mwongozo wa Utekelezaji wa Huduma ya Wakunga wa Jadi Tanzania. Training manual written with the assistance of the WHO and UNICEF. Dar es Salaam: Ministry of Health, 1998.

National Museum of Tanzania, Dar es Salaam

J. A. R. Wembah-Rashid, "The Traditional Religions of the People of Masasi District: Ethnographic Field Research Report." Occasional Paper No. 1, National Museum of Tanzania, 1974.

J. A. R. Wembah-Rashid, "Social, Political, & Economic Organization of the People of Masasi District: Ethnographic Field Research Project." Occasional Paper No. 2, National Museum of Tanzania, 1976.

Tanzanian National Archives (TNA), Dar es Salaam

Newala District Books, 1928–1955

Accession no. 16
  16/1/14: Tribal History
  16/5/7: Witchcraft vol. II
  16/11/77: Noxious and Poisonous Plant Fees
  16/37/105: Sociology
  16/37/29: Native Revolt of 1905 (Maji Maji)
  16/37/28: Lindi, Noxious and Poisonous Plants, Trees, etc.
Accession no. 567
  567/M.10/24: Midwifery and Clinical Centres (1959–68)
  567/M.10/28: Native Medicines General Examinations—Permits
World Health Organization Library, WHO Headquarters, Geneva, Switzerland
  "Safe Motherhood Initiative," THE/SMI/88.2

Books, Articles, Theses, and Papers

Abrahams, R. G., ed. 1994. *Witchcraft in Contemporary Tanzania*. Cambridge: African Studies Centre, University of Cambridge.

Adams, Vincanne. 2001. "The Sacred in the Scientific: Ambiguous Practices of Science in Tibetan Medicine." *Cultural Anthropology* 16(4): 542–575.

———. 2002. "Randomized Controlled Crime: Postcolonial Sciences in Alternative Medicine Research." *Social Studies of Science* 32(5–6): 659–690.

Ademuwagun, Z. A., J. Ayoade, J. Harrison, and D. M. Warren, eds. 1978. *African Therapeutic Systems*. Waltham, Mass.: Crossroads Press.

Akerele, Olayiwola. 1987. "The Best of Both Worlds: Bringing Traditional Medicine up to Date." *Social Science and Medicine* 24: 177–181.

———. 1991. *The Conservation of Medicinal Plants: Proceedings of an International Consultation, 21–27 March 1988 Held at Chiang Mai, Thailand*. Cambridge: Cambridge University Press.

———. 1998. *Medicinal Plants: Their Role in Health and Biodiversity*. Philadelphia: University of Pennsylvania Press.

Akhahenda, Elijah Fraylor. 1984. "A Content Analysis of Zambian and Tanzanian Newspapers during the period of Nationalization." Ph.D. diss., School of Journalism, Southern Illinois University.

Alpers, Edward. 1968. "Enlargement of Scale among the Yao in the Nineteenth Century." Paper presented at the University of East Africa Social Sciences Conference, Dar es Salaam, January 2–5.

———. 1972. "Toward a History of the Expansion of Islam in East Africa: The Matrilineal Peoples of the Southern Interior." In *The Historical Study of African Religion*, ed. T. O. Ranger and I. N. Kimambo, 172–201. Berkeley: University of California Press.

Althusser, Louis. 1971. "Ideology and Ideological State Apparatuses. Notes Toward an Investigation." In Althusser, *Lenin and Philosophy and Other Essays*, 127–186. New York: Monthly Review Press.

Anderson, Neil, and Shula Marks. 1989. "In State, Class and the Allocation of Health Resources in Southern Africa." *Social Science and Medicine* 28(5): 515–530.

Anderson, Warwick. 2001. "Excremental Colonialism: Public Health and the Poetics of Pollution." In *Contagion: Historical and Cultural Studies,* ed. Alison Bashford and Claire Hooker, 76–105. London: Routledge.

———. 2002. "Introduction: Postcolonial Technoscience." *Social Studies of Science* 32(5–6): 643–658.

———. 2006. *Colonial Pathologies: American Tropical Medicine, Race and Hygiene in the Philippines.* Durham, N.C.: Duke University Press.

Appadurai, Arjun. 1996. *Modernity at Large: Cultural Dimensions of Globalization.* London and Minneapolis: University of Minnesota Press.

Arnold, David. 1993. *Colonizing the Body: State Medicine and Epidemic Disease in Nineteenth-Century India.* Berkeley: University of California Press.

Austen, Ralph A. 1993. "The Moral Economy of Witchcraft: An Essay in Comparative History." In *Modernity and Its Malcontents: Ritual and Power in Postcolonial Africa,* ed. John Comaroff and Jean Comaroff, 89–110. Chicago: University of Chicago Press.

Baer, Hans. 2006. "The Drive for Legitimation in Australian Naturopathy: Successes and Dilemmas." *Social Science and Medicine* 63: 1771–1783.

Baer, Hans, Cindy Jen, Lucia M. Tanassi, Christopher Tsia, and Helen Wahbeh. 1998. "The Drive for Professionalization in Acupuncture: A Preliminary View from the San Francisco Bay Area." *Social Science and Medicine* 46(4–5): 533–537.

Barad, Karen. 1999. "Agential Realism: Feminist Interventions in Understanding Scientific Practices." In *The Science Studies Reader,* ed. M. Biagioli, 1–11. New York: Routledge.

Barkan, Joel D. 1984. "Introduction: Comparing Politics and Public Policy in Kenya and Tanzania." In *Politics and Public Policy in Kenya and Tanzania,* ed. Joel D. Barkan, 3–42. Rev. ed. New York: Praeger.

Barnes, Barry, and David Bloor. 1982. "Relativism, Rationalism and the Sociology of Knowledge." In *Rationality and Relativism,* ed. M. Hollis and S. Lukes, 21–47. Oxford: Blackwell.

Barthes, Roland. 1988. "Semiology and Medicine." In Barthes, *The Semiotic Challenge.* Trans. Richard Howard. New York: Hill and Wang.

Bashford, Alison. 2003. *Imperil Hygiene: A Critical History of Colonialism, Nationalism, and Public Health.* London: Palgrave.

Bastian, Misty L. 1993. "'Bloodhounds Who Have No Friends': Witchcraft and Locality in the Nigerian Popular Press." In *Modernity and Its Malcontents: Ritual and Power in Postcolonial Africa,* ed. John Comaroff and Jean Comaroff, 129–166. Chicago: University of Chicago Press.

Becker, Felicitas. 2004. "Traders, 'Big Men,' and Prophets": Political Continuity and Crisis in the Maji Maji Rebellion in Southeast Tanzania." *Journal of African History* 45: 1–22.

Berg, Marc, and Annemarie Mol. 1998. *Differences in Medicine: Unraveling Practices, Techniques, and Bodies.* Durham, N.C.: Duke University Press.

Berlant, Lauren. 1997. *The Queen of America Goes to Washington City: Essays on Sex and Citizenship.* Durham, N.C.: Duke University Press.

Bhabha, Homi. 1994. *The Location of Culture.* London: Routledge.

Bielawski, Ellen. 1996. "Inuit Indigenous Knowledge and Science in the Arctic." In *Naked Science: Anthropological Inquiry into Boundaries, Power, and Knowledge,* ed. Laura Nader, 216–227. New York: Routledge.

Bloch, Maurice. 1968. "Astrology and Writing in Madagascar." In *Literacy in Traditional Societies,* ed. Jack Goody. Cambridge: Cambridge University Press.

Bourdieu, Pierre. 1977. *Outline of a Theory of Practice.* Cambridge: Cambridge University Press.

Bolam, A., et al. 1999. "Factors Affecting Home Delivery in Kathmandu Valley, Nepal." *Health Policy and Planning* 13(2): 152–158.

Brautigam, Deborah. 2003. "Close Encounters: Chinese Business Networks as Industrial Catalysts in Sub-Saharan Africa." *African Affairs* 102: 447–467.

Browner, C. H., and Nancy A. Press. 1996. "The Production of Authoritative Knowledge in American Prenatal Care." *Medical Anthropology Quarterly* 10: 141–156.

Burke, Timothy. 1996. *Lifebuoy Men, Lux Women: Commodification, Consumption, and Cleanliness in Modern Zimbabwe.* Durham, N.C.: Duke University Press.

Butler, Judith. 1993. *Bodies That Matter: On the Discursive Limits of "Sex."* New York: Routledge.

Callon, Michel. 1986/1999. "Some Elements of a Sociology of Translation: Domestication of the Scallops and the Fisherman of St. Brieuc Bay." In *The Science Studies Reader,* ed. M. Biagioli, 67–83. New York: Routledge.

Castaneda, Claudia. 2002. *Figurations: Child, Bodies, World.* Durham, N.C.: Duke University Press.

Chachage, Chachage S. L., and Marjorie Mbilinyi, eds. 2003. *Against Neoliberalism: Gender, Democracy, and Development.* Dar es Salaam: E & D Limited.

Chakrabarty, Dipesh. 2000. *Provincializing Europe.* Princeton, N.J.: University of Princeton Press.

Chanock, Martin. 1998. *Law, Custom, and Social Order: The Colonial Experience in Malawi and Zambia.* London: Heinemann.

Chavunduka, G. L. 1978. *Traditional Healers and the Shona Patient.* Gwelo: Mambo Press.

Cho, Byong-Hee. 2000a. "The Politics of Herbal Drugs in Korea." *Social Science and Medicine* 51: 505–509.

———. 2000b. "Traditional Medicine, Professional Monopoly, and Structural Interests: A Korean Case." *Social Science and Medicine* 50: 123–135.

Choy, Timothy. Forthcoming. *Ecologies of Comparison.* Durham, N.C.: Duke University Press.

Ciekawy, Diane. 1998. "Witchcraft in Statecraft: Five Technologies of Power in Colonial and Postcolonial Kenya." *African Studies Review* 41(3): 119–141.

Cocks, Michelle, and Anthony Dold. 2000. "The Role of 'African Chemists' in the Health Care System of the Eastern Cape Province of South Africa." *Social Science and Medicine* 51: 1505–1515.

Cohen, Lawrence. 1998. *No Aging in India: Alzheimer's, the Bad Family, and Other Modern Things.* Berkeley: University of California.

Colson, Elizabeth. 2000. "The Father as Witch." *Africa* 70(3): 333–358.

Comaroff, Jean. 1985. *Body of Power, Spirit of Resistance: The Culture and History of a South African People.* Chicago: University of Chicago Press.

———. 1993. "The Diseased Heart of Africa: Medicine, Colonialism, and the Black Body." In *Knowledge, Power, and Practice: The Anthropology of Medicine and Everyday Life*, ed. Shirley Lindenbaum and Margaret M. Locke, 305–329. Berkeley: University of California Press.

———, and John Comaroff. 1997. *Of Revelation and Revolution: The Dialectics of Modernity on a South African Frontier*. Vol. 2. Chicago: University of Chicago Press.

Comaroff, John, and Jean Comaroff, eds. 1993. *Modernity and Its Malcontents: Ritual and Power in Postcolonial Africa*. Chicago: University of Chicago Press.

Crawford, Robert. 1984. "A Cultural Account of 'Health': Control, Release, and the Social Body." In *Issues in the Political Economy of Health Care*, ed. John B. McKinlay, 60–103. New York: Tavistock.

Croizier, Ralph. 1968. *Traditional Medicine in Modern China: Science, Nationalism, and the Tensions of Cultural Change*. Cambridge, Mass.: Harvard University Press.

Curtin, P. 1992. "Medical Knowledge and Urban Planning in Colonial Tropical Africa." In *The Social Basis of Health and Healing in Africa*, ed. Steven Feierman and John M. Janzen, 235–255. Berkeley: University of California Press.

Cussins, Charis M. 1998. "Ontological Choreography: Agency for Women Patients in an Infertility Clinic." In *Difference in Medicine: Unraveling Practices, Techniques, and Bodies*, ed. Marc Berg and Annemarie Mol, 166–201. Durham, N.C.: Duke University Press.

Daston, Lorraine, ed. 2000. *Biographies of Scientific Objects*. Chicago: University of Chicago Press.

De Laet, Marianne, ed. 2002. "Introduction: Knowledge and Technology Transfer or the Travel of Thoughts and Things." In *Research in Science and Technology Studies: Knowledge and Technology Transfer*, vol. 13, ed. Marianne de Laet. Amsterdam: JAI/Elsevier Science.

Dehne, K. L., et al. 1995. "Training Birth Attendants in the Sahel." *World Health Forum* 16: 415–419.

Devisch, Rene. 1993. *Weaving the Threads of Life*. Chicago: University of Chicago.

Downey, Gary Lee, and Joseph Dumit, eds. 1998. *Cyborgs & Citadels: Anthropological Interventions in Emerging Sciences and Technologies*. Santa Fe, Calif.: School of American Research Press.

Dumit, Joseph. 2003. *Picturing Personhood: Brain Scans and Biomedical Identity*. Princeton, N.J.: Princeton University Press.

———, and Kaushik Sunder Rajan. 2007. "Biocapital, Surplus Health and Clinical Trials: Toward a Health Theory of Value." Paper presented at the conference Experimental Systems, States, and Speculations: Anthropology at the Intersection of Life, Science and Capital, University of California, Irvine, April 13–14.

Du Toit, Brian, and I. Abdallah, eds. 1985. *African Healing Systems*. New York: Trado-Medic Books.

Eisenman, Joshua, Eric Heginbotham, and Derek Mitchell, eds. 2007. *China and the Developing World: Beijing's Strategy for the Twenty-First Century*. New York: M. E. Sharpe.

Englund, Harri. 1996. "Witchcraft, Modernity, and the Person: The Morality of Accumulation in Central Malawi." *Critique of Anthropology* 16(3): 257–279.

Erdtsieck, Jessica. 1997. *Pepo as an Inner Healing Force: Practices of a Female Spiritual Healer in Tanzania.* Amsterdam: Royal Tropical Institute.

Evans-Pritchard, E. E. 1937/1976. *Witchcraft, Oracles, and Magic among the Azande.* Abridged with an introduction by Eva Gillies. Oxford: Clarendon Press.

Fabricius, Andreas. 1999. *Capacity Assessment of the Laboratories in Mtwara Region in Tanzania and the Clinicians' Perception of the Laboratory Services.* Report to the Regional Medical Doctor and the District Health Improvement Programme. Edinburgh: Queen Margaret University College.

Farquhar, Judith. 1994a. *Knowing Practice: The Clinical Encounter in Chinese Medicine.* Boulder, Colo.: Westview.

——. 1994b. "Multiplicity, Point of View, and Responsibility in Traditional Chinese Healing." In *Body, Subject, and Power in China,* ed. A. Zito and T. E. Barlow, 78–99. Chicago: University of Chicago Press.

——. 2002. *Appetites: Food and Sex in Post-Socialist China.* Durham, N.C.: Duke University Press.

Feierman, Steven. 1974. *The Shambaa Kingdom.* Madison: University of Wisconsin Press.

—— 1981. "Therapy as a System-in-Action in Northern Tanzania." *Social Science and Medicine* 15(3): 353–360.

——. 1985. "Struggles for Control: The Social Roots of Health and Healing in Modern Africa." *African Studies Review* 28(2/3): 73–147.

——. 1986. "Popular Control over the Institutions of Health: A Historical Study." In *The Professionalisation of African Medicine,* ed. Murray Last and G. L. Chavunduka, 205–220. Manchester: Manchester University Press.

——. 1990. *Peasant Intellectuals: Anthropology and History in Tanzania.* Madison: University of Wisconsin Press.

——. 1999. "Colonizers, Scholars, and the Creation of Invisible Histories." In *Beyond the Cultural Turn: New Directions in the Study of Society and Culture,* ed. V. Bonnell and L. Hunt, 182–216. Berkeley: University of California Press.

——. 2000. "Explanation and Uncertainty in the Medical World of the Ghaambo." *Bulletin of the History of Medicine* 74(2): 317–344.

Feierman, Steven, and John M. Janzen, eds. 1992. *The Social Basis of Health and Healing in Africa.* Berkeley: University of California Press.

Ferguson, James. 1999. *Expectation of Modernity: Myths and Meanings of Urban Life on the Zambian Copperbelt.* Berkeley: University of California Press.

——. 2002. "Of Mimicry and Membership: African and the 'New World Society.'" *Cultural Anthropology* 17(4): 551–569.

Flint, Karen. 2008. *Healing Traditions: African Medicine, Cultural Exchange, and Competition in South Africa, 1820–1948.* Athens: Ohio University Press.

Franklin, Sarah. 1997. *Embodied Progress: A Cultural Account of Assisted Conception.* London: Routledge.

Galison, Peter. 1997. *Image and Logic: A Material Culture of Microphysics.* Chicago: University of Chicago Press.

——. 1999. "Trading Zones: Coordinating Action and Belief." In *The Science Studies Reader,* ed. Mario Biagioli, 137–160. New York: Routledge.

Gaonkar, Dilip Parameshwar, ed. 2001. *Alternative Modernities*. Durham, N.C.: Duke University Press.

Geissler, P. Wenzel, and Ruth Prince. 2009. "Active Compounds and Atoms of Society: Plants, Bodies, Minds and Cultures in the Work of Kenyan Ethnobotanical Knowledge." *Social Studies of Science* 39(4): 599–634.

Geschiere, Peter. 1995/1997. *The Modernity of Witchcraft: Politics and the Occult in Postcolonial Africa*. Charlottesville: University of Virginia Press.

Gessler, M., D. Msuya, M. Nkunya, A. Schar, M. Henrich, and M. Tanner. 1995. "Traditional Healers in Tanzania: Sociocultural Profile and Three Short Portraits." *Journal of Ethnopharmacology* 48: 145–160.

Giles, Linda L. 1987. "Possession Cults on the Swahili Coast: A Re-examination of the Theories of Marginality." *Africa* 57(2): 234–258.

———. 1999. "Spirit Possession and the Symbolic Construction of Swahili Society." In *Spirit Possession, Modernity, and Power in Africa*, ed. Heike Behrend and Ute Luig, 142–164. Oxford: James Currey.

Good, Byron. 1994. *Medicine, Rationality, and Experience: An Anthropological Perspective*. Cambridge: Cambridge University Press.

Good, Charles M. 1987. *Ethnomedical Systems in Africa: Patterns of Traditional Medicine in Rural and Urban Kenya*. New York: Guilford.

Gordon, David. 1984. "Foreign Relations Dilemmas of Independence and Development." In *Politics and Public Policy in Kenya and Tanzania*, ed. Joel D. Barkan, 297–335. Rev. ed. New York: Praeger.

Goscinny, Yves, ed. 2001. *Tribute to George Lilanga*. Dar es Salaam: East African Movies Ltd.

Gottlieb, Alma. 2004. *The Afterlife Is Where We Come From*. Chicago: University of Chicago Press.

Gould, Stephen Jay. 1993. "American Polygeny and Craniometry before Darwin: Blacks and Indians as Separate, Inferior Species." In *The "Racial" Economy of Science: Toward a Democratic Future*, ed. Sandra Harding, 84–115. Bloomington: Indiana University Press.

Green, Edward C. 1989. "Mystical Black Power: The Calling to Diviner-Mediumship in Southern Africa." In *Women as Healers in Cross-Cultural Perspectives*, ed. Carol Shepherd McClain, 186–203. New Brunswick, N.J.: Rutgers University Press.

Green, Maia. 1996. "Medicines and the Embodiment of Substances among Pogoro Catholics, Southern Tanzania." *The Journal of Royal Anthropological Institute* 2(3): 485–498.

———. 2000. "Public Reform and the Privatisation of Poverty: Some Institutional Determinants of Health Seeking Behavior in Southern Tanzania." *Culture, Medicine and Psychiatry* 24: 403–430.

———. 2003. "The Birth of the 'Salon': Poverty, 'Modernization' and Dealing with Witchcraft in Southern Tanzania." Paper presented at the annual meeting of the American Anthropological Association, Chicago, Illinois.

———, and Simeon Mesaki. 2005. "The Birth of the 'Salon': Poverty, 'Modernization' and Dealing with Witchcraft in Southern Tanzania." *American Ethnologist* 32(3): 371–388.

Hailey, W. M. 1938. *An African Survey: A Study of Problems Arising in Africa South of the Sahara*. London: Oxford University Press.

Hall, Stuart. 1996. "When Was the Postcolonial? Thinking at the Limit." In *The Postcolonial Question: Common Skies, Divided Horizons,* ed. Iain Chambers and Lidia Curti, 242–260. London: Routledge.

Hamza, M. H., and M. M. Segall. 1973. *Care of the Newborn Baby in Tanzania.* Dar es Salaam: Tanzania Publishing House.

Haraway, Donna. 1988. "Situated Knowledges: The Science Question in Feminism and the Privilege of Partial Perspective," *Feminist Studies* 14(3): 575–599.

———. 1989. *Primate Visions: Gender, Race, and Nature in the World of Modern Science.* New York: Routledge.

———. 1991. *Simians, Cyborgs, and Women: The Reinvention of Nature.* London: Free Association.

———. 1993. "The Biopolitics of Postmodern Bodies: Determinations of the Self in Immune System Discourse." In *Knowledge, Power, & Practice: The Anthropology of Everyday Life,* ed. Shirley Lindenbaum and Margaret M. Lock, 364–410. Berkeley: University of California.

———. 1997. *Modest_Witness@Second_Millennium.FemaleMan©_Meets_Oncomouse^{TM}: Feminism and Technoscience.* New York: Routledge.

Harding, Sandra. 1994. "Is Science Multicultural?" with three commentaries by Judith Farquhar, Shigehisa Kuriyama, and Lawrence Cohen as well as Sandra Harding's response. *Configurations* 2(2): 301–330.

———. 2006. *Science and Social Inequality: Feminist and Postcolonial Issues.* Urbana: University of Illinois Press.

Harries, Lyndon. 1944. "The Initiation Rites of the Makonde Tribe." *Rhodes-Livingstone Institute Communications,* no. 3.

Harvey, David. 2005. *A Brief History of Neoliberalism.* Oxford: Oxford University Press.

Hayden, Cori. 2003. *When Nature Goes Public: The Making and the Unmaking of Bioprospecting in Mexico.* Princeton, N.J.: Princeton University Press.

Hecht, Gabrielle. 2006. "Uranium and Its Travels: African Geographies in the Making, Marketing, and Flow of 'Nuclear' Materials." Paper presented at the annual meeting of the Society for the Social Studies of Science, Vancouver, November 1–5.

Hedberg, I., O. Hedberg, P. J. Madati, K. E. Mshigeni, E. N. Mshiu, and G. Samuelsson. 1983. "Inventory of Plants Used in Traditional medicine in Tanzania. II. Plants of the Families Dilleniaceae—Opiliaceae." *Journal of Ethnopharmacology* 9(2–3): 237–260.

Hess, David. 1994. "Parallel Universes: Anthropology in the World of Technoscience." *Anthropology Today* 10(2): 16–18.

———. 2004. "Organic Food and Agriculture in the US: Object Conflicts in a Health-Environmental Social Movement." *Science as Culture* 13(4): 493–513.

Hetherwick, A. 1902. "Some Animistic Beliefs among the Yaos of British Central Africa." *Journal of the Anthropological Institute of Great Britain and Ireland* 32: 89–95.

Hsu, Elisabeth. 2002. "'The Medicine from China Has Rapid Effects': Chinese Medicine Patients in Tanzania." *Anthropology & Medicine* 9(3): 291–313.

Hunt, Nancy Rose. 1999. *A Colonial Lexicon of Birth Ritual, Medicalization, and Mobility in the Congo.* Durham, N.C.: Duke University Press.

Ibhawoh, Bonny, and J. I. Dibua. 2003. "Deconstructing Ujamaa: The Legacy of Julius Nyerere in the Quest for Social and Economic Development in Africa." *African Journal of Political Science* 8(1): 59–83.

Ihde, Don. 2003. "If Phenomenology Is an Albatross, Is *Post-Phenomenology* Possible?" In *Chasing Technoscience: Matrix for Materiality,* ed. Don Idhe and Evan Selinger, 131–145. Bloomington: Indiana University Press.

———, and Evan Selinger, eds. 2003. *Chasing Technoscience: Matrix for Materiality.* Bloomington: Indiana University Press.

Ikingura, J. K., M. Kruger, and W. Zeleke. 2007. "Health Research Ethics Review and Needs of Institutional Ethics Committees in Tanzania." *Tanzania Health Research Bulletin* 9(3): 154–158.

Iliffe, John. 1969. *Tanganyika under German Rule, 1905–1912.* Cambridge: Cambridge University Press.

———. 1979. *A Modern History of Tanganyika.* Cambridge: Cambridge University Press.

———. 1998. *East African Doctors: A History of the Modern Profession.* Cambridge: Cambridge University Press.

Ingham, Kenneth. 1962. *The History of East Africa.* London: Longmans.

Ivy, Marilyn. 1995. *Discourses of the Vanishing: Modernity, Phantasm, Japan.* Chicago: University of Chicago Press.

Janes, Craig. 1999. "The Health Transition, Global Modernity, and the Crisis of Traditional Medicine: The Tibetan Case." *Social Science and Medicine* 48: 1803–1820.

Janzen, John M. 1978. *The Quest for Therapy: Medical Pluralism in Lower Zaire.* Berkeley: University of California Press.

———. 1982. *Lemba, 1650–1930: A Drum of Affliction in Africa and the New World.* New York: Garland.

———. 1992. *Ngoma: Discourses of Healing in Central and Southern Africa.* Berkeley: University of California Press.

Johnson, Frederick. 1939/1999. *A Standard Swahili-English Dictionary.* London: Oxford University Press.

Jones, D. 2000. "Visions of a Cure: Visualization, Clinical Trials, and Controversies in Cardiac Therapeutics, 1968–1998." *Isis* 91: 504–541.

Kasembe, J. N. R. 1968. *Report on the Symposium of African Medicinal Plants.* Dar es Salaam: Tanzanian Ministry of Agriculture and Cooperative Development.

Kaufert, Patricia. 1998. "Women, Resistance, and the Breast Cancer Movement." In *Pragmatic Women and Body Politics,* ed. Margaret Lock and Patricia Kaufert. Cambridge: Cambridge University Press.

Kayombo, Edmund J. 1999. "Traditional Healers and Treatment of HIV/AIDS Patients in Tanzania: A Case of Njombe Rural District, Iringa Region." Ph.D. thesis, University of Wien, Austria.

Kilewo, J., I. Semali, I. Msuya, E. Mshiu, D. DoAmsi, C. Makwaya, and E. Muhondwa. 1987. "The Patterns of Illness and the Utilization of Available Health Services in Two Regions of Tanzania." *Tanzanian Medical Journal* 4(1): 25–30.

Kingsley, David. 1996. *Health, Healing, and Religion: A Cross-Cultural Perspective.* Upper Saddle River, N.J.: Prentice Hall.

Kitua, Andrew, Yohana Mashalla, and Joseph Shija. 2000. "Coordinating Health Research to Promote Action: The Tanzanian Experience." *British Medical Journal* 321: 821–823.

Kitua, A. Y., T. Smith, P. L. Alonso, H. Masanja, H. Urassa, C. Menendez, J. Kimario, and M. Tanner. 1996. "*Plasmodium falciparum* Malaria in the First Year of Life in an Area of Intense and Perennial Transmission." *Tropical Medicine and International Health* 1(4): 475–484.

———, T. A. Smith, P. L. Alonso, H. Urassa, H. Masanja, J. Kimario, and M. Tanner. 1997. "The Role of Low Level *Plasmodium falciparum* Parasitaemia in Anaemia among Infants Living in an Area of Intense and Perennial Transmission." *Tropical Medicine and International Health* 2(4): 325–333.

Klaits, Frederick. 2002. "Housing the Spirit, Hearing the Voice: Care, Kinship, and Faith in Botswana during the Time of AIDS." Ph.D. diss., Johns Hopkins University.

Kluckhohn, Clyde. 1944(1982). "Navajo Witchcraft." In *Witchcraft and Sorcery,* ed. Max Marwick, 246–262. Harmondsworth: Penguin Books.

Knauft, Bruce M. 2002. *Critically Modern: Alternatives, Alterities, Anthropologies.* Bloomington: Indiana University Press.

Koch, Ellen. 1993. "In the Image of Science? Negotiating the Development of Diagnostic Ultrasound in the Cultures of Surgery and Radiology." *Technology and Culture* 34: 858–893.

Krige, J. D. 1947/1982. "The Social Function of Witchcraft." In *Witchcraft and Sorcery.* Harmondsworth, ed. Max Marwick, 263–275. Harmondsworth: Penguin Books.

Lambert, Sylvie, and David Sahn. 2002. "Incidence of Public Spending in the Health and Education Sectors in Tanzania." In *Education and Health Expenditure and Poverty Reducation in East Africa: Madagascar and Tanzania*, ed. Christian Morrisson. Paris: Development Centre of the Organisation for Economic Co-operation and Development.

Langford, Jean. 2002. *Fluent Bodies: Ayurvedic Remedies for Postcolonial Imbalance.* Durham, N.C.: Duke University Press.

Langwick, Stacey. 2001. "Devils and Development." Ph.D. diss., University of North Carolina–Chapel Hill.

———. 2006. "Geographies of Medicine: Interrogating the Boundary between 'Traditional' and 'Modern' Medicine in Colonial Tanganyika." In *Borders and Healers: Brokering Therapeutic Resources in Southeast Africa,* ed. Tracy J. Luedke and Harry G. West, 143–165. Bloomington: Indiana University Press.

———. 2007. "Devils, Parasites and Fierce Needles: Healing and the Politics of Translation in Southeastern Tanzania." *Science, Technology and Human Values* 32(1): 88–117.

———. 2008a. "Articulate(d) Bodies: Traditional Medicine in a Tanzanian Hospital." *American Ethnologist* 35(3): 428–439.

———. 2008b. "New Publics of Traditional Medicine in Tanzania." Paper presented at the conference Regimes of Care, Relations of Care: Exploring the Changing Order of Public Health in Africa, Cambridge University, UK, June 7.

———. 2010. "From Non-Aligned Medicines to Market-Based Herbals: China's Relationship to the Shifting Politics of Traditional Medicine in Tanzania." *Medical Anthropology* 29(1): 1–29.

———. Forthcoming a. "The Choreography of Global Subjection: The Traditional Birth Attendant in Contemporary Configurations of World Health." In *Medicine, Mobility, and Power in Global Africa: Transnational Health and Healing*, eds. Hansjörg Dilger, Abdoulaye Kane, and Stacey Langwick. Bloomington: Indiana University Press.

———. Forthcoming b. "Healers and Scientists: The Epistemological Politics of Research about Medicinal Plants in Tanzania, *or* 'Moving Away from Traditional Medicine.'" In *Evidence, Ethics and Ethnography: Medical Research in Africa*, ed. Wenzel Geissler. New York & Oxford: Berghahn Books.

Larkin, Brian. 1997. "Indian Films and Nigerian Lovers: Media and the Creation of Parallel Modernities." *Africa* 67 (3): 406–440.

Larson, L. E. 1976. "A History of the Mhenge (Ulanga) District, c. 1860–1957." Ph.D. thesis, University of Dar es Salaam.

Last, Murray. 1992. "The Importance of Knowing about Not Knowing: Observations from Hausaland." In *The Social Basis of Health and Healing in Africa*, ed. Steven Feireman and John M. Janzen, 393–406. Berkeley: University of California Press.

———, and G. L. Chavunduka. 1986. *The Professionalisation of African Medicine*. Manchester: Manchester University Press in association with the International African Institute.

Latour, Bruno. 1987. *Science in Action*. Cambridge, Mass.: Harvard University Press.

———. 1988. *The Pasteurization of France*. Trans. Alan Sheridan and John Law. Cambridge, Mass.: Harvard University Press.

———. 1993. *We Have Never Been Modern*. Cambridge, Mass.: Harvard University.

———. 1999. *Pandora's Hope: Essays on the Reality of Science Studies*. Cambridge, Mass.: Harvard University Press.

———. 2004. "How to Talk About the Body? The Normative Dimension of Science Studies." *Body and Society* 10(2–3): 205–229.

———, and Steve Woolgar. 1979. *Laboratory Life: The Construction of Scientific Facts*. Princeton, N.J.: Princeton University Press.

Law, John. 1999. "After ANT: Complexity, Naming, and Topology." In *Actor Network Theory and After*, ed. John Law and John Hassard. Oxford: Blackwell.

———. 2004. *After Method: Mess in Social Science Research*. London and New York: Routledge.

Law, John, and Annemarie Mol, eds. 2002. *Complexities: Social Studies of Knowledge Practices*. Durham, N.C.: Duke University Press.

———, and John Urry. 2002. "Enacting the Social." Available at http://www.lancs.ac.uk /fass/sociology/papers/law-urry-enacting-the-social.pdf.

Laws of Tanzania. 2002. Rev. ed. 21 vols. Cape Town: Juta.

Liebenow, J. Gus. 1971. *Colonial Rule and Political Development in Tanzania: The Case of the Makonde*. Evanston, Ill.: Northwestern University Press.

Livingston, Julie. 2005. *Debility and the Moral Imagination in Botswana*. Bloomington: Indiana University Press.

Lock, Margaret. 1993a. "Cultivating the Body: Anthropology and Epistemologies of Bodily Practice and Knowledge." *Annual Review of Anthropology* 22: 133–155.

———. 1993b. *Encounters with Aging: Mythologies of Menopause in Japan and North America*. Berkeley: University of California Press.

———. 1993c. "The Politics of Mid-Life and Menopause: Ideologies for the Second Sex in North America and Japan." In *Knowledge, Power, & Practice: The Anthropology of Medicine in Everyday Life*, ed. Shirley Lindenbaum and Margaret Lock, 330–363. Berkeley: University of California Press.

———. 1998. "Perfecting Society: Reproductive Technologies, Genetic Testing, and the Planned Family in Japan." In *Pragmatic Women and Body Politics*, ed. Margaret Lock and Patricia Kaufert. Cambridge: Cambridge University Press.

———. 2002. *Twice Dead: Organ Transplants and the Reinvention of Death*. Berkeley: University of California Press.

Lock, Margaret, Allan Young, and Alberto Cambrosio, eds. 2000. *Living and Working with the New Medical Technologies: Intersections of Inquiry*. Cambridge: Cambridge University Press.

Madoffe, Seif, A. Dino, and F. Mombo. 2008. "A Potentially Valuable Medicinal Plant for Sustainable Income Generation in Tanzania." Paper presented at the 13th Research on Poverty Alleviation (REPOA) Research Workshop, Dar es Salaam, April 2–3.

Mahunnah, R. L. A., and K. E. Mshigeni. 1996. "Tanzania's Policy on Biodiversity Prospecting and Drug Discovery Programs." *Journal of Ethnopharmacology* 51: 221–228.

Makemba, A. M., et al. 1996. "Treatment Practices for *Degedege*, a Local Recognized Febrile Illness, and Implications for Strategies to Decrease Mortality from Severe Malaria in Bagamoyo District, Tanzania." *Tropical Medicine and International Health* 1: 305–313.

Malinowski, Bronislaw. 1925/1982. "Sorcery and Mimetic Representation." In *Witchcraft and Sorcery*, ed. Max Marwick, 240–245. Harmondsworth: Penguin Books.

Martin, Emily. 1990. "Toward an Anthropology of Immunology: The Body as Nation State." *Medical Anthropology Quarterly* 4, no. 4: 410–426.

———. 1994. *Flexible Bodies: Tracking Immunity in American Culture from the Days of Polio to the Age of AIDS*. Boston: Beacon Press.

Marwick, Max, ed. 1970/1982. *Witchcraft and Sorcery*. Harmondsworth: Penguin Books.

Masquelier, Adeline. 1993. "Narratives of Power, Images of Wealth: The Ritual Economy of Bori in the Market." In *Modernity and its Malcontents: Ritual and Power in Postcolonial Africa*, ed. John Comaroff and Jean Comaroff, 3–33. Chicago: University of Chicago Press.

Matthew, M. K., et al. 1995. "Training Traditional Birth Attendants in Nigeria—a Pictorial Method." *World Health Forum* 16: 409–414.

Mauss, Marcel. 1933/1973. "Techniques of the Body." Economy and Society 2: 70–88.

McMillen, H. Heather. 2004. "The Adapting Healer: Pioneering through Shifting Epidemiological and Sociocultural Landscapes." *Social Science & Medicine* 59(5): 889–902.

McNeil, Maureen. 2005. "Introduction: Postcolonial Technoscience." *Science as Culture* 14(2): 105–112.

Meena, Ruth. 2008. *Social Policy Regime, Care Policies and Programmes in the Context of HIV/AIDS, Tanzania*. Political and Social Economy of Care, Tanzania Research Report 3. Geneva: United Nations Research Institute for Social Development.

Mesaki, Simeon. 1993. "Witchcraft and Witch-Killings in Tanzania: Paradox and Dilemma." Ph.D. diss., University of Minnesota.

Meyer, Birgit. 1992. "'If You Are a Devil, You Are a Witch and, If You Are a Witch, You Are a Devil': The Integration of 'Pagan' Ideas into the Conceptual Universe of Ewe Christians in Southeastern Ghana." *Journal of Religion in Africa* 22(2): 98–132.

Mhame, Paulo P. 2000. "The Role of Traditional Knowledge (TK) in the National Economy: The Importance and Scope of TK, Particularly Traditional Medicine in Tanzania." Paper prepared for UNCTAD Expert Meeting on Systems and National Experiences for Protecting Traditional Knowledge, Innovations and Practices, Geneva. Available at http://www.unctad.org/trade_env/docs/tanzania.pdf.

Middleton, J., and E. H. Winter, eds. 1963. *Witchcraft and Sorcery in East Africa.* New York: Frederick A. Praeger.

Mitchell, Timothy. 1988. *Colonizing Egypt.* New York: Cambridge University Press.

Mol, Annemarie. 2002. *The Body Multiple: Ontology in Medical Practice.* Durham, N.C.: Duke University Press.

———, and John Law. 1994. "Regions, Networks and Fluids: Anemia and Social Topology." *Social Studies of Science* 24: 641–671.

———, and Jessica Mesman. 1996. "Neonatal Food and the Politics of Theory: Some Questions of Method." *Social Studies of Science* 26(2): 419–444.

Monson, Jamie. 1998. "Relocating Maji Maji: The Politics of Alliance and Authority in the Southern Highlands of Tanzania, 1870–1918." *Journal of African History* 39: 95–120.

Nader, Laura. 1996. "Introduction: Anthropological Inquiry into Boundaries, Power, and Knowledge." In *Naked Science: Anthropological Inquiry into Boundaries, Power, and Knowledge,* ed. Laura Nader, 1–25. New York: Routledge.

Napier, A. David. 2003. *Age of Immunology: Conceiving a Future in an Alienating World.* Chicago: University of Chicago.

Needham, Rodney. 1972. *Belief, Language, and Experience.* Chicago: University of Chicago Press.

Nelson, Kenrad, Carolyn Masters Williams, and Neil M. H. Graham. 2001. *Infectious Disease Epidemiology: Theory and Practice.* Gaithersburg, Md.: Aspen Publishers.

Ngubane, Harriet. 1981/1992. "Clinical Practice and Organization of Indigenous Healers in South Africa." In *The Social Basis of Health and Healing in Africa,* ed. Steven Feierman and John Janzen, 366–375. Berkeley: University of California Press.

Oberlander, Lars, and Beth Elverdan. 2000. "Malaria in the United Republic of Tanzania: Cultural Considerations and Health-Seeking Behavior." *Bulletin of the World Health Organization* 78: 1352–1357.

Ong, Aihwa. 2005. "Ecologies of Expertise: Governmentality in Asian Knowledge Societies." In *Global Assemblages: Technology, Politics and Ethics as Anthropological Problems,* ed. Aihwa Ong and Stephen Collier. Malden, Mass.: Wiley-Blackwell.

———. 2007. *Neoliberalism as Exception: Mutations in Citizenship and Sovereignty.* Durham, N.C.: Duke University Press.

Packard, Randall. 1989. "Industrial Production, Health and Disease in Sub-Saharan Africa." *Social Science and Medicine* 28(5): 475–496.

Pickering, Andrew. 1995. *The Mangle of Practice: Time, Agency, and Science.* Chicago: University of Chicago Press.

Pigg, Stacy Leigh. 1995. "Acronyms and Effacement: Traditional Medical Practitioners (TMP) in International Health Development." *Social Science and Medicine* 41(1): 47–68.

———. 1996. "The Credible and the Credulous: The Questions of 'Villagers' Beliefs' in Nepal." *Cultural Anthropology* 11(2): 160–201.

———. 1997a. "'Found in Most Traditional Societies': Traditional Medical Practitioners between Culture and Development." In *International Development and the Social Sciences,* ed. Fredrick Cooper and Randall Packard, 259–290. Berkeley: University of California Press.

———. 1997b. "Authority in Translation: Finding Knowing, Naming and Training 'Traditional Birth Attendants' in Nepal." In *Childbirth and Authoritative Knowledge: Cross-Cultural Perspectives,* ed. Robbie Davis-Floyd and Carolyn Sargent, 233–262. Berkeley: University of California Press.

———. 2001. "Languages of Sex and AIDS in Nepal: Notes on the Social Production of Commensurability." *Cultural Anthropology* 16(4): 481–541.

Prakash, Gyan. 1999. *Another Reason: Science and the Imagination of Modern India.* Princeton, N.J.: Princeton University Press.

Prentice, Rachel. Forthcoming. *Bodies In Formation: An Ethnography of Anatomy and Surgical Training.* Durham: Duke University Press.

Rabinow, Paul. 1992. "Studies in the Anthropology of Reason." *Anthropology Today* 8(5): 7–10.

———. 1996. "Artificiality and Enlightenment: From Sociobiology to Biosociality." In Rabinow, *Essays on the Anthropology of Reason.* Princeton: Princeton University Press.

Raikes, A. 1989. "Women's Health in East Africa." *Social Science and Medicine* 28(5): 447–459.

Rajani, Rakesh, and Gitte Robinson. 1999. *The State of Education in Tanzania: Crisis and Opportunity.* Mwanza: Kuleana Centre for Children's Rights.

———. 1992. "Godly Medicine: The Ambiguities of Medical Mission in Southeastern Tanzanian, 1900–1945." In *The Social Basis of Health and Healing in Africa,* ed. Steven Feierman and John M. Janzen, 256–284. Berkeley: University of California Press.

Rasmussen, N. 1997. *Picture Control: The Electron Microscope and the Transformation of Biology in America, 1940–1960.* Stanford, Calif.: Stanford University Press.

Redfield, Peter. 2002. "The Half-Life of Empire in Outer Space." *Social Studies of Science* 32(5–6): 791–825.

Reid, Marlene B. 1982. "Patient/Healer Interactions in Sukuma Medicine." In *African Health and Healing Systems: Proceedings of a Symposium,* ed. P. S. Yoder, 121–158. Los Angeles: Crossroads Press.

Rekdal, Ole Bjorn. 1999. "Cross-Cultural Healing in East African Ethnography." *Medical Anthropology Quarterly* 13(4): 458–482.

Reynolds, Pamela. 1996. *Traditional Healers and Childhood in Zimbabwe.* Athens: Ohio University Press.

Rheinberger, Hans-Jorg. 1997. *Toward a History of Epistemic Things: Synthesizing Proteins in the Test Tube.* Stanford, Calif.: Stanford University Press.

———. 2000. "Cytoplasmic Particles: The Trajectory of a Scientific Object." In *Biographies of Scientific Objects,* ed. Lorraine Daston, 270–294. Chicago: University of Chicago Press.

Roitt, Ivan. 1997. *Roitt's Essential Immunology*. Berlin: Blackwell Science.

Richey, Lisa Ann. 2003. "Women's Reproductive Health and Population Policy: Tanzania." *Review of African Political Economy* 96: 273–292.

Rofel, Lisa. 1999. *Other Modernities: Gendered Yearnings in China after Socialism*. Berkeley: University of California Press.

Rosario, S. 1995. "Traditional Birth Attendants in Bangladeshi Villages: Cultural and Sociological Factors." *International Journal of Gynecology & Obstetrics* 50 (Supplement 2): S145–S152.

Rowlands, Michael, and J. P. Warnier. 1988. "Sorcery, Power and the Modern State in Cameroon." *Man* 23: 118–132.

Safe Motherhood Task Force. 1992. "Safe Motherhood Strategy for Tanzania." Prepared by Safe Motherhood Task Force with the assistance of Family Care International (March). Dar es Salaam: Safe Motherhood Task Force.

Sanders, Todd. 2001. "Save Our Skins: Structural Adjustment, Morality, and the Occult in Tanzania." In *Magical Interpretations, Material Realities: Modernity, Witchcraft and the Occult in Postcolonial Africa*, ed. Henrietta L. Moore and Todd Sanders, 160–183. London: Routledge.

———. 2003. "Reconsidering Witchcraft: Postcolonial Africa and Analytic (Un)Certainties." *American Anthropologist* 105(2): 338–352.

Scheid, Volker. 2002. *Chinese Medicine in Contemporary China: Plurality and Synthesis*. Durham, N.C.: Duke University Press.

Scott, James. 1998. *Seeing Like a State: How Certain Schemes to Improve the Human Condition Have Failed*. New Haven, Conn.: Yale University Press.

Selinger, Evan. 2003. "Introduction, Part II." In *Chasing Technoscience: Matrix for Materiality*, ed. Don Ihde and Evan Selinger, 11–14. Bloomington: Indiana University Press.

Semali, I. A. J. 1982. "The Opinions of Allopathic Health Workers on Traditional Medicine/ Healers and Degree of Contact between the Two in Tanzania." Diploma in Public Health diss., University of Dar es Salaam.

Shapin, Steven, and Simon Schaffer. 1985. *Leviathan and the Air-Pump: Hobbes, Boyle, and the Experimental Life*. Princeton, N.J.: Princeton University Press.

Shivji, Issa. 2008. "Accumulation in an African Periphery: A Theoretical Framework." Paper presented at the thirteenth Research on Poverty Alleviation (REPOA) Research Workshop, Dar es Salaam. April 2–3, 2008.

Sindiga, Isaac. 1995. "Traditional Medicine in Africa: An Introduction." In *Traditional Medicine in Africa*, ed. Isaac Sindiga, Chacha Nyaigotti-Chacha, and Mary Peter Kanunah, 1–15. Nairobi, Kenya: East African Educational Publishers Ltd.

Sindzingre, N., and A. Zempleni. 1992. "Causality of Disease among the Senufo." In *The Social Basis of Health and Healing in Africa*, ed. Steven Feierman and John Janzen, trans. John Janzen. Berkeley: University of California Press.

Smith, Barbara Herrnstein. 1997. *Belief and Resistance: Dynamics of Contemporary Intellectual Controversy*. Cambridge, Mass.: Harvard University Press.

Smith, J., et al. 1997. *The Impact of TBA Training on the Health of Mothers and Newborns in Brong-Ahafo, Ghana*. Research Triangle Park, N.C.: Family Health International.

Spivak, Gayatri Chakravorty. 1987. *In Other Worlds: Essays in Cultural Studies*. New York: Methuen.

———. 1990. *The Post-Colonial Critic: Essays, Strategies, Dialogues.* New York: Routledge.

Star, Susan Leigh, and James R. Griesemer. 1989. "Institutional Ecology, 'Translations' and Boundary Objects: Amateurs and Professionals in Berkeley's Museum of Vertebrate Zoology, 1907–39." *Social Studies of Science* 19: 387–420.

Stirling, Leader. 1947. *Bush Doctor: Being Letters from Dr. Stirling, Tanganyika Territory.* Westminster, England: Parrett & Neves, Ltd.

———. 1977. *Tanzanian Doctor.* London: Heinemann.

Stoler, Ann L. 1991. "Carnal Knowledge and Imperial Power: Gender, Race, and Morality in Colonial Asia." In *Gender at the Crossroads of Knowledge: Feminist Anthropology in the Postmodern Era,* ed. Micaela di Leonardo, 51–101. Berkeley: University of California Press.

Stoller, Paul. 1995. *Embodying Colonial Memories: Spirit Possession, Power, and the Hauka in West Africa.* New York and London: Routledge.

Strathern, Marilyn. 1991/2004. *Partial Connections.* Updated edition. Walnut Creek, Calif.: AltaMira Press.

———. 1999a. "The New Modernities." In Strathern, *Property, Substance, Effect: Anthropological Essays on Persons and Things,* 117–135. London: Athlone Press.

———. 1999b. "What Is Intellectual Property After?" In *Actor Network Theory and After,* ed. John Law and John Hassard, 156–180. Oxford: Blackwell.

———. Forthcoming. "Can One Rely on Knowledge?" In *African Trial Communities: Ethnographies and Histories of Medical Research in Africa,* ed. Wenzel Geissler. New York & Oxford: Berghahn Books.

Sturmer, Martin. 1999. *The Media History of Tanzania.* Ndanda, Tanzania: Ndanda Mission Publishing.

Swantz, Lloyd. 1974. "The Role of the Medicine Man among the Zaramo of Dar es Salaam." Ph.D. thesis, University of Dar es Salaam.

Tanganyika Standard. 1946. "We Told Him Why He Had Been Killed: Morogoro Story of Self-Confessed Witch." *Tanganyika Standard,* November 27. Also in File 13401, Witchcraft Ordinance, Vol. II, Tanzanian National Archives.

Tantala, Rene. 1989. "The Early History of Kitara in Western Uganda: Process Models of Religious and Political Change." Ph.D. diss., University of Wisconsin, Madison.

Taylor, Ian. 1998. "China's Foreign Policy towards Africa in the 1990s." *Journal of Modern African Studies* 36(3): 443–460.

Taylor, Kim. 2005. *Chinese Medicine in Early Communist China, 1945–63: A Medicine of Revolution.* London: Routledge Curzon.

Thomas, Lynn M. 2003. *Politics of the Womb: Women, Reproduction, and the State in Kenya.* Berkeley: University of California Press.

Thompson, Charis. 2005. *Making Parents: The Ontological Choreography of Reproductive Technologies.* Cambridge, Mass.: MIT Press.

Tiffany, Daniel. 2000. *Toy Medium: Materialism and Modern Lyric.* Berkeley: University of California Press.

Trimingham, S. J. 1964. *Islam in East Africa.* Oxford: Clarendon Press.

Tsing, Anna Loweenhaupt. 2005. *Friction: An Ethnography of Global Connection.* Princeton, N.J.: Princeton University Press.

Turnbull, David. 2000. *Masons, Tricksters and Cartographers: Comparative Studies in the Sociology of Scientific and Indigenous Knowledge*. Amsterdam: Harwood Academic.

Turner, Victor. 1967. *The Forest of Symbols: Aspects of Ndembu Ritual*. Ithaca, N.Y.: Cornell University Press.

———. 1968. *The Drums of Affliction: A Study of Religious Processes among the Ndembu of Zambia*. Oxford: Clarendon Press.

———. 1975. *Revelation and Divination in Ndembu Ritual*. Ithaca, N.Y.: Cornell University Press.

Turshen, Meredith. 1984. *The Political Ecology of Disease in Tanzania*. New Brunswick, N.J.: Rutgers University Press.

———. 1989. *The Politics of Public Health*. New Brunswick, N.J.: Rutgers University Press.

———, ed. 1991. *Women and Health in Africa*. Trenton, N.J.: Africa World Press.

Vansina, Jan. 1972. *The Tio Kingdom of the Middle Congo, 1880–1892*. London: Oxford University Press.

Vaughan, Megan. 1991. *Curing Their Ills: Colonial Power and African Illness*. Stanford, Calif.: Stanford University Press.

Verran, Helen. 2001. *Science and African Logic*. Chicago: University of Chicago.

———. 2002. "Transferring Strategies of Land Management: Indigenous Land Owners and Environmental Scientists." In *Research in Science and Technology Studies: Knowledge and Society*, ed. Marianne de Laet, 155–181. Oxford: Elsevier & JAI Press.

Vounatsou, P., T. Smith, A. Y. Kitua, P. L. Alonso, and M. Tanner. 2000. "Apparent Tolerance of *Plasmodium falciparum* in Infants in a Highly Endemic Area." *Parasitology* 120: 1–9.

Waite, Gloria. 1992. "Public Health in Pre-Colonial East Central Africa." In *The Social Basis of Health and Healing in Africa*, ed. Steven Feierman and John M. Janzen, 212–234. Berkeley: University of California Press.

Waldram, James B. 2000. "Efficacy of Traditional Medicine: Current Theoretical and Methodological Issues." *Medical Anthropology Quarterly* 14(4): 603–625.

Weiss, Brad. 1992. "Plastic Teeth Extraction: The Iconography of Haya Gastro-Sexual Affliction." *American Ethnologist* 19(3): 538–552.

———. 1997. "Forgetting Your Dead: Alienable and Inalienable Objects in Northwest Tanzania." *Anthropological Quarterly* 70(4): 164–172.

———. 1998. "Electric Vampires: Haya Rumors of the Commodified Body." In *Bodies and Persons: Comparative Perspectives from Africa and Melanesia*, ed. Michael Lambek and Andrew Strathern, 172–194. Cambridge: Cambridge University Press.

Wembah-Rashid, J. A. R. 1975. *The Ethno-History of the Matrilineal Peoples of Southeast Tanzania*. Wien, Austria: E. Stiglmayer.

West, Harry. 2001. "Sorcery of Construction and Socialist Modernization: Ways of Understanding Power in Post-Colonial Mozambique." *American Ethnologist* 28(1): 119–150.

———. 2005. *Kupilikula: Governance and the Invisible Realm in Mozambique*. Chicago: University of Chicago Press.

White, Luise. 2000. *Speaking with Vampires: Rumor and History in Colonial Africa*. Berkeley: University of California Press.

Whyte, Susan Reynolds. 1997. *Questioning Misfortune: The Pragmatics of Uncertainty in Eastern Uganda*. Cambridge: Cambridge University Press.

————. 2005. "Uncertain Undertakings: Practicing Health Care in the Subjunctive Mood." In *Managing Uncertainty: Ethnographic Studies of Illness, Risk and the Struggle for Control,* ed. Vibeke Steffen, Richard Jenkins, and Hanne Jessen, 245–264. Copenhagen: Museum Tusculanum Press.

Wiener, Margaret. 2003. "Hidden Forces: Colonialism and the Politics of Magic in the Netherlands Indies." In *Magic and Modernity: Interfaces of Revelation and Concealment,* ed. Birgit Meyer and Peter Pels. Stanford, Calif.: Stanford University Press.

Williamson, John. 1990. "What Washington Means by Policy Reform." In *Latin American Adjustment: How Much Has Happened?* ed. John Williamson. Washington, D.C.: Institute for International Economics.

Winch, Peter. 1999. "The Role of Anthropological Methods in a Community-Based Mosquito Net Intervention in Bagamoyo District, Tanzania." In *Anthropology in Public and International Health: Bridging Differences in Culture and Society,* ed. Robert A. Hahn, 44–62. Cambridge: Oxford University Press.

World Bank. 1980. *Health Sector Policy Paper.* Washington, D.C.: World Bank.

World Health Organization. 1978a. *Primary Health Care: Report of the International Conference on Primary Health Care, Alma-Ata, U.S.S.R., 6–12 September.* Geneva: World Health Organization.

————. 1978b. *The Promotion and Development of Traditional Medicine: A Report of a WHO Meeting.* Geneva: World Health Organization Technical Report Series 622.

————. 1983. *Traditional Medicine and Health Care Coverage.* Geneva: World Health Organization.

————. 2002. *WHO Traditional Medicine Strategy 2002–2005.* Geneva: World Health Organization. Available at http://whqlibdoc.who.int/hq/2002/WHO_EDM_TRM _2002.1.pdf.

Young, Allan. 1995. *The Harmony of Illusions: Inventing Post-Traumatic Stress Disorder.* Princeton, N.J.: Princeton University Press.

————. 2004. "How Narratives Work in Psychiatric Science: An Example from the Biological Psychiatry of PTSD." In *Narrative Research in Health and Illness,* ed. Brian Hurwitz, Trisha Greenhalgh, and Vieda Skultans. Malden, Mass.: Blackwell BMJ Books.

Yu, George T. 1988. "Africa in Chinese Foreign Policy." *Asian Survey* 28(8): 849–862.

Zhan, Mei. 2001. "Does It Take a Miracle? Negotiating Knowledges, Identities, and Communities of Traditional Chinese Medicine." *Cultural Anthropology* 16(4): 453–480.

Index

accountability, 11–12, 76, 78, 172–73
actants, 21, 204
actors, 6, 21, 25, 35, 67, 78, 99, 119, 145, 172, 175, 181, 191, 198, 204–205, 207, 227, 229, 249n20; biomedical, 122, 124, 129, 135, 137, 143, 168, 210; nonhuman, 5, 20–21, 78, 93–96, 98, 102–11, 113, 116, 118–19, 129, 136, 157–58, 202, 204–205, 214, 236, 250n28, 263n8. *See also majini* (nonhuman spirits); *mashetani* (devils or demons)
acupuncture, 75, 261n56
Adams, Vincanne, 262n1
agency, 21, 106, 118, 126, 153, 264n17
AIDS. *See* HIV/AIDS
amulets, 52, 90, 92, 93, 97, 102, 159, 163–65, 190, 224
ancestors, 3, 4, 5, 7, 8, 17, 23, 24, 41, 95, 108, 109, 110, 119, 157, 159, 163, 207, 237, 238, 263n8, 271n4. *See also mahoka* (ancestral shade)
anthropology, 8, 16, 20, 27, 34, 173, 181, 201, 234–36, 240, 262n3, 269n5; medical, 22, 248n6, 249n21, 251n30
Arabic language, 89–93, 98, 109, 162, 165
Athusser, Louis, 126
Awadhi, Shehe, 91–92, 112, 264n10

Barthes, Roland, 201–203
biomedicine, 2, 6–11, 16–18, 21–22, 24, 31, 34–35, 60–61, 67–68, 71–72, 74–75, 80, 82, 88, 90, 97, 121–23, 125–26, 128–34, 137, 139, 141, 145–47, 151–54, 159, 161, 166, 170, 172–73, 175, 177–81, 188, 191, 200, 202–205, 207–10, 212–13, 219–21, 223–24, 226–27, 230–31, 232–35, 238–39, 249nn17,21, 251n30, 262n3,

263n6, 268n18, 269n5. *See also* actors, biomedical; body, biomedical; diagnoses, biomedical; disease, biomedical; health care, biomedical; hegemony, biomedical; practitioners, biomedical; therapy, biomedical
birth attendants, traditional (TBAs), 16, 32–33, 88–89, 103, 121–47, 233, 260n45, 271n3; National Traditional and Birth Attendants Implementation Policy Guidelines, 74; training of, 24, 121–46, 146, 230, 233, 265n1, 266n10. *See also* midwives
Bloor, David, 34
body: biological, 10, 131, 134, 159; biomedical, 24, 159, 204; boundedness of, 189–91, 203, 224; corporeality, 210, 224–25, 228; physical, 11–12, 18, 22–25, 107, 132–33, 146, 152–53, 161, 165, 170–72, 177, 181, 189, 198, 200–201, 203, 205, 207, 210, 219, 223–26, 228–30, 235, 251n30, 253n11, 264n17, 271n4. *See also* enactment, of body; healers, physical body of; materiality, bodily
breast milk, 35, 100, 107, 133–34,163, 207, 212, 220–21, 224, 228–30
Butler, Judith, 207

Callon, Michel, 21
cancer, 12, 16, 251n30
capital, 235; capitalism, 7, 58
causality, 201–202, 269n5
Chanock, Martin, 44, 47
Chenga, Fatu, 94–97, 106, 108, 112, 115, 155, 264n13
Chiduo, Aaron, 66, 68

Stacey A. Langwick (M.P.H., Ph.D.) is Assistant Professor in the Department of Anthropology at Cornell University. Her research sits at the intersection of ethnography, history, and medicine. Her courses on healing and medicine, anthropology of the body, and postcolonial science are cross-listed with Global Health, Africana Studies, and Science and Technology Studies at Cornell. She currently holds an associateship with the Max Planck Institute of Social Anthropology in Germany. She has published in *American Ethnologist; Science, Technology & Human Values; Medical Anthropology;* and in several edited volumes on healing in Africa.